THE SCIENTIFIC AND CLINICAL APPLICATION OF ELASTIC RESISTANCE

Phillip Page, MS, PT, ATC, CSCS
Benchmark Physical Therapy, Baton Rouge, LA
The Hygenic Corporation

Todd S. Ellenbecker, MS, PT, SCS, OCS, CSCS
Physiotherapy Associates, Scottsdale Sports Clinic
Scottsdale, Arizona

Human Kinetics

Library of Congress Cataloging-in-Publication Data

The scientific and clinical application of elastic resistance / Phillip
Page, Todd S. Ellenbecker, editors.
    p. ; cm.
Includes bibliographical references and index.
  ISBN 0-7360-3688-1
  1. Stretching exercises 2. Rubber bands. 3. Exercise--Equipment and
supplies.
  [DNLM: 1. Exercise Therapy--methods. 2. Physical Fitness. 3.
Rehabilitation--methods. WB 541 S4155 2003] I. Page, Phillip, 1967-
II. Ellenbecker, Todd S., 1962-
  RA781.63 .S356 2003
  613.7'1--dc21   2002004502

ISBN: 0-7360-3688-1

Acquisitions Editor: Loarn D. Robertson, PhD; **Developmental Editor:** Jennifer Clark; **Assistant Editor:** Amanda Gunn; **Copyeditor:** Julie Anderson; **Proofreader:** Anne Meyer Byler; **Indexer:** Susan Danzi Hernandez; **Permissions Manager:** Dalene Reeder; **Graphic Designer:** Fred Starbird; **Graphic Artist:** Angela K. Snyder; **Photo Manager:** Leslie A. Woodrum; **Cover Designer:** Jack W. Davis; **Photographer (cover):** The Hygenic Corporation; **Photographer (interior):** Leslie A. Woodrum, unless otherwise noted; **Art Manager:** Kelly Hendren; **Illustrator:** Roberto Sabas; **Printer:** Sheridan Books, Inc.

Printed in the United States of America   10 9 8 7 6 5 4 3 2

Human Kinetics
Web site: www.HumanKinetics.com

United States: Human Kinetics, P.O. Box 5076, Champaign, IL 61825-5076
800-747-4457
e-mail: humank@hkusa.com

Canada: Human Kinetics, 475 Devonshire Road, Unit 100, Windsor, ON N8Y 2L5
800-465-7301 (in Canada only)
e-mail: orders@hkcanada.com

Europe: Human Kinetics, 107 Bradford Road, Stanningley
Leeds LS28 6AT, United Kingdom
+44 (0) 113 255 5665
e-mail: hk@hkeurope.com

Australia: Human Kinetics, 57A Price Avenue, Lower Mitcham, South Australia 5062
08 8277 1555
e-mail: liahka@senet.com.au

New Zealand: Human Kinetics, P.O. Box 105-231, Auckland Central
09-523-3462
e-mail: hkp@ihug.co.nz

This book is dedicated to our patients who provide us invaluable experience and
countless learning opportunities, and for whom we are in this profession,
with hopes that this book will help other patients.
We would also like to dedicate this book to our teachers, mentors, colleagues,
and students, in hopes that this book will continue to be a tool
for teaching well into the future.

Contents

PART II EXERCISE APPLICATIONS 39

Chapter 4 Upper Extremity Exercises With Elastic Resistance 41

Todd S. Ellenbecker

Chapter 5 Lower Extremity Exercises With Elastic Resistance 69

Jill Thein-Nissenbaum and Jill C. Orzehoskie

Chapter 6 Spinal Exercises With Elastic Resistance 99

Andre Labbe

Chapter 22   Sport-Specific Training for Skiing   281

Burt Johson and Jeff Carlson

PART V   SPECIAL POPULATIONS   287

Chapter 23   Elastic Resistance Training for Older Adults   289

Robert Topp

Chapter 24   Rehabilitation of Persons With Physical Disabilities   309

Mark A. Anderson, Kathleen Curtis, and James Laskin

Chapter 25 Elastic Resistance Exercise for Chronic Disease   327

Phillip Page and Melvin Manning

Contributors

Mark A. Anderson, PhD, PT, ATC
University of Oklahoma Health Sciences Center

Ray Barile, MS, ATC, CSCS, LMT
St. Louis Blues Hockey Club, St. Louis, Missouri

Greg Brittenham, MS
New York Knickerbockers

Jeff Carlson, PT
Howard Head Sports Medicine Centers

Michael A. Clark, MS, PT, CSCS, PES
National Academy of Sports Medicine

Randy Craig, MS, PT, ATC
PRORehab, PC, St. Louis, Missouri

Kathleen Curtis, PhD, PT
California State University at Fresno

George J. Davies, MEd, PT, SCS, ATC, CSCS
University of Wisconsin at La Crosse

Todd S. Ellenbecker, MS, PT, SCS, OCS, CSCS
Physiotherapy Associates, Scottsdale Sports Clinic, Scottsdale, Arizona

Scott Gallant, MS, PT, ATC
PRORehab, PC, St. Louis, Missouri

Chris Hughes, PT, PhD, CSCS
Slippery Rock University, Slippery Rock, Pennsylvania

Vladimir Janda, MD, DSc
Charles University Hospital, Prague, Czech Republic

Burt Johson, ATC
Howard Head Sports Medicine Centers

Andre Labbe, PT, MOMT
Advantage Physical Therapy, New Orleans, Louisiana

James Laskin, PhD, PT
University of Montana at Missoula

Melvin Manning, MD
Texas Sports Medicine Group, Dallas, Texas

James W. Matheson, MS, PT, CSCS
University of Montana Physical Therapy Clinic

Malachy P. McHugh, PhD
The Nicholas Institute of Sports Medicine and Athletic Trauma

Terri Mitchell, PTA
Austin, Texas

Timothy C. Murphy, MA, PT, ATC
Concorde Therapy Group, Canton, Ohio

Jill C. Orzehoskie, MPT, ATC
Sheboygan Memorial Hospital, Sheboygan, Wisconsin

Phillip Page, MS, PT, ATC, CSCS
Benchmark Physical Therapy, Baton Rouge, Louisiana
The Hygenic Corporation

E. Paul Roetert, PhD, FACSM
USA Tennis High Performannce, Key Biscayne, Florida

Jill Thein-Nissenbaum, MPT, SCS, ATC
University of Wisconsin at Madison

Robert Topp, PhD, RN
School of Nursing, Medical College of Georgia

Timothy F. Tyler, MS, PT, ATC
The Nicholas Institute of Sports Medicine and Athletic Trauma

Tyler W.A. Wallace, BS, CPT, PES
National Academy of Sports Medicine

Robert Wood, Chartered Physiotherapist
Active Life Physiotherapy Center, Norfolk, United Kingdom

Preface

Elastic resistance has been used over the last 100 years for strength training. As early as 1901, the elastic "Whitely Exerciser" (produced in Chicago, IL) was used for "Strength for Men, Grace and Beauty for Women, Perfect Development for Children." Several other personal fitness products using elastic resistance were marketed through the 1950's, including the "Whitely Elastic Rubber Cable Chest Pull" and the "Stretch Rope" by Paige Palmer in Cleveland, OH.

In the 1960s and 1970s, the benefits of elastic resistance exercise for strength training in rehabilitation were noted by therapists and athletic trainers. Surgical tubing and bicycle inner tubes were used to strengthen injured or weak muscles. In 1978, two physical therapists approached The Hygenic Corporation (Akron, OH) with a general concept of using their Dental Dam product for physical therapy, from which the company developed the Thera-Band® color-coded system of progressive elastic resistance. The original Dental Dam product was manufactured in bulk rolls of 5 3/4 inches, which led to the standard length and colors today.

Because of its physical properties, elastic resistance was incorporated into a strengthening and cardiovascular conditioning machine designed for an orbiting space station in the 1960s. Ultimately, in 1987, the Shuttle horizontal leg press was developed in Seattle, WA, and although it never made it into space, it is frequently found in athletic training rooms and therapy clinics today. Elastic resistance has also been used in several other strength-training machines, including the Soloflex multi-joint home strengthening machine, and the Pro Fitter device initially designed for training and rehabilitation of skiing athletes in Canada.

Obviously, elastic resistance has quite a history and presence in professional rehabilitation as well as home fitness. Unfortunately, elastic resistance was essentially taken for granted in the research community, and was never placed under scientific scrutiny, as for example, the isokinetic devices were in the 1970s and 1980s. It was commonly accepted that elastic resistance increased strength, and little was devoted to its properties or applications in the literature. This ultimately filtered into the professional schools, as elastic resistance was only offered as an option for a strength training modality, along with free weights, springs, or machines. However, many clinicians continued to prescribe elastic resistance to their patients. Only recently has elastic resistance become closely studied. For example, the first peer-reviewed article evaluating the clinical effects of elastic resistance was published in 1984 by Annianson.

Elastic bands and tubing have been used by a wide range of persons, from young to old, and sick to healthy. Because of its wide use in a variety of populations, elastic resistance has been used around the world for both therapy and fitness. Professionals from around the world have different applications for elastic resistance. This book was conceived as a result of a need for an objective and practical review of the use of elastic resistance exercise. Because of it's versatility, ideas for elastic resistance applications should be shared between professions.

Hopefully, this book can be used by the seasoned clinician as a new way to look at an old tool, as well as by the new student just learning about the properties of elastic resistance. For example, the therapist can learn how elastic resistance can be adapted to a certain patient based on applications from fitness. The exercises in the book can be used as a reference for clinicians interested in using new exercises or adapting older ones. This book will also serve as a reference for researchers developing programs for elastic resistance exercise. Most importantly, we hope this book fosters more creative uses of this versatile product, as well as more clinical research outcomes.

Part I of this book reviews the current literature regarding elastic resistance from a basic and applied science approach, as well as the outcomes of clinical trials involving elastic resistance. Part II reviews the basic applications of elastic resistance to the upper body, lower body, and spine. In Part III the various training methods involving elastic resistance are discussed. Part IV describes the specific uses of elastic resistance in a variety of sports. Finally, Part V provides the application of elastic resistance for special populations, such as older adults, and those with chronic disease or disability.

Acknowledgments

Special thanks to our contributors for their time and for sharing their experience and knowledge in each chapter. We would also like to thank Human Kinetics for their support and patience on this project, in particular Loarn Robertson (Big Bear), Jennifer Clark, Amanda Gunn, and Dalene Reeder (for her help with permissions), and to all the other great people behind the scenes at HK for their help. And thanks to everyone at Hygenic Corporation for their support in this project.

Most importantly, we would like to thank our wives, Angela and Gail, and our families for their support, patience, and understanding. Finally, thanks to God for giving us the opportunity and ability to share this with the world.

PART 1

SCIENTIFIC BASIS

E lastic resistance exercise has been used for almost a century. It began as a fitness device and progressed to a rehabilitation device. Although a commonly accepted and widely used method, elastic resistance has not been evaluated as scientifically as other types of resistance exercise devices. Instead, elastic resistance exercise has been used based on clinical experience rather than scientific evidence. The following chapters provide the scientific basis for the use of elastic resistance exercise. First, the basic and applied science of elastic resistance exercise is reviewed. Outcomes of clinical research on elastic resistance are then presented, followed by the scientific rationale for elastic resistance exercise prescription.

CHAPTER 1

Scientific Basis of Elastic Resistance

• • • • •

Chris Hughes, PT, PhD, CSCS
Slippery Rock University, Slippery Rock, Pennsylvania

Phillip Page, MS, PT, ATC, CSCS
Benchmark Physical Therapy, Baton Rouge, LA
The Hygenic Corporation

Many methods are available to the rehabilitation specialist to increase muscle strength in patients, athletes, and the general population. All of these methods are based on providing enough resistance to stimulate adaptation in muscle at the cellular level in order to alter the muscle's contractility. The choice of training depends on the athlete's or patient's current level of fitness or ability, goals, and time commitment. Some training methods require the use of expensive exercise machines, whereas others rely on simple devices to provide resistance. A popular and simple form of exercise uses elastic tubing or bands as a form of resistance. Elastic resistance is used commonly for training because of its low cost, simplicity, portability, and versatility and because it does not rely on gravity for resistance.

Despite the popularity of elastic resistance training and its success in increasing strength, little attention has been devoted in the literature to understanding the resistive properties provided by elastic bands or tubing. Athletic trainers, therapists, and strength and conditioning specialists must understand the fundamental differences among these methods and also must understand the requirements and constraints of the musculoskeletal system in exerting effort. The interplay between the training method used and the physiological and mechanical interactions of the musculoskeletal system will determine what results are achieved. This chapter discusses the basic principles of resistance training, the basic material properties governing elastic resistance, the biomechanics of elastic materials, and electromyography of muscles during elastic resistance exercise.

Scientific Basis of Resistance Training

Muscle strengthening methods commonly fall under the category of isotonic, isokinetic, or isometric exercise (Atha 1981; Fox 1979; Morrissey, Harman, and Johnson 1995). Operational definitions are associated with each form of training. Isotonic exercise requires that an individual lift or move a constant weight through a range of movement. Free weights are the most common and popular form of isotonic exercise. Isokinetic exercise requires a dynamometer to ensure that segment motion occurs at a preset and controlled velocity. With isokinetic exercise, a varied and accommodating resistance is provided in direct relationship to changing levels of torque output that are evident throughout the range of motion to allow a constant velocity when the load is lifted (Rodgers and Cavanagh 1984). Isometric exercise uses a submaximal or maximal muscle effort without joint motion. Isometric exercise does not require the use of special equipment.

Various research studies have compared strength gains resulting from various methods of training but have not conclusively determined the superiority of one particular method (Bandy, Lovelace-Chandler, and McKitrick-Bandy 1990). According to the principle of specific adaptations to imposed demands (SAID), human tissue including skeletal muscle incurs specific adaptations in response to the stimulus imposed. Therefore, it seems logical to infer that different methods may be suitable for different training goals (Morrissey, Harman, and Johnson 1995). Surprisingly, elastic resistance exercise does not display typical characteristics of any of the three previously mentioned exercise classifications (isotonic, isokinetic, and isometric). Resistance training with elastic is unique. The variability in force when elastic bands or tubing is stretched negates classifying elastic exercise as a form of isotonic training, and the accompanying change in stretch rate (velocity) prohibits classification as isokinetic exercise. A summary of the load, moment, and speed characteristics of each method of training appears in Table 1.01.

Table 1.01   Load, Moment, and Speed Characteristics of Each Method of Training

Training method	Load	Torque (moment)	Speed of movement
Isotonic	Constant	Variable	Variable
Isokinetic	Accommodative	Variable	Constant
Isometric	Accommodative	Variable	None
Elastic	Variable	Variable	Variable

Reprinted, by permission, from C. Hughes, P. Page, and D. Maurice, 2000. "Elastic exercise training," *Orthopaedic Physical Therapy Clinics of North America* 9(4): 581-95.

Resistance exercise and human motion in general are also categorized based on the mechanics of muscle contraction. Concentric, eccentric, and isometric contractions are described commonly in the literature. A concentric muscle effort is defined as an increase in muscle tension that results in muscle shortening and, consequently, limb movement. This type of contraction is highly dependent on the leverage changes between the resistance or load provided and the net effort from the agonist muscles. Torque or moment of force represents the net effect of the forces acting through the lever system that cause rotation about the joint axis. When the net moment or torque from muscle contraction exceeds the moment generated by an external resistive force, a concentric action takes place.

When the moment generated by muscles attempting to rotate a skeletal segment is less than the moment generated by an external resistive force, an eccentric contraction occurs. Eccentric contractions occur when the muscle lengthens during contraction and the limb segment moves in a direction opposite of the muscle effort. Eccentric contractions commonly are generated in opposition to inertial or gravitational forces. When the net moment from internal (muscle contraction) and external (weight, gravity) forces acting on a skeletal segment is zero, the moment generated by the muscles acting on the segment is equal to the opposing resistive moment. This event characterizes an isometric condition. An isometric condition occurs when there is no joint movement although forces and moments are acting on the segment. Training with elastic bands and tubing can include all three mechanical conditions of muscle contraction (concentric, eccentric, isometric), similar to isotonic exercise.

Regardless of the method of training, all forms of resistance exercise must adhere to the overload principle to increase strength. If contractions are strong or prolonged and if they are repeated regularly, then adaptive changes will take place, which allow the muscle to handle greater amounts of work (Atha 1981). A muscle must be overloaded to a certain threshold before it will respond and adapt to training (Bandy, Lovelace-Chandler, and McKitrick-Bandy 1990). Increases in muscle size (hypertrophy) also may occur. Exercise against maximal resistance must be performed to stimulate physiological adaptations that can increase muscle strength (Atha 1981; Bandy, Lovelace-Chandler, and McKitrick-Bandy 1990; Fox 1979). A muscle exercising against resistances that are normally encountered will be maintained but will not increase. The choice of exercise appears to influence the amount and rate of strength gain and also the adaptations that occur in skeletal muscle (Bandy, Lovelace-Chandler, and McKitrick-Bandy, 1990; Morrissey, Harman, and Johnson 1995; Tesch 1988). Regardless of the choice of exercise, the resistance must also be progressive for the greatest rate of strength gains to occur (Kisner and Colby 1996). Similar to other methods of training, exercise regimens using elastic bands or tubing as a form of resistance have been shown to increase muscle strength 10% to 20% (Anderson et al. 1992; Fornataro et al. 1994; Mikesky et al. 1994; Page et al. 1993).

Basic Properties of Elastic Materials

The distinguishing characteristic of elastic materials (elastomers) is that the resistance provided changes as the material is elongated or stretched. The resistance provided by elastic exercise is often simplistically compared to the dynamics of a spring. The relationship between force and length can be summarized by the formula proposed by Robert Hooke (Hooke's law):

$$F = k \times s$$

where F, force, or in the case of elastomers, resistance, is the product of the given change in length (s) times k, which is the numerical constant representing the stiffness of the material. Elastomers remain elastic even at great elongations, and their stress-strain behavior is nearly linear, making their response to elongation quite predictable. Elastic material stores energy when it is stretched or deformed (McCrum, Buckley, and Bucknall 1988; Schultz 1974; Young 1983). The change in length as a function of the applied force, the modulus of elasticity of the material, and the cross-sectional area all dictate the level of resistance and the amount of potential energy stored by elastic (Ozkaya and Nordin 1991).

Two consequences of this stress-elongation behavior are important to the rehabilitation specialist. First, because resistance is a function of how much the elastic material is elongated, it is important to ensure that the patient grasp the band or tubing in the same place each time. If the patient takes a shorter section of band than in the previous session, the resistance will increase relative to the previous session, which may make the movement too hard and may mislead the patient and clinician to think that the patient has experienced a setback. Conversely, if the patient takes a longer length of band than in the previous session, the resistance will

decrease relative to the previous session. This may make the movement seem easy and may mislead the patient and clinician to think that the patient has made more progress than really has been made.

Second, as the range of motion through which the patient can move increases, it may be appropriate to increase the length of the band or tubing used. If a band has been used over a range of 60° and the patient is now capable of 75°, then continuing to use that same band length will mean that those final 15° of motion, over which the patient is weakest or most tentative, will have the greatest resistance. Overall, both the length of the band and the position of the patient can dictate changes in the resistance encountered during elastic exercise. Other factors to consider include the size of the elastic material, rate or velocity of stretch, and cyclic loading and deformation.

Size of Elastic Material

Given that elastic material's resistance to stretch is proportional to its original cross-sectional area, a thin piece of elastic band or tubing can be doubled, which doubles the effective cross-sectional area and doubles the resistance. With sufficient elastic material, the therapist or patient can make any desired multiple of the original resistance. If a suitable device for securing the ends of the elastic is available, it is even feasible to combine elastic bands or tubing of different thicknesses. Thus, a variety of methods can be used to vary resistance with elastic bands or tubing.

Rate (Velocity) of Stretch

Like many other materials, elastomers have stress responses that are influenced by the rate at which the imposed elongation is applied. As the rate at which elastomers deform increases, their resistance to further elongation increases as well. Elastic left under tension or stored under load for an extended duration can undergo permanent changes called viscoelastic creep. *Creep* is defined as a continued deformation in material under a constant and sustaining load. This condition ultimately will change the force elongation properties of the material. Signs of excessive viscoelastic creep (i.e., brittleness, wrinkled appearance) indicate that the elastic product may need to be replaced.

Cyclic Loading and Deformation

Repeatedly stretching and relaxing elastic material is considered cyclic deformation. Cyclic deformation causes fatigue, or cumulative damage to the material, which eventually will result in failure. Unfortunately, there is no practical way to avoid this; elastic resistive products should be replaced periodically.

Simoneau et al. (2001) found that elastic bands and tubing decrease in force by 5% to 12% when stretched to 100% for 500 cycles. The researchers noted that most of the change occurred within the first 50 pulls. Patterson et al. (2001) noted consistent force production of elastic tubing after 20 initial elongations to prestretch the material. This prestretching caused an initial "setting" or slight plastic deformation of the elastic material with the first few elongations out of the box that actually lengthened the material from the initial resting length. Therefore, absolute force production will decrease because the resting length of the material increases, but relative force production will remain the same (based on percentage of elongation). Finally, Patterson et al. (2001) also noted consistent force production after 5,700 cycles up to 250% elongation.

Biomechanics of Elastic Resistance Exercise

Although elastic resistance has been accepted as a standard mode of resistance training, some clinicians may not understand the biomechanical principles of elastic resistance.

Force-Elongation Characteristics

Knowing the actual variation of force as a function of length is important when prescribing exercise that uses elastic resistance. Researchers have attempted to quantify the amount of force generated during stretching of elastic material (Hughes et al. 1999; Jones et al. 1998; Page, Labbe, and Topp 2000; Simoneau et al. 2001). Different types of elastic material (such as bands or tubing) from different manufacturers may provide different amounts of force (Simoneau et al. 2001). Regardless of the form of the elastic material (bands or tubing), the physical characteristics of force-elongation will remain the same. The resistance provided by the elastic band or tubing is based on the amount of elastic material; thicker bands and tubing provide more resistance than thinner ones.

The force of elastic resistance depends on percentage of elongation, regardless of initial length. For example, if a 1-ft length of band or tubing were elongated to 2 ft (100% elongation), the force exerted would be the same as if a 2-ft length of the same color band or tubing were elongated to 4 ft. The percentage of elongation (change in length) is calculated with the following formula:

$$\text{Percentage of elongation} = [(\text{final length}) - (\text{resting length}) / (\text{resting length})] \times 100$$

Figure 1.01 shows force-elongation curves (Page, Labbe, and Topp 2000) for various resistances of Thera-Band elastic bands (Hygenic Corporation, Akron, OH).

As shown in figure 1.01, the slope of the resistance curve varies with changes in the stiffness and diameter of the material. Because elastic resistance normally is prescribed categorically only by color, one must not assume that changes in resistance are of equal increment when moving from color to color. As figure 1.01 indicates, there is a considerable difference in the slope of the curve representing the yellow-colored elastic bands versus the silver-colored elastic bands. There is generally a 20% to 30% increase in force between each color (yellow, red, green, blue, black, and silver) of Thera-Band elastic bands (Page, Labbe, and Topp 2000).

Typical clinical elongations rarely exceed 200%. Hughes et al. (1999) found tubing length changes of 18% to 160% from starting length during shoulder abduction exercise. Table 1.02 provides force-elongation data for Thera-Band elastic bands (Page, Labbe, and Topp 2000).

Researchers (Hughes et al. 1999; Page, Labbe, and Topp 2000) also have developed linear regression equations to predict force at different stages of elongation (table 1.03).

The resistance has to be sufficient and accommodative within the range of motion to maximize training gains in accordance with the overload principle and SAID principle. Therefore, the resting length of the band can be adjusted to meet the amount of elongation required to complete the range of motion of various exercises.

The Role of Torque Generation in Resistance Exercise

In reviewing skeletal muscle mechanics, Lieber and Bodine-Fowler (1993) stated that strength must be evaluated in relation to torque to understand the true strength requirements and effect of the exercise on the musculoskeletal system. They stated that resistance training must include variables that

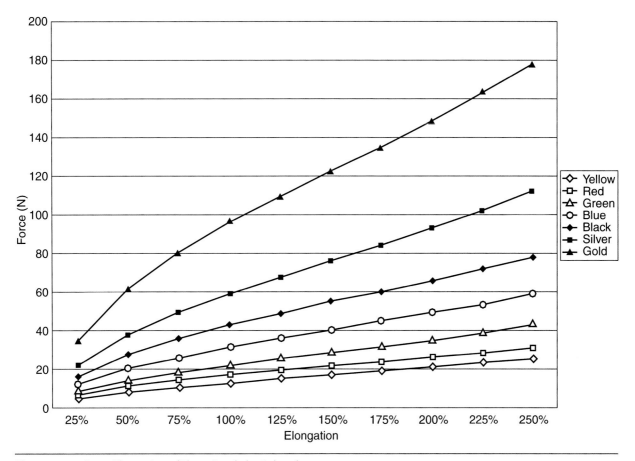

Figure 1.01 Force-Elongation of Thera-Band elastic bands.

Data from P. Page, A. Labbe, and R. Topp, 2000, "Clinical force production at Thera-Band elastic bands," *Journal of Orthopaedic and Sports Physical Therapy* 30(1):A47-8.

Table 1.02   Force-Elongation for Thera-Band Elastic Bands (Force in Pounds)

Elongation (%)	Yellow	Red	Green	Blue	Black	Silver	Gold
25	1.1	1.5	2	2.8	3.6	5	7.9
50	1.8	2.6	3.2	4.6	6.3	8.5	13.9
75	2.4	3.3	4.2	5.9	8.1	11.1	18.1
100	2.9	3.9	5	7.1	9.7	13.2	21.6
125	3.4	4.4	5.7	8.1	11	15.2	24.6
150	3.9	4.9	6.5	9.1	12.3	17.1	27.5
175	4.3	5.4	7.2	10.1	13.5	18.9	30.3
200	4.8	5.9	7.9	11.1	14.8	21	33.4
225	5.3	6.4	8.8	12.1	16.2	23	36.6
250	5.8	7	9.6	13.3	17.6	25.3	40.1

Data from P. Page, A. Labbe, and R. Topp, 2000, "Clinical force production at Thera-Band elastic bands," *Journal of Orthopaedic and Sports Physical Therapy* 30(1):A47-8.

Table 1.03 Prediction Equations for Thera-Band Elastic Bands in Pounds

Band color	Regression equation
Yellow	$R = 0.788 + .0202\ (E)$
Red	$R = 1.367 + .0229\ (E)$
Green	$R = 1.525 + .0325\ (E)$
Blue	$R = 2.323 + .0443\ (E)$
Black	$R = 3.223 + .0587\ (E)$
Silver	$R = 4.053 + .0856\ (E)$
Gold	$R = 6.882 + .1350\ (E)$

R = resistance in pounds; E = percent elongation from initial length; $p < .000$ for all band colors.
Data from P. Page, A. Labbe and R. Topp, 2000, "Clinical force production of Thera-Band elastic bands," *Journal of Orthopaedic and Sports Physical Therapy* 30(1):A47-48.

identify magnitude of force, moment arm, and angle between the moving segment and the direction in which the resistance is acting. If the culmination of these variables is considered, then load effects can be displayed graphically with a torque versus joint angle curve. A torque versus joint angle curve is otherwise known as a *strength curve*.

Three common patterns of strength curves are associated with single-joint exercises: ascending, descending, and ascending-descending (Kulig, Andrews, and Hay 1984). An ascending curve portrays strength or torque increasing as the joint angle of movement increases. A descending curve shows an inverse relationship between strength and joint angle. An ascending-descending curve is a pattern of effort that first shows an increase in strength as joint angle increases and then displays strength decreases with further increases in joint angle. An ascending-descending strength curve is the most common pattern exhibited for a majority of joints. Factors such as the mechanics of contraction (concentric, eccentric, or isometric), type of contraction, speed of contraction, and body position can influence the form of strength curve presented. Ultimately, muscle force output will vary throughout the joint range of motion and depends on training mode, interaction of the resistance provided, and the changing mechanical advantage of the musculoskeletal system. With elastic resistance training, as with other types of resistance training, clinicians should consider the applied and resistive torque generated throughout the range of motion as a factor in determining whether an exercise is appropriate and effectively overloads the muscle.

Elastic resistance offers some of the advantages of isotonic resistance and minimizes its disadvantages. Similar to isotonic resistance, elastic resistance provides a constant load, requiring the muscle to recruit more motor units to complete the motion. However, elastic resistance exercise requires muscle activation throughout the range of motion because patients cannot "cheat" by using momentum to complete the exercise (Hughes, Page, and Maurice 2000). Also, unlike an athlete using free weights or machines, the patient using elastic resistance is not influenced by the considerable inertia of the weight and is free to move outside a predetermined range of motion. This allows for exercise patterns without concern for gravity, such as diagonal patterns. This attribute also may be beneficial for using elastic as a form of resistance for plyometric exercise. Some authors have described the use of elastic resistance in plyometrics (Davies and Dickoff-Hoffman 1993; Pezzullo, Karas, and Irrgang 1995; Wilk and Arrigo 1993).

Although gravity does not significantly affect the resistive characteristics of elastic products, other factors need to be considered. The rate of stretch and overall elongation of the elastic band or tubing, the point of the application, the distance of the resistance from the joint axis, and the orientation (angle) of the elastic band or tubing to the moving limb all affect the torque required by the muscles to move the limb segment. With elastic products, it is possible to have a linear change in resistance throughout the range of movement but to have a variable resistive torque pattern, because of the changing angle of pull. Previous research investigating the resistance properties of elastic tubing during shoulder abduction exercise revealed a linear resistance pattern as the tubing length increased (Hughes et al. 1999). However, when the resistance torque pattern was calculated for tubing, the resistance curves resembled an ascending-descending pattern (figure 1.02) similar to that obtained when a constant load was used (isotonic training).

Elastic resistance training that loads muscle to its limits throughout the range of motion should result in maximal muscle activation and greater strength gains. Furthermore, the attachment points of the band or tubing to the moving body segment will influence the resistive torque curve. This point of attachment can be referred to as the *resistance arm angle* (RAA). The RAA is the angle formed by the interaction of the resistive device and lever arm (figure 1.03).

As the RAA changes, the effective torque on the exercised joint changes as well. This is based on the

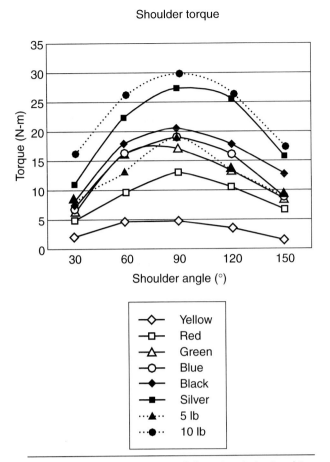

Figure 1.02   Strength curves of Thera-Band elastic tubing compared to free weights.

Reprinted, by permission, from C.J. Hughes, K. Hurd, A. Jones, and S. Sprigle, 1999, "Resistance properties of Thera-Band tubing during shoulder abduction exercise," *Journal of Orthopaedic and Sports Physical Therapy* 29(7):413-20.

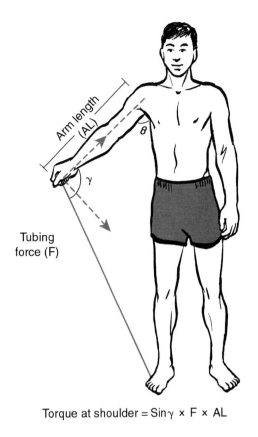

Torque at shoulder = Sin γ × F × AL

Figure 1.03   Resistance-arm angle (γ) is formed by the interaction of the lever arm and elastic tubing.

Adapted, by permission, from C.J. Hughes, K. Hurd, A. Jones, and S. Sprigle, 1999, "Resistance properties of Thera-Band tubing during shoulder abduction exercise," *Journal of Orthopaedic and Sports Physical Therapy* 29(7):413-20.

following formula, where joint torque equals the product of the sine of the RAA, the force of the resistance, and the length of the lever arm:

$$Torque = sin(RAA) \times force \times lever\ arm$$

Recently, the torque production of elastic resistance was compared with pulley system resistance. Page and Labbe (2000) studied the torque produced by a weight-and-pulley system and elastic tubing. The researchers used an isokinetic dynamometer in the continuous passive mode (CPM) to determine torque production (foot-pounds) throughout 180° of motion. Torque data were collected during both lengthening (concentric phase) and shortening (eccentric phase) of the tubing. Samples were tested at 60°/s and 120°/s. The researchers found that elastic tubing demonstrated symmetrical concentric and eccentric

torque curves with peak torque occurring near the middle range of motion (figures 1.04 and 1.05).

The pulley resistance demonstrated asymmetrical concentric/eccentric torque curves with the eccentric torque values approximately half of the concentric values (figures 1.06 and 1.07).

Additionally, the peak torque provided by pulleys occurred earlier in the motion, and torque tended to decrease toward the end range. Speed did not affect the peak torque values of either resistive mode, but speed did affect the overall pulley curve characteristics, demonstrating more rapid and variable torque production early in the concentric motion. Tubing and pulley systems represent different forms of resistance exercise patterns. In this study, the inertial properties of the pulley system with isotonic loading influenced the pattern of resistance.

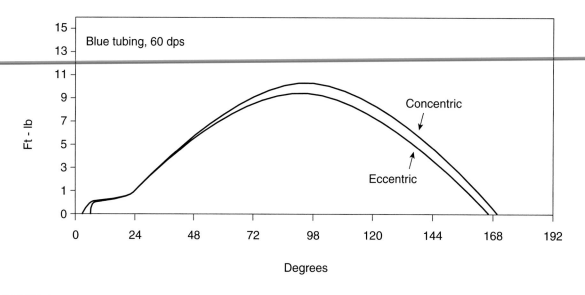

Figure 1.04 Torque curves over 180° for Thera-Band resistive tubing at 60° × s⁻¹.

Data from P. Page and A. Labbe, 2000, "Torque Characteristics of Elastic Resistance and Weight-and-Pulley Exercise," (Abstract). *Medicine and Science in Sports and Exercise* 32(5) (Suppl.):S151.

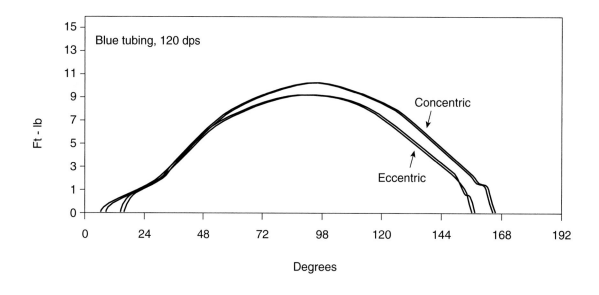

Figure 1.05 Torque curves over 180° for Thera-Band resistive tubing at 120° × s⁻¹.

Data from P. Page and A. Labbe, 2000, "Torque Characteristics of Elastic Resistance and Weight-and-Pulley Exercise," (Abstract). *Medicine and Science in Sports and Exercise* 32(5) (Suppl.):S151.

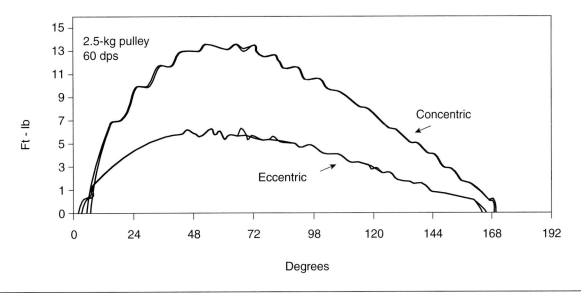

Figure 1.06 Torque curves over 180° for 2.5 kg LOJER pulley system at 60° × s⁻¹.

Data from P. Page and A. Labbe, 2000, "Torque Characteristics of Elastic Resistance and Weight-and-Pulley Exercise," (Abstract). *Medicine and Science in Sports and Exercise* 32(5) (Suppl.):S151.

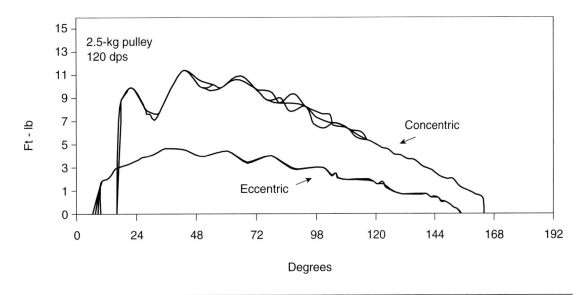

Figure 1.07 Torque curves over 180° for 2.5 kg LOJER pulley system at 120° × s⁻¹.

Data from P, Page and A. Labbe, 2000, "Torque Characteristics of Elastic Resistance and Weight-and-Pulley Exercise," (Abstract). *Medicine and Science in Sports and Exercise* 32(5) (Suppl.):S151.

Electromyographic Research on Elastic Resistance Exercise

Several researchers have investigated electromyographic activity in muscles during elastic resistance exercise (Cordova, Jutte, and Hopkins 1999; Decker et al. 1999; Hintermeister, Bey, et al. 1998; Hintermeister, Lange, et al. 1998; Hopkins et al. 1999; McCann et al. 1993; Schulthies et al. 1998; Willett et al. 1998). Willett et al. (1998) found that closed-chain terminal knee extensions against elastic resistance were superior to no resistance in activating the vastus medialis oblique (VMO) and vastus lateralis (VL). Electromyographic activity for the VMO and VL ranged from 44% to 48% maximal voluntary isometric contraction (MVIC). Hintermeister, Bey, et al. (1998) quantified muscle activation levels by using electromyography of the lower extremity muscles during five knee rehabilitation exercises. They found that elastic tubing provides suitable progressive resistance in the lower extremity muscles for patients beginning a typical rehabilitation program. In another study, Hintermeister, Lange, et al. (1998) found that shoulder exercises that used elastic resistance could effectively target the rotator cuff muscles for postinjury and postoperative patients. Unfortunately, none of the studies cited compared the electromyographic activity of elastic resistance with other forms of resistance.

An interesting observation can be made when comparing isotonic exercise with elastic exercise for shoulder rehabilitation. In a study by Hughes and McBride (2000), 12 noninjured subjects compared shoulder rehabilitation exercises that used free weights and elastic tubing. Surface electromyographic activity was collected for the shoulder and scapular muscles while four different exercises were performed with both elastic tubing and dumbbells. The researchers noted distinct differences for muscle activation that were dependent on load and method of resistance. As an example, figure 1.08 shows almost twice the amount of peak muscle activation in the posterior deltoid during the scaption exercise when red, green, and blue Thera-Band elastic tubing was used compared with isotonic loads of 1, 3, and 5 lb with a dumbbell.

In addition, infraspinatus activity was significantly greater when tubing was used versus free (isotonic) weights during the external rotation exercise in side-lying (free weights) and standing (tubing) positions. Factors relating to these differences included postural stabilization, force-elongation changes, direction of resistance application (gravity-dependent vs. non-gravity-dependent), load equivalencies, and changes in resistive torque.

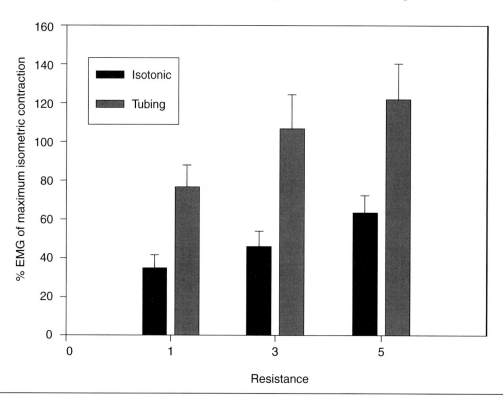

Figure 1.08 EMG comparison of posterior deltoid during scaption exercise between isotonic and elastic resistance.

Data from C.J. Hughes, and A. McBride, 2000, "A Comparative Electromographic Analysis of Shoulder Rehabilitation Excercises Using Isotonic and Elastic Resistances." In review.

Conclusion

Despite considerable research on various topics in resistance training, the effects and implications of elastic exercise training largely have been ignored. This brief discussion is an attempt to highlight some of the important characteristics associated with using elastic as a form of resistance in exercise programs. Future research should investigate the clinical validity of elastic exercise and distinguish it from other forms of exercise. This area of clinical research will help guide the rehabilitation specialist in prescribing the proper exercise and the proper amount of exercise for patients with various pathologies.

References

Anderson, L., R. Rush, L. Shearer, and C.J. Hughes. 1992. "The Effects of a Thera-Band® Exercise Program on Shoulder Internal Rotation Strength" (Abstract). *Physical Therapy* 72 (Suppl.): 540.

Atha, J. 1981. "Strengthening Muscle." *Exercise and Sport Sciences Reviews* 9: 1-73.

Bandy, W.D., V. Lovelace-Chandler, and B. McKitrick-Bandy. 1990. "Adaptation of Skeletal Muscle to Resistance Training." *Journal of Orthopaedic and Sports Physical Therapy* 12(6): 248-55.

Cordova, M.L., L.S. Jutte, and J.T. Hopkins. 1999. "EMG Comparison of Selected Ankle Rehabilitation Exercises." *Journal of Sport Rehabilitation* 8: 209-18.

Davies, G.J., and S. Dickoff-Hoffman. 1993. "Neuromuscular Testing and Rehabilitation of the Shoulder Complex." *Journal of Orthopaedic and Sports Physical Therapy* 18(2): 449-58.

Decker, M.J., R.A. Hintermeister, K. Faber, and R.J. Hawkins. 1999. "Serratus Anterior Muscle Activity During Selected Rehabilitation Exercises." *American Journal of Sports Medicine* 27(6): 784-91.

Fornataro, S., M. Green, D. Martz, K. Masneri, and C.J. Hughes. 1994. "Investigation to Determine Differences in Strength Gains Using Thera-Band at Fast and Slow Training Speeds" (Abstract). *Physical Therapy* 74(5) (Suppl.): S53.

Fox, E.L. 1979. *Sports physiology.* Philadelphia: Saunders.

Hintermeister, R.A., M.J. Bey, G.W. Lange, J.R. Steadman, and C.J. Dillman. 1998. "Quantification of Elastic Resistance Knee Rehabilitation Exercises." *Journal of Orthopaedic and Sports Physical Therapy* 28(1): 40-50.

Hintermeister, R.A., G.W. Lange, J.M. Schulthies, M.J. Bey, and R.J. Hawkins. 1998. "Electromyographic Activity and Applied Load During Shoulder Rehabilitation Exercises Using Elastic Resistance." *American Journal of Sports Medicine* 26(2): 210-20.

Hopkins, J.T., C.D. Ingersoll, M.A. Sandrey, and S.D. Bleggi. 1999. "An Electromyographic Comparison of 4 Closed Chain Exercises." *Journal of Athletic Training* 34(4): 353-7.

Hughes, C.J., K. Hurd, A. Jones, and S. Sprigle. 1999. "Resistance Properties of Thera-Band Tubing During Shoulder Abduction Exercise." *Journal of Orthopaedic and Sports Physical Therapy* 29(7): 413-20.

Hughes, C.J., and A. McBride. 2000. "A Comparative Electromyographic Analysis of Shoulder Rehabilitation Exercises Using Isotonic and Elastic Resistances." In review.

Hughes, C.J., P. Page, and D. Maurice. 2000. "Elastic Exercise Training." *Orthopaedic Physical Therapy Clinics of North America* 9(4): 581-95.

Jones, K.W., D.S. Sims Jr, A.M. Prebish, J.D. Cornelius, M.L. Kvamme, T.L. Morneault, and R.A. Schmieg. 1998. "Predicting Forces Applied by Thera-Band Tubing During Resistive Exercises" (Abstract). *Journal of Orthopaedic and Sports Physical Therapy* 27(1): 65.

Kisner, C., and L.A. Colby. 1996. *Therapeutic exercise: Foundations and techniques.* 3rd ed. Philadelphia: Davis.

Kulig, K., J.G. Andrews, and J.G. Hay. 1984. "Human Strength Curves." *Exercise and Sport Sciences Reviews* 12: 417-66.

Lieber, R.L., and S.C. Bodine-Fowler. 1993. "Skeletal Muscle Mechanics: Implications for Rehabilitation." *Physical Therapy* 73(12): 844-56.

McCann, P.D., M.E. Wootten, M.P. Kadaba, and L.U. Bigliani LU. 1993. "A Kinematic and Electromyographic Study of Shoulder Rehabilitation Exercises." *Clinical Orthopaedics* 288: 179-88.

McCrum, N.G., C.P. Buckley, and C.B. Bucknall. 1988. *Principles of polymer engineering.* New York: Oxford University Press.

Mikesky, A.E., R. Topp, J.K. Wigglesworth, D.M. Harsha, and J.E. Edwards. 1994. "Efficacy of a Home-Based Training Program for Older Adults Using Elastic Tubing." *European Journal of Applied Physiology* 69: 316-20.

Morrissey, M.C., E.A. Harman, and M.J. Johnson. 1995. "Resistance Training Modes: Specificity and Effectiveness." *Medicine and Science in Sports and Exercise* 27(5): 648-60.

Ozkaya, N., and M. Nordin. 1991. *Fundamentals of biomechanics: Equilibrium, motion, and deformation.* New York: Van Nostrand Reinhold.

Page, P., and A. Labbe. 2000. "Torque Characteristics of Elastic Resistance and Weight-and-Pulley Exercise" (Abstract). *Medicine and Science in Sports and Exercise* 32(5) (Suppl.): S151.

Page, P., A. Labbe, and R. Topp. 2000. "Clinical Force Production of Thera-Band Elastic Bands" (Abstract). *Journal of Orthopaedic and Sports Physical Therapy* 30(1): A47-8.

Page, P.A., J. Lamberth, B. Abadie, R. Boling, R. Collins, and R. Linton. 1993. "Posterior Rotator Cuff Strengthening Using Thera-Band, in a Functional Diagonal Pattern in Collegiate Baseball Pitchers." *Journal of Athletic Training* 28(4): 346-54.

Patterson, R.M., C.W.S. Jansen, H.A. Hogan, and M.D. Nassif. 2001. "Material Properties of Thera-Band® Tubing." *Physical Therapy* 81(8): 1437-45.

Pezzullo, D.J., S. Karas, and J.J. Irrgang. 1995. "Functional Plyometric Exercises for the Throwing Athlete." *Journal of Athletic Training* 30(1): 22-6.

Rodgers, M.M., and P.R. Cavanagh. 1984. "Glossary of, Biomechanical Terms Concepts, and Units." *Physical Therapy* 64(12): 1886-902.

Schulthies, S.S., M.D. Ricard, K.J. Alexander, and J.W. Myrer. 1998. "An Electromyographic Investigation of 4 Elastic Tubing Closed Kinetic Chain Exercises After Anterior Cruciate Ligament Reconstruction." *Journal of Athletic Training* 33(4): 328-35.

Schultz, J.M. 1974. *Polymer materials science.* Englewood Cliffs, NJ: Prentice Hall.

Simoneau, G.G., S.M. Bereda, D.C. Sobush, and A.J. Starsky. 2001. "Biomechanics of Elastic Resistance in Therapeutic Exercise Programs." *Journal of Orthopaedic and Sports Physical Therapy* 31(1): 16-24.

Tesch, P.A. 1988. "Skeletal Muscle Adaptations Conse-quent to Long-Term Heavy Resistance Exercise." *Medicine and Science in Sports and Exercise* 20(5) (Suppl.): S132-4.

Wilk, K.E., and C. Arrigo. 1993. "Current Concepts in the Rehabilitation of the Athletic Shoulder." *Journal of Orthopaedic and Sports Physical Therapy* 18(1): 365-78.

Willett, G.M., J.B. Paladino, K.M. Barr, J.N. Korta, and G.M Karst. 1998. "Medial and Lateral Quadriceps Muscle Activity During Weight-Bearing Knee Extension Exercise." *Journal of Sport Rehabilitation* 7: 248-57.

Young, R.J. 1983. *Introduction to polymers.* London: Chapman & Hall.

CHAPTER 2

Clinical Research on Elastic Resistance

• • • • •

Phillip Page, MS, PT, ATC, CSCS
Benchmark Physical Therapy, Baton Rouge, LA
The Hygenic Corporation

In the past 20 years, elastic resistance has gained tremendous popularity in therapy and fitness settings around the world. Because of its general acceptance among clinicians as an effective mode of strengthening, there is limited research on the use of elastic resistance. Clinicians have relied on the premise of "biologic plausibility" regarding the efficacy of elastic resistance, understanding that any device that imparts resistive force to muscle will increase strength. However, clinicians realize other benefits of using elastic resistance in many different populations.

Recently, there has been an emphasis on evidence-based practice in health care, where clinicians must be able to show in the literature that their interventions are effective. For purposes of insurance, it is particularly important for health care professionals to validate their use of interventions. Randomized controlled trials (RCTs) offer the best evidence to support these interventions and outcomes.

The basis of evidence-based practice is the use of protocols and outcomes. Protocols must be scientifically evaluated through RCTs to validate clinical outcomes. Clinicians tend to avoid using protocols and instead rely on clinical experiences to guide their intervention. However, clinicians should use protocols as part of a rehabilitation program to provide consistency in treatments and to scientifically demonstrate efficacy and outcomes. Although many articles regarding elastic resistance are available in the literature, most are anecdotal applications and descriptive studies. The purpose of this chapter is to review the available RCTs on elastic resistance, including different outcomes in several populations.

A literature search of elastic resistance is difficult for several reasons. Most reference to elastic resistance in the literature is anecdotal and observational, noting mostly clinical applications. Few research titles or abstracts use the term *elastic*, making MEDLINE searches very difficult. Therefore, for this review, each potential article was read for its use of elastic resistance and each study cross-referenced.

At least 62 clinical trials on elastic resistance have been published in the literature. More than half (35) of these trials were RCTs. Of those, 12 were abstracts of presentations at national meetings and were excluded from this review. The remaining 23 studies (table 2.01) are reviewed in this chapter.

Traditionally, the literature evaluating any therapeutic intervention has focused on ameliorating

Table 2.01   Clinical Randomized Controlled Trials of Elastic Resistance

Author	Population	Frequencies (days/week)	Duration (weeks)	Outcomes
Anainsson et al. 1984	Older adults with "moderate disorders"	2	40	↑ Knee strength 6-13%[a]
Baker, Webright, and Perrin 1998	Young, healthy athletes	3	6	↓ Postural sway
Bang and Deyle 2000	Shoulder impingement patients	2	3	↓ Pain[a] ↑ Function[a] ↑ Strength 16%[a] (combined with manual therapy)
Curtis et al. 1999	Wheelchair users with shoulder pain	7	24	↓ Shoulder pain[a]
Damush and Damush 1999	Older adults, untrained	2	8	↑ Strength 16-28%[a] ↑ Functional score
Deyle et al. 2000	Older adults, knee osteoarthritis	2	4	↑ Gait[a] ↑ Function[a]
Docherty, Moore, and Arnold 1998	Young subjects with functionally unstable ankle	3	6	↑ Ankle strength 50%[a] ↑ Ankle joint position sense[a]
Duncan et al. 1998	Mild to moderate stroke patients	3	8	↑ Gait velocity[a] ↑ Functional score[a] ↑ Balance
Hanson et al. 1992	Healthy older adults	3	6	No change in strength
Hartigan et al. 2000	Lower back pain patients	3	8	↓ Disability[a] ↓ Pain[a]
Jette et al. 1996	Older adults, nondisabled	3	15	↑ Knee strength 10%[a]
Jette et al. 1996	Older adults, disabled	3	24	↑ Lower extremity strength 6-12%[a] ↑ Gait ↓ Disability[a]
Krebs, Jette, and Assman 1998	Older adults, disabled	3	24	↑ Lower extremity strength 18%[a] ↑ Gait
Mikesky et al. 1994	Older adults	3	12	↑ Knee strength 10-12%[a]
Page et al. 1993	Young, healthy baseball pitchers	3	6	↑ Shoulder strength 19%[a]
Ruhland and Shields 1997	Peripheral neuropathy patients	7	6	↑ Strength 5%[a] ↑ Grip strength ↑ Gait
Skelton and McLaughlin 1996	Older adults, healthy	3	8	↑ Knee strength 20%[a] ↑ Grip strength[a] ↑ Balance[a] ↑ Flexibility[a] ↑ Function[a]
Skelton et al. 1995	Older adults, healthy	3	12	↑ Strength 22-27% ↑ Grip strength[a] ↑ Leg power 18%[a]
Tinetti et al. 1999	Older adults	7	12	↓ Risk of falls[a]
Topp et al. 1996	Older adults, healthy	3	14	↑ Ankle strength 3-16%[a] ↑ Gait velocity[a]
Topp et al. 1993	Older adults, healthy	3	12	↑ Gait ↑ Balance
Treiber et al. 1998	Young, healthy tennis players	3	4	↑ Shoulder strength 17-24%[a] ↑ Serve velocity (function)[a]

[a]Statistically significant difference.

impairments such as decreased strength, decreased range of motion, or poor balance. Although lessening these impairments is important, many persons can still function with impairments. Health care recently has focused more on "functional ability"; subsequently, researchers have started investigating improvements in function and reductions in disability rather than improvements in impairment alone. Obviously, more research is needed on the reduction of disability with any therapeutic intervention.

Strength Impairments

Elastic resistance has been used primarily for strengthening exercise. There is strong evidence from several RCTs that elastic resistance improves strength in a number of populations. Most RCTs on elastic resistance training are performed on older adults because of its popularity in community exercise programs. In untrained, nondisabled older adults, moderate strength training with elastic resistance improves strength from 3% to 27% (Damush and Damush 1999; Jette et al. 1999; Mikesky et al. 1994; Skelton and McLaughlin 1996; Skelton et al. 1995; Topp et al. 1996). In disabled older adults, strength improves from 6% to 18% (Aniansson et al. 1984; Jette et al. 1999; Krebs, Jette, and Assmann 1998; Ruhland and Shields 1997). An added benefit of elastic resistance training is an improvement in grip strength (Ruhland and Shields 1997; Skelton and McLaughlin 1996; Skelton et al. 1995). One study on healthy older adults did not find any significant increase in strength when participants used bands (Hanson et al. 1992); however, the investigators did not individualize resistance to each subject at the beginning of the study. Instead they provided all subjects with the lowest level of resistance before the intervention regardless of baseline strength.

Trained athletes also have experienced improvements in strength when using elastic resistance. Page et al. (1993) noted a 19% increase in eccentric deceleration strength of the rotator cuff in baseball pitchers who used elastic resistance, significantly more than the control group, which used traditional isotonic resistance training. Subjects performed exercise 3 times per week for 6 weeks at 3 sets of 10 to 25 repetitions.

Treiber et al. (1998) also noted a 17% to 24% increase in shoulder strength, as well as an improvement in serve velocity, in collegiate tennis players. Subjects exercised for 4 weeks using 2 sets of 20 repetitions at two different speeds with elastic bands.

Pain Impairments

Three RCTs investigated the use of elastic resistance in subjects who experienced chronic pain. Curtis et al. (1999) reported a significant reduction in shoulder pain among wheelchair users over 6 months. Bang and Deyle (2000) noted significant reductions in shoulder impingement pain in 3 weeks. Hartigan and colleagues (2000), investigating patients with low back pain, reported a significant reduction in pain in 8 weeks when elastic resistance was part of a comprehensive exercise program.

Balance and Proprioception Outcomes

Strength training of the lower extremities with elastic resistance also may improve balance and proprioception. Elastic resistance can be used to improve balance indirectly or directly. General strengthening of the lower extremities and trunk (with open-chain exercise) can improve individual joint strength and improve neuromuscular connections, thus indirectly improving postural stability. A more direct method of balance training involves closed-chain strengthening, in which the lower extremity is challenged to maintain postural stability. A common method of closed-chain strengthening is for the participant to perform resisted kicks with one leg while balancing on the other, called *Thera-Band (T-Band) kicks*.

Topp et al. (1993) and Skelton and McLaughlin (1996) found that older adults improved in postural stability after 12 and 8 weeks of elastic resistance training, respectively. Duncan et al. (1998) also noted nonsignificant improvements in balance in stroke patients. These investigators used general strengthening routines to indirectly improve balance.

Investigation of direct methods (T-Band kicks) to improve balance and proprioception is relatively new. Kicking with elastic bands has become a very popular therapeutic exercise, particularly with patients who have lower extremity impairments. One study (Baker, Webright, and Perrin 1998) found improvements in postural sway with young, healthy athletes, although the findings were not statistically significant. This lack of significance may have been attributed to several factors: lack of technology to evaluate improvements in balance, insufficient protocol to challenge balance, or a ceiling effect with healthy individuals.

Function and Disability Outcomes

Several RCTs have investigated the effect of elastic resistance exercise on functional ability in subjects with disabilities. Subjects showing improvements in functional scales with elastic resistance include those with shoulder impingement (Bang and Deyle 2000), knee osteoarthritis (Deyle et al. 2000), stroke (Duncan et al. 1998), and low back pain (Hartigan et al. 2000).

Gait also can be considered a measure of functional ability. Topp and colleagues (1996, 1993) found that healthy, older adults improved their gait after 12 to 14 weeks of strengthening. Several other studies have shown that elastic resistance training improves gait in subjects with disability (Jette et al. 1999; Krebs, Jette, and Assmann 1998), including knee osteoarthritis (Deyle et al. 2000), stroke (Duncan et al. 1998), and peripheral neuropathy (Ruhland and Shields 1997).

Preventive Outcomes

Health care is experiencing a shift from focusing solely on treatment to focusing on prevention as well. Much research has yet to be done on the preventive effect of exercise that uses elastic resistance. Tinetti and colleagues (1999) investigated the effect of a multifactorial intervention to reduce the risk of falling in older adults. Elastic resistance exercises for the lower extremities were included with behavioral interventions, education, and gait, balance, and transfer training. The investigators noted a significant reduction in the risk of falling among those in the multifactorial intervention group during 1 year of follow-up.

Conclusion

Several RCTs have shown that elastic resistance reduces pain as well as impairments in strength and balance among several different populations. In addition, elastic resistance improves function and reduces disability. Elastic resistance is a cost-effective and clinically proven mode of therapeutic exercise with favorable outcomes.

References

Aniansson, A., P. Ljungberg, A. Rundgren, and H. Wetterqvist. 1984. "Effect of a Training Programme for Pensioners on Condition and Muscular Strength." *Archives of Gerontology and Geriatrics* 3: 229-41.

Baker, A.G., W.G. Webright, and D.H. Perrin. 1998. "Effect of a 'T-Band' Kick Training Protocol on Postural Sway." *Journal of Sport Rehabilitation* 7: 122-7.

Bang, M.D., and G.D. Deyle. 2000. "Comparison of Supervised Exercise With and Without Manual Physical Therapy for Patients With Shoulder Impingement Syndrome." *Journal of Orthopedic and Sports Physical Therapy* 30(3): 126-37.

Curtis, K.A., T.M. Tyner, L. Zachary, G. Lentell, D. Brink, T. Didyk, K. Gean, J. Hall, M. Hopper, J. Klos, S. Lesina, and B. Pacillas. 1999. "Effect of a Standard Exercise Protocol on Shoulder Pain in Long-Term Wheelchair Users." *Spinal Cord* 37: 421-9.

Damush, T.M., and J.G. Damush. 1999. "The Effects of Strength Training on Strength and Health-Related Quality of Life in Older Adult Women." *Gerontologist* 39(6): 705-10.

Deyle, G.D., N.E. Henderson, R.L. Matekel, M.G. Ryder, M.B. Garber, and S.C. Allison. 2000. "Effectiveness of Manual Physical Therapy and Exercise in Osteoarthritis of the Knee." *Annals of Internal Medicine* 132(3): 173-81.

Docherty, C.L., J.H. Moore, and B.L. Arnold. 1998. "Effects of Strength Training on Strength Development and Joint Position Sense in Functionally Unstable Ankles." *Journal of Athletic Training* 33(4): 310-4.

Duncan, P., L. Richards, D. Wallace, J. Stoker-Yates, P. Pohl, C. Luchies, A. Ogle, and S. Studenski. 1998. "A Randomized, Controlled Pilot Study of a Home-Based Exercise Program for Individuals With Mild and Moderate Stroke." *Stroke* 29: 2055-60.

Hanson, C.S., J. Agostinucci, P.J. Dasler, and G. Creel. 1992. "The effect of Short Term, Light Resistive Exercise on Well Elders." *Physical and Occupational Therapy in Geriatrics* 10(3): 73-81.

Hartigan, C., J. Rainville, J.B. Sobel, and M. Hipona. 2000. "Long-Term Exercise Adherence After Intensive Rehabilitation for Chronic Low Back Pain." *Medicine and Science in Sports Exercise* 32(3): 551-7.

Jette, A.M., B.A. Harris, L. Sleeper, M.E. Lachman, D. Heislein, M. Giorgetti, and C. Levenson. 1996. "A Home-Based Exercise Program for Nondisabled Older Adults." *Journal of the American Geriatric Society* 44(6): 644-9.

Jette, A.M., M. Lachman, M.M. Giorgetti, S.F. Assmann, B.A. Harris, C. Levenson, M. Wernick, and D. Krebs. 1999. "Exercise—It's Never Too Late: The Strong for Life Program." *American Journal of Public Health* 89(1): 66-72.

Krebs, D.E., A.M. Jette, and S.F. Assmann. 1998. "Moderate Exercise Improves Gait Stability in Disabled Elders." *Archives of Physical Medicine and Rehabilitation* 79(12): 1489-95.

Mikesky, A.E., R. Topp, J.K. Wigglesworth, D.M. Harsha, and J.E. Edwards. 1994. "Efficacy of a Home-Based Training Program for Older Adults Using Elastic Tubing." *European Journal of Applied Physiology* 69: 316-20.

Page, P.A., J. Lamberth, B. Abadie, R. Boling, R. Collins, and R. Linton. 1993. "Posterior Rotator Cuff Strengthening Using Thera-Band in a Functional Diagonal Pattern in Collegiate Baseball Pitchers." *Journal of Athletic Training* 28(4): 346-54.

Ruhland, J.L., and R.K. Shields. 1997. "The Effects of a Home Exercise Program on Impairment and Health-Related Quality of Life in Persons With Chronic Peripheral Neuropathies." *Physical Therapy* 77(10): 1026-37.

Skelton, D.A., and A.W. McLaughlin. 1996. "Training Functional Ability in Old Age." *Physiotherapy* 82(3): 159-67.

Skelton, D.A., A. Young, C.A. Greig, and K.E. Malbut. 1995. "Effects of Resistance Training on Strength, Power, and Selected Functional Abilities of Women Aged 75 and Older." *Journal of the American Geriatric Society* 43(10): 1081-7.

Tinetti, M.E., D.I. Baker, M. Gottschalk, C.S. Williams, D. Pollack, P. Garrett, T.M. Gill, R.A. Marottoli, and D. Acampora. 1999. "Home-Based Multicomponent Rehabilitation Program for Older Persons After Hip Fracture: A Randomized Trial." *Archives of Physical Medicine and Rehabilitation* 80: 916-22.

Topp, R., A. Mikesky, N.E. Dayhoff, and W. Holt. 1996. "Effect of Resistance Training on Strength, Postural Control, and Gait Velocity Among Older Adults." *Clinical Nursing Research* 5(4): 407-27.

Topp, R.A., A. Mikesky, J. Wigglesworth, W. Holt, and J.E. Edwards. 1993. "The Effect of a 12-Week Dynamic Resistance Strength Training Program on Gait Velocity and Balance of Older Adults." *Gerontologist* 33(4): 501-6.

Treiber, F.A., J. Lott, J. Duncan, G. Slavens, and H. Davis. 1998. "Effects of Thera-Band and Lightweight Dumbbell Training on Shoulder Rotation Torque and Serve Performance in College Tennis Players." *American Journal of Sports Medicine* 26(4): 510-5.

CHAPTER 3

Dosing of Elastic Resistance Exercise

• • • • •

Phillip Page, MS, PT, ATC, CSCS
Benchmark Physical Therapy, Baton Rouge, LA
The Hygenic Corporation

The ultimate goal of any rehabilitation program is to provide an optimal environment for healing without causing inflammation. Therapeutic exercise should be specifically prescribed to achieve this goal. Unfortunately, existing outcome studies offer very little information on specific exercise dosage parameters, including initial exercise prescription and progression. Most only describe exercise interventions as "progressive resistance exercise."

Clinicians tend to rely on clinical experiences to guide intervention, avoiding protocols and a "cookbook" approach. Davies (1995), however, suggested that clinicians and researchers should use detailed rehabilitation protocols to provide consistency in treatments and to demonstrate treatment efficacy.

Unfortunately, therapeutic exercise prescription is also based on clinical experience. This is particularly true of elastic resistance exercise, because clinicians have developed strengthening programs based on the color of an elastic band rather than the patient's actual strength capacities. The lack of specific protocols defining exercise prescription in outcome studies compounds this problem. Therapeutic exercise should be prescribed specifically to elicit a dose-response. Each type of tissue responds specifically to different exercise stimuli. Concomitant injury or disease is also a factor to consider in determining a dose-response to exercise.

The purpose of this chapter is to introduce the concept of exercise dosing, discuss the dose-response of resistance exercise, describe resistance exercise prescription, and provide biomechanical principles of patient positioning with elastic resistance exercise.

The Dosing Concept

Orthopedic manual physical therapists have popularized dosing of therapeutic exercise in rehabilitation. Scandinavian therapists were among the first to use this concept and believed that specifically dosed therapeutic exercise was a key component of any treatment. They advocated specific dosing of exercises, combined with manual therapy, to improve muscular strength, endurance, and coordination (Grimsby 1994).

In the management of disease or injury, therapeutic exercise should be dosed just as medication is.

The key is to provide the optimal dose for optimal results; therefore, exercise should be specifically dosed for the individual patient and for the individual tissues. For example, bone grows in response to compression or weight bearing, muscle responds best to tension, and cartilage responds best to compression (Engles 1994). Table 3.01 summarizes the optimal biomechanical forces for specific tissue healing.

Therapeutic Exercise Dose-Response

Exercise imparts forces to connective tissue, including tension, compression, and shear forces. Normal tissue requires a certain amount of physiologic force for normal tissue health and function. Specifically dosed amounts and types of forces will elicit specific results.

The exercise dose-response assumes that tissue responds to a specific exercise with a specific adaptation based on the amount and type of exercise performed. This is also known as the SAID principle: specific adaptation to imposed demands. The exercise stimulus must be strong enough to elicit a

Table 3.01   Tissue-Specific Optimal Biomechanical Forces

Tissue type	Optimal force
Bone	Compression (weight-bearing)
Muscle	Tension
Cartilage	Compression/decompression
Ligament	Tension

response. To avoid over- or underdosing of exercise, clinicians need reliable, accurate, and predictable means of prescribing exercise for both clinical and home exercise programs. The overall goal of any resistance exercise program is to increase the tissue tolerance to activity, including tissue-specific increases in load production, shock absorption, flexibility, coordination, and endurance. This tissue tolerance is related to load and frequency, or the total ability to perform work.

Tissue tolerance can be demonstrated graphically through the establishment of load and frequency. All human tissue can be considered to have an "envelope of function" (figure 3.01; Dye 1996).

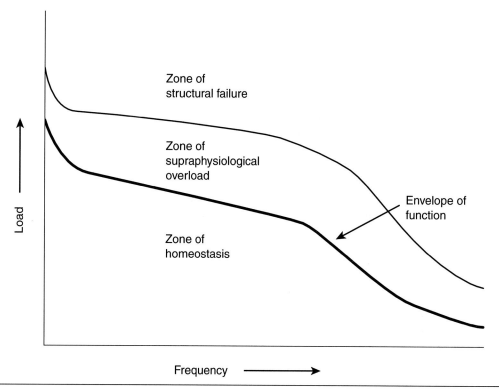

Figure 3.01   Envelope of function.

Reprinted, by permission, from S. Dye, 1996, "The Knee as a Biologic Transmission With an Envelope of Function," *Clinical Orthopaedics and Related Research* 325: 10-18.

This envelope of function is a theoretical barrier between normal tissue tolerance and function (zone of homeostasis), exercise adaptation (zone of supraphysiologic overload), and injury (zone of structural failure). The zones are direct functions of load and frequency. For example, higher loads at low frequencies of occurrence cause injury (e.g., trauma); lower loads over high frequencies can cause injury (e.g., repetitive strain injury) as well. The goal of exercise dosing is to increase tissue tolerance by stressing tissues within the zone of supraphysiological overload without causing inflammation.

Tissue injury and healing directly affect this envelope of function, shifting it down and to the left, essentially decreasing the tissue tolerance to load and frequency. Therefore, the amount of load or repetitions to further injure already-injured tissue is much less than for healthy tissue. This has direct implications for therapeutic exercise dosing and prescription. The appropriate resistance and number of repetitions must be applied to healing tissue just above the envelope of function to increase tissue tolerance and avoid subsequent injury. Therefore, clinicians must know the load characteristics (force and torque) of any activity to safely prescribe exercise.

Dose-Response to Resistance Exercise

The dose-response to resistance exercise has been studied extensively in healthy, untrained and trained individuals in many age groups (Franklin 2000). Unfortunately, few studies have evaluated the specific dose-response of resistive exercise on injured or healing tissue. Illness, injury, or disease significantly affects the tissue tolerance, thus requiring modifications to a typical exercise prescription. The most critical time to appropriately dose therapeutic exercise is very early in the rehabilitation process.

Table 3.02 provides the phases of the healing process.

Table 3.02   Phases of Healing

Phase	Time frame
Inflammatory	0-2 days
Repair	2 days to 6 weeks
Remodeling	6 weeks to 6 months

During the early repair phase (2 days to 6 weeks after injury or surgery), collagen is deposited randomly to repair damaged structures (Engles 1994). Healing collagen must be realigned along the lines of tensile stress, particularly in musculotendinous tissue, to avoid excessive scarring and contractures. Therefore, range of motion (ROM) and gentle strengthening exercises are indicated to place tension on the musculotendinous tissues and align collagen fibers.

Neuromuscular connections also are being reestablished during the first 4 to 6 weeks after injury. During this time, it is particularly important to emphasize normal movement patterns. Therefore, it is vital that patients have normal timing of muscular contraction, adequate neuromuscular control, and the ability to perform a particular movement without resistance before using any resistance exercise. Finally, it is essential that muscular strength balance between antagonistic groups be properly developed to prevent further dysfunction (Janda and Jull 1987).

Physiologically, resistance exercise has many benefits in regard to tissue healing and repair; therefore, therapeutic resistance exercise typically is prescribed for several different impairments.

Strength Impairments

Obviously, progressive resistance exercise increases muscular strength. Increases in strength depend on several factors, including dosage, initial strength levels, and experience. Strength training with elastic resistance improves strength in several different populations. Untrained individuals, both younger (Anderson et al. 1992; Fornataro et al. 1994; Leiby et al. 1995) and older (Damush and Damush 1999; Jette et al. 1996; Skelton et al. 1995) subjects, generally improve 10% to 28%. Disabled older adults have shown 6% to 18% improvements in strength (Aniansson et al. 1984; Jette et al. 1999; Krebs, Jette, and Assmann 1998), whereas trained younger adults demonstrate 19% to 24% improvements in strength (Page et al. 1993; Treiber et al. 1998). The initial improvements in strength, particularly early in the training program, also are associated with improvements in neuromuscular coordination (Sale 1988). Increases in strength may carry over into improvements in functional activities (Topp, Mikesky, and Thompson 1998; Treiber et al. 1998), but research is needed on the relationship of strength and function.

Balance Impairments

Theoretically, improvements in strength and neuromuscular coordination should improve postural stability and balance. Although some studies have shown that elastic resistance exercise improves balance in older individuals (Duncan et al. 1998; Skelton and McLaughlin 1996; Topp et al. 1993), more research is needed on the dose-response of strength training on balance. Strength training with elastic resistance may improve balance to prevent falls in older adults (Tinetti et al. 1994).

Cardiovascular Impairments

Strength training may indirectly influence the cardiovascular system. Exercising muscle increases local blood flow to the working muscles. This localized increase in blood flow is associated with a systemic cardiovascular adaptation. The cardiovascular adaptations to resistance exercise include lowered blood pressure, increased stroke volume, and improved peak oxygen uptake (Fleck and Kramer 1997).

Resistance Exercise Prescription and Progression

Several steps are necessary to determine an appropriate dosage of exercise for a desired response (table 3.03).

The first step in any exercise prescription involves assessment and goal setting. Goals should be directed at reducing impairments, improving function, and decreasing disability. Specific interventions then are determined to accomplish these goals by following the SAID principle. When determining specific interventions, one must first consider the tissue tolerance and its relative position on the envelope of function. The effects of the exercise on the target tissue as well as other associated tissues should be considered. Once the specific joint and target tissues have been established, acute variables are defined in the exercise prescription.

Mode of Exercise

The mode of exercise is directly related to the specific exercise goal. Different modes of elastic exercise may include strengthening exercises, balance activities, cardiovascular conditioning, or functional training.

Range of Motion

The clinician should next determine the appropriate ROM. Typically, smaller ranges are performed first; these protected motions then are gradually increased to include the outer ROMs before full ROM exercises are performed.

Type of Contraction

The type of muscular contraction (isometric, concentric, eccentric, or plyometric) is an important functional consideration. Clinicians should always remember that the most basic function of resistance exercise is to facilitate muscle contraction or to enhance neural recruitment for function. Therefore, based on the force-velocity curve (figure 3.02), the continuum of force production is eccentric → isometric → concentric.

Elastic resistance also can be used effectively for plyometric training. A plyometric contraction is an advanced series of muscular contractions involving rapid transition from eccentric to concentric contraction within the same muscle. Clinicians also should consider associated contractions of neutralizers, stabilizers, and antagonists during the exercise.

Speed of Movement

In general, slower movements precede faster movements during resistance training. The type of contraction also is related to the speed of movement. The force-velocity relationship (figure 3.02) indicates higher force production with eccentric contractions as speed increases, whereas concentric contractions decrease in force with increasing speed of movement.

Intensity of Exercise

The intensity (resistance) must be dosed appropriately for optimal stimulus of healing tissue. Resistance is the most important stimulus for strength gains and endurance (McDonagh and Davies 1984). Too much resistance may result in injury, whereas too little may result in inadequate strength gains. When dosing elastic resistance exercise, clinicians must match the appropriate resistance levels with the individual's specific strength capabilities. Preliminary strength can be determined by using manual muscle testing, dynamometry, or repetition maximums (RM). DeLorme and Watkins (1948) first used the RM concept in 1948 to prescribe resistances that could be lifted only a specific number of times.

There are many ways to determine appropriate resistance intensity. Although percentage of one RM (1RM) is used commonly in strength training,

Table 3.03 Acute Dosing Variables

Variable	Consideration
Exercise goal	Reduce impairments Improve function Decrease disability
Target tissue	Determine specific tissue to be exercised Consider other effects on bone, muscle, ligament, tendon, cartilage Consider tissue tolerance (low → high) Consider forces imposed (shear, compression, tension)
Mode of exercise	Strength training, stretching, balance training, cardiovascular
Motion	Smaller ranges → larger ranges Inner ranges → outer ranges Isolated → functional patterns Protected → unprotected ranges
Contraction	Passive → isometric → eccentric → concentric → plyometric Consider associated contractions (cocontractions, neutralizers, stabilizers, antagonists)
Speed	Velocity of movement (slow → fast)
Intensity	Resistance levels (RM, RPE) Torque effects (lever arm, resistance-arm angle)
Volume	Sets and repetitions Time RPE Rest periods between sets and exercises
Frequency	Times per week Rest periods between workouts/recovery
Duration	Total length of treatment for goals
Order	Large/small muscle groups Isolated/compound movements Proximal/distal Phasic/tonic Anaerobic/aerobic

RM = repetition maximum; RPE = rating of perceived exertion.

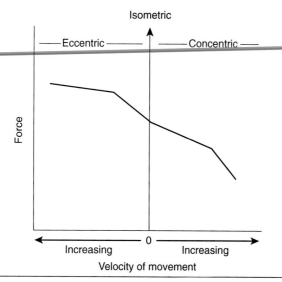

Figure 3.02 Force-velocity curve.

Adapted, by permission, from S.J. Fleck and W.J. Kraemer, 1997. *Designing resistance training programs,* Champaign, IL: Human Kinetics, 53.

research shows that the number of repetitions at a particular percentage of RM varies greatly by exercise, gender, and experience (Hoeger et al. 1987, 1990). In addition, formulas to predict 1RM (Arnold et al. 1995; Mayhew, Ball, and Arnold 1989) usually are based on healthy trained individuals using exercises such as bench press and squat. Because of the limitations in using percent of 1RM, a multiple RM approach to resistance dosing in therapeutic exercise is recommended. This involves having the patient complete as many correct repetitions (generally 8-12 repetitions for fitness and 20-25 for rehabilitation) to fatigue by using a particular resistance. Fatigue is recognized as the point where the patient begins to experience a burning sensation in the muscle or begins to alter his or her mechanics by compensating motion to complete the repetition. Several studies have demonstrated improved strength with elastic resistance training at 8 to 12RM (Jette et al. 1996, 1999; Mikesky et al. 1994; Skelton et al. 1995; Skelton and McLaughlin 1996).

The starting resistance to determine the appropriate intensity can be estimated by using a rating of perceived exertion (RPE) from Borg's Scale (1982, 1998). RPE is particularly useful to teach patients how to progress as they transition to home exercise programs. Relatively few studies that use the Borg scales in force production have been performed (Jackson and Dishman 2000). Although several elastic exercise training studies have successfully used Borg's RPE scale in older adults and subjects with chronic disease (Aniansson et al. 1984; Damush and Damush 1999; Heislein,

Harris, and Jette 1994), no clear relationship between resistance intensity dosing and the RPE scale has been established. Nevertheless, the RPE scale can be used as a general tool to estimate the appropriate starting resistance.

As the intensity of elastic resistance exercise increases, it is important to increase to the next larger size of band or tubing rather than "shorten up." Typically, patients are told to grasp the band closer to the origin as they improve in strength to increase the resistance. When tension is added to an elastic resistive device, the effective force increases greatly, which changes the torque curve of the exercise and alters the biomechanics of the motion (Simoneau et al. 2001). Therefore, the next level of resistance should be used to progress exercise intensity. Page, Labbe, and Topp (2000) showed a 20% to 30% increase in force production between colors of Thera-Band resistive bands.

Volume

Volume and intensity are inversely related; high-volume training requires low intensities, whereas low-volume training can sustain much higher intensities. The volume of training is defined as the total number of sets and repetitions at a particular resistance.

Single sets are appropriate for beginners, whereas multiple sets that improve strength and power faster than single sets may be more appropriate for experienced individuals. As patients progress, volume should be increased before intensity. Once a patient has attained a certain volume at a set intensity, the intensity is increased and the volume decreased. This ensures that the tissue has the metabolic capability for activities of daily life.

Table 3.04 provides guidelines for prescribing appropriate intensities (resistance) and volumes (sets and repetitions) of resistance exercise.

In general, higher intensity and lower volume (6RM or less) are appropriate for strength and power gains; lower intensity and higher volume improve muscular endurance (20RM or more; Fleck and Kraemer 1997). Typically, 2 to 3 sets of 25 repetitions are used for rehabilitation. This corresponds to an RPE of 9 to 10. Volume also can be dosed by setting a certain time frame to complete exercise. For example, a set of 10 to 12RM resistance should be performed in approximately 30 s for anaerobic training. Adequate rest and recovery of the tissue between sets and training sessions are necessary to repair and improve strength. Rest should be proportional to activity and based on the metabolism

Table 3.04   Resistance Exercise Dosing

Goal	Metabolism (s)	Intensity (% 1RM)	Intensity (multiple RM)	Rating of Perceived Exertion
				20 Maximal Exertion
				19 Extremely Hard
Strength and power	ATP-CP	90	3	18
	10 s	85	6	17 Very Hard
				16
				15 Hard (heavy)
High-intensity endurance and speed	Anaerobic	75	10	14
	30-90 s	70	12	13 Somewhat Hard
				12
				11 Light
Low-intensity endurance	Aerobic	60	20	10
	>120 s	55	25	9 Very Light
				8
				7 Extremely Light
				6 No exertion at all

RM = repetition maximum; ATP – CP = adenosine triphosphate – creatine phosphate

Part of this table reprinted, by permission, from G. Borg. 1998. *Borg's Perceived Exertion and Pain Scales,* Champaign, IL: Human Kinetics, 47.

Part of this table was created from data in S.J. Fleck and W.J. Kraemer. 1997. *Designing Resistance Training Programs.* 2nd ed. Champaign, IL: Human Kinetics.

used during the exercise. For example, for quick exercises that use the adenosine triphosphate-creatine phosphate system, the work/rest ratio should be 1:3 to 1:5 (3-5RM); for anaerobic exercise, 1:2 to 1:3 (10-12RM); and for aerobic exercise, 1:1 (20-25RM).

Frequency and Duration of Exercise

Two to three sessions a week improve strength, whereas one session per week maintains strength (Graves et al. 1988). Typically, 4 to 6 weeks of resistance exercise are necessary to see improvements in strength. Interestingly, the strength gains noted in the first 4 weeks of a resistance training program are related to improved recruitment and neuromuscular coordination rather than muscular hypertrophy (Sale 1988). Clinical trials have shown that, similar to other types of resistance exercise training, elastic resistance programs performed 6 to 12 weeks, 3 times a week, for 2 to 3 sets at 8 to 12RM resistance, significantly improve strength when progressed with increasing volume and intensity of elastic resistance.

Order of Exercises

The optimal order of exercise is determined by the functional and metabolic capabilities of the tissue.

Within a single session, large muscle groups should be exercised before smaller groups so that the smaller stabilizing muscles aren't fatigued during more heavily resisted movements. Metabolically, tissues prone to fatigue should be exercised last in order to prevent injury.

American College of Sports Medicine (ACSM) Guidelines

The ACSM (Franklin, 2000) recommends specific guidelines for cardiorespiratory fitness, musculoskeletal fitness, and flexibility in an apparently healthy population. These guidelines define specific volumes, intensity, frequency, and duration, and they are slightly modified for older adults or special populations.

Strength Index of Elastic Bands

For functional strength testing, Topp, Mikesky, and Thompson (1998) described a "strength index" that established an objective measure of strength by having patients perform a particular exercise with a certain resistance. The total number of repetitions to fatigue was multiplied by the force of Thera-Band elastic bands at full elongation. This provides a repeatable measurement of any movement or functional activity that can be used in the overall assessment process. The appendix (page 339) provides the strength index for all colors of Thera-Band elastic bands. Mikesky et al. (1996) reported that techniques to assess muscular strength by using elastic resistance yielded correlations from .48 to .93. Topp, Mikesky, and Thompson (1998) further noted that the seated row, squats, and hip flexion strength indexes with elastic resistance correlated well with functional tasks in older individuals.

Biomechanical Principles of Elastic Resistance Exercise

Patient positioning during exercise sometimes is taken for granted or is determined out of convenience rather than according to biomechanical principles. Clinicians must be aware of the effects of gravity, torque, specificity, and positioning during exercise. The basic science of elastic resistance has been presented earlier in this book. It is important for the clinician to understand the difference between force and torque when positioning a patient for elastic resistance exercise.

Force

As noted previously, elastic resistance offers increasing force with elongation. Clinically, elongations with elastic resistance rarely exceed 300%. All elastic products have characteristic force-elongation curves, which are typically three-phased (figure 3.03). The first phase is marked by an exponential increase in the first 25% elongation. Next, there is a linear increase between 25% and 500% and finally a sharp exponential increase until failure (Klippel et al. 1999).

Therefore, it is recommended that patients work between 25% and 250% elongation and increase resistance by progressing to the next color, rather than increasing the stretch on the band or tubing. Increasing the stretch on the elastic band or tubing to increase the force before exercising may change the biomechanics of the exercise as well (Simoneau et al. 2001).

Torque

Torque, or moment of force, expresses the effectiveness of a force in turning a lever system; therefore, torque is related directly to strength. A particular joint movement possesses a torque versus joint angle curve, otherwise known as a *strength curve*. Strength curves result from the interaction of resistance and changing mechanical advantage of the musculoskeletal system. The strength curve of a joint is related to the length-tension relationship of muscles crossing the joint. Typically, force production of a muscle is greatest at its resting length; if the muscle is lengthened or shortened, it has less capability to produce force. Therefore, the length-tension relationship of muscle produces an ascending-descending force curve, similar to the strength curves of joints. Ramsey and Street (1940) defined the physiologically useful portion of the length-tension curve as approximately 70% to 110% of resting length (figure 3.04).

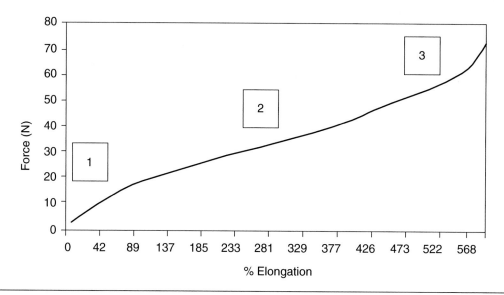

Figure 3.03 Three regions of elastic resistance.

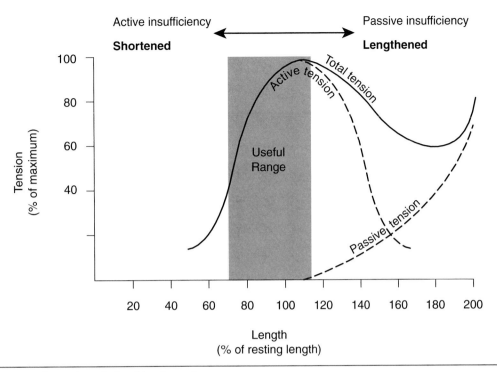

Figure 3.04   Length-tension relationship of muscle.

Adapted from R.W. Ramsey, and S.F. Street 1940."Isometric Length-Tension Diagram of Isolated Skeletal Muscle Fibers of Frog." *Journal of Cell Composition and Physiology* 15:11.

This curve indicates that the least amount of strength is produced from shortened muscle lengths. This corresponds to ending ROM, where joints are typically their weakest.

When applied correctly, elastic resistance exercise provides ascending and descending torque curves (Hughes et al. 1999; Page, McNeil, and Labbe 2000), demonstrating characteristics similar to human strength curves. Thus, elastic resistance allows individuals to complete the ROM. Resistance exercise should provide an amount of torque throughout the ROM that is correct for the strength capacity of the joint. The torque production (moment) of the resistance exercise should equal the torque capability (moment, or M) of the joint ($M_{exercise} = M_{joint}$) This has been termed the *muscular strength utilization ratio* (Arborelius and Ekholm 1978). The goal of any strengthening exercise is to stimulate the maximal number of muscle fibers. Elastic resistance training that loads muscle to its limits throughout the ROM should result in maximal muscle activation and greater strength gains.

Positioning for Elastic Resistance Exercise

Muscular strength gains are specific to the demands placed on the muscles. Positioning is a critical fac-

tor in any resistance exercise because of its importance in developing resistive torque. Improper positioning can preclude an adequate muscular-strength utilization ratio (Arborelius and Ekholm 1978) because of inadequate torque production.

Until recently, there was no literature on proper positioning during elastic resistance exercise. Hughes et al. (1999) first described the biomechanical implications of patient positioning by describing the torque production during shoulder abduction with elastic resistance. Simoneau and colleagues (2001) provided a similar biomechanical analysis of elastic resistance exercise, noting the importance of proper positioning and its effect on torque.

Several biomechanical variables must be considered for proper positioning (figure 3.05). In addition to the resistive force of the band or tubing, the distance of the origin to the axis (DOA), the angle of origin to axis (AOA), and the angle of the resistance to the lever arm (resistance arm angle, or RAA) affect the resultant torque curve of the exercise (Arborelius and Ekholm 1978).

Length of Band or Tubing

The first step in positioning for elastic resistance exercise is to define the axis of rotation and the lever arm. Arborelius and Ekholm (1978) found that

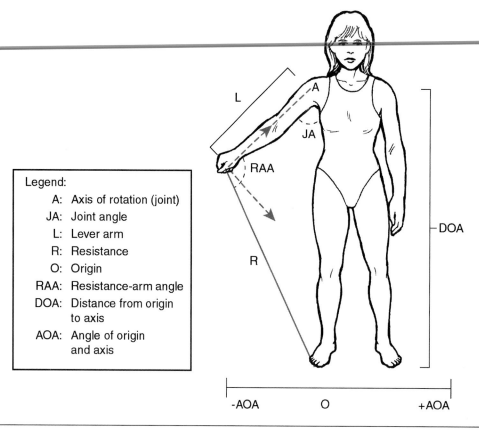

Figure 3.05 Positioning variables. Adapted, by permission, from C.J. Hughes, K. Hurd, A. Jones, and S. Sprigle, 1999, "Resistance properties of Thera-Band tubing during shoulder abduction exercise," *Journal of Orthopaedic and Sports Physical Therapy* 29(7):413-20.

the DOA should be twice the lever arm for an optimal ascending-descending torque curve. Therefore, the starting length of tubing or band should be equal to the length of the lever arm. This will provide a DOA of twice the lever arm length and will ensure that elongations remain below 200% (figures 3.06 and 3.07).

For example, if the length of the patient's arm from shoulder to fist measures 25 in., then a 25-in. length of band would be used for the shoulder abduction exercise in figure 3.06. This band would then be elongated 200% at the end of 180° of shoulder abduction (figure 3.07).

Origin of Elastic Resistance

Once the ROM for exercise and the starting length of the band or tubing have been established, the origin of the tubing or band must be determined. The origin should place the band or tubing in the plane of the axis of rotation and in the direction of motion. The position of the origin affects the resulting torque curve of the exercise (figures 3.08-3.10).

Increasing the AOA (figure 3.10) increases and shifts the torque curve to the left; conversely, de-

creasing the AOA (figure 3.08) decreases and shifts the torque curve to the right (Arborelius and Ekholm 1978). The torque curves are affected by the AOA because it directly affects the RAA. The optimal angle of the origin to the axis is zero (figure 3.09)

Resistance Arm Angle

The most important angle to consider in effective torque production is the RAA: the angle produced by the band or tubing and the lever arm. The RAA is directly related to the torque production of the resistive exercise. Torque is defined as follows:

Force × Lever arm × Sine of the RAA

During 180° of shoulder flexion, for example, the RAA decreases from 180° to 0° as joint ROM increases from 0° to 180° (figure 3.11), producing an ascending-descending torque curve while the resistance of the band or tubing increases.

Because the least amount of torque is available at the ending physiological range (shortest muscle

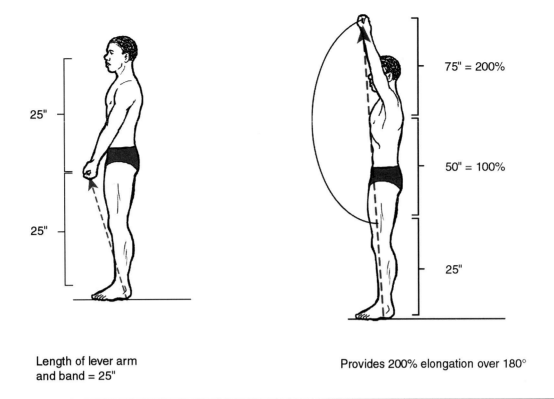

25"

25"

75" = 200%

50" = 100%

25"

Length of lever arm
and band = 25"

Provides 200% elongation over 180°

Figures 3.06 and 3.07 Starting length of band equal to lever arm. The length of the lever arm and the band should be 25 inches. This provides 200% elongation over 180 degrees of shoulder flexion.

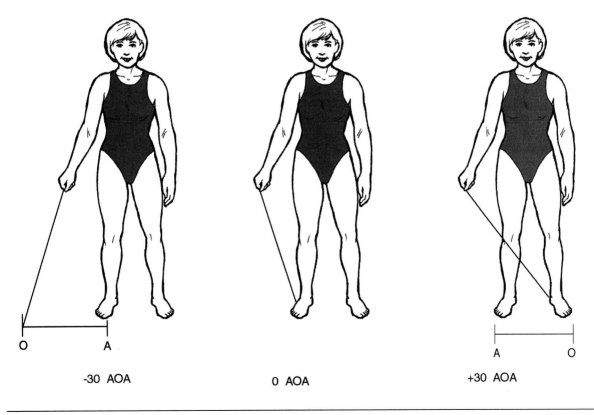

O   A

-30 AOA

0 AOA

A   O

+30 AOA

Figures 3.08-3.10 Effect of angle of origin to axis (AOA). (3.08) shifts strength curve to right; (3.09) provides optimal strength curve; (3.10) shifts strength curve to left.

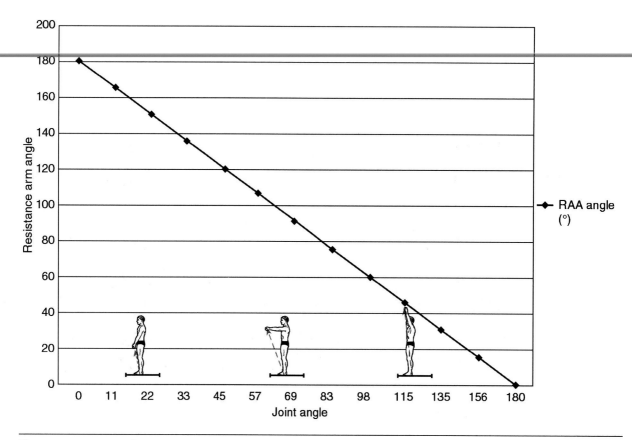

Figure 3.11   Joint angle versus resistance-arm angle.

length), the band or tubing should be aligned with the ending lever arm at an RAA of 15° to 0° to minimize torque at end range (figure 3.12).

This allows exercise throughout the ROM. Therefore, the end position of the limb during physiological ROM ultimately will determine the origin of the band. Partial ROM exercise (such as 0-90°) should still be aligned with the physiological ending lever to ensure a physiologically correct torque curve during the exercise (figure 3.13). Figures 3.14 through 3.19 demonstrate examples of proper positioning for common exercises to provide a physiological ascending-descending torque curve.

Precautions for Using Elastic Resistance

- Avoid long fingernails.
- Remove jewelry before exercise.
- Check bands and tubing for wear, tears, and rubbing before use; replace as needed.

- Check connections and secure attachments before use.
- Protect the eyes during exercise.
- Avoid stretching the band or tubing more than 300% elongation to prevent breakage.
- Persons with latex allergies should use latex-free resistive bands or tubing.

Home Program Considerations

In today's health care environment, there is an increased need for home exercise prescription. Elastic resistance is ideal for the home setting because of its portability. It is especially important to instruct patients on proper technique and precautions when they use elastic resistance at home. The most important factor in any exercise program is compliance, and patients are more likely to continue exercise programs that are easy to understand and that demonstrate progression toward goals. Many

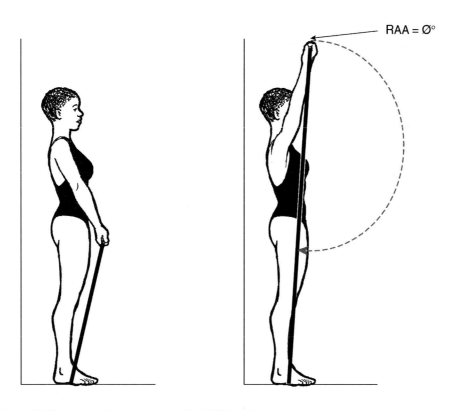

Figure 3.12   Physiologic range of motion (shoulder flexion).

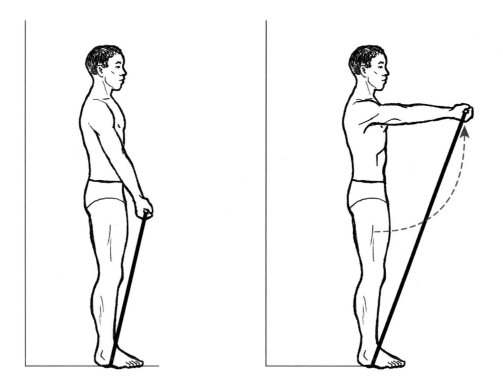

Figure 3.13   Partial range of motion (shoulder flexion).

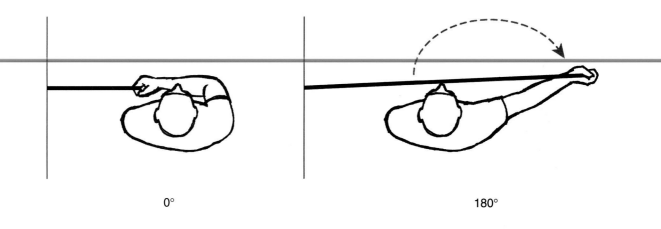

0°   180°

Figure 3.14-3.15 Proper positioning for shoulder external rotation.

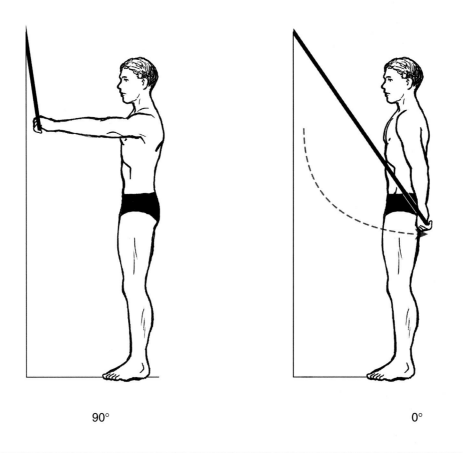

90°   0°

Figure 3.16-3.17 Proper positioning for shoulder extension.

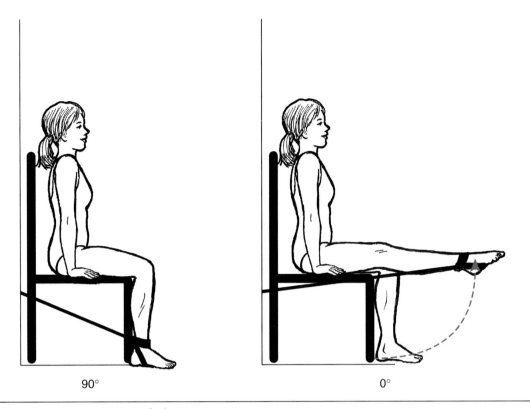

90°   0°

Figure 3.18-3.19 Proper positioning for knee extension.

patients continue their clinical exercises as part of a maintenance program. Clinicians also should instruct their patients on proper progression of sets, repetitions, and resistance.

Conclusion

The following summarizes the elastic resistance exercise dosing process:

1. Determine ROM to be exercised and establish the physiological end lever. Remember that the end position of the exercise may not be the physiological end position.
2. Approximate the starting amount of resistance desired and the appropriate band color.
3. Use a starting length of band or tubing approximately equal to the length of the lever arm (e.g., a 12-in. forearm length requires a 12-in. length of band for shoulder internal rotation).
4. Place the origin of the band or tubing in the plane of the axis of rotation and align the band or tubing with the physiological ending lever

(may not be the ending lever of the exercise) so that RAA is between 15° and 0°.
5. Begin the motion with a slight stretch on the band, approximately 25% elongation.
6. Ask the patient to perform two repetitions and rate the resistance on a scale of 0 to 10, and then modify resistance level according to goals (refer to table 3.04). Perform multiple RMs. Be sure patient positioning is correct.
7. To increase the resistance, do not increase tension on the band or tubing to increase force; proceed to the next color or add additional bands or tubing for resistance.

It is important for clinicians to use appropriate biomechanical principles and to understand physiological function when applying elastic resistance exercise to healing tissue. Resistance exercise should be dosed specifically to individual tissues for optimal healing. Acute variables such as volume, intensity, duration, and frequency should be prescribed specific to the goals of the patient. Finally, positioning of the patient is vital to provide an optimal dose of resistance throughout the ROM.

References

Anderson, L., R. Rush, L. Shearer, and C.J. Hughes. 1992. "The Effects of a Thera-Band Exercise Program on Shoulder Internal Rotation Strength" (Abstract). *Physical Therapy* 72(6): S40.

Aniansson, A., P. Ljungberg, A. Rundgren, and H. Wetterqvist. 1984. "Effect of a Training Programme for Pensioners on Condition and Muscular Strength." *Archives of Gerontology and Geriatrics* 3: 229-41.

Arborelius, U.F., and J. Ekholm. 1978. "Mechanics of Shoulder Locomotor System During Exercises Resisted by Weight-and-Pulley-Circuit." *Scandinavian Journal of Rehabilitation Medicine* 10: 171-7.

Arnold, M.D., J.L. Mayhew, D. LeSeur, and M. McCormick. 1995. "Accuracy of Predicting Bench Press and Squat Performance From Repetitions as Low and High Intensity." *Journal of Strength and Conditioning Research* 9(3): 205.

Borg G. 1982. "Psychophysical Bases of Perceived Exertion." *Medicine and Science in Sports and Exercise* 14(4): 377-81.

Borg G. 1998. *Borg's Perceived Exertion and Pain Scales.* Champaign, IL: Human Kinetics

Damush, T.M., and J.G. Damush. 1999. "The Effects of Strength Training on Strength and Health-Related Quality of Life in Older Adult Women." *Gerontologist* 39(6): 705-10.

Davies, G.J. 1995. "The Need for Critical Thinking in Rehabilitation." *Journal of Sport Rehabilitation* 4: 1-22.

DeLorme, T.L., and A.L. Watkins. 1948. "Techniques of Progressive Resistive Exercise." *Archives of Physical Medicine* 29: 263-73.

Duncan, P., L. Richards, D. Wallace, J. Stoker-Yates, P. Pohl, C. Luchies, A. Ogle, and S. Studenski. 1998. "A Randomized, Controlled Pilot Study of a Home-Based Exercise Program for Individuals With Mild and Moderate Stroke." *Stroke* 29:2055-60.

Dye, S. 1996. "The Knee as a Biologic Transmission With an Envelope of Function." *Clinical Orthopaedics and Related Research* 325: 10-18.

Engles, M. 1994. "Tissue Response." Pp. 1-31 in *Orthopaedic Physical Therapy,* ed. R.A. Donatelli and M.J. Wooden. New York: Churchill Livingstone.

Fleck, S.J., and W.J. Kraemer. 1997. *Designing Resistance Training Programs.* 2nd ed. Champaign, IL: Human Kinetics.

Fornataro, S., M. Green, D. Martz, K. Masneri, and C.J. Hughes. 1994. "Investigation to Determine Differences in Strength Gains Using Thera-Band" at Fast and Slow Training Speeds" (Abstract). *Physical Therapy* 74(5) (Suppl.): S53.

Franklin, B.A., ed. 2000. *ACSM's Guidelines for Exercise Testing and Prescription.* 6th ed. Philadelphia: Lippincott Williams & Wilkins.

Graves, J.E., M.L. Pollock, S.H. Leggett, R.W. Braith, D.M. Carpenter, and L.E. Bishop. 1988. "Effect of Reduced Training Frequency on Muscular Strength." *International Journal of Sports Medicine* 9(5): 316-9

Grimsby, O. 1994. "Scientific Therapeutic Exercise Progressions." *Journal of Manual and Manipulative Therapy* 2: 94-101.

Heislein, D.M., B.A. Harris, and A.M. Jette. 1994. "A Strength Training Program for Postmenopausal Women: A Pilot Study." *Archives of Physical Medicine and Rehabilitation* 75(2): 198-204.

Hoeger, W.W.K., S.L. Barette, D.F. Hale, and D.R. Hopkins. 1987. "Relationship Between Repetitions and Selected Percentages of One Repetition Maximum." *Journal of Applied Sports Science Research* 1:11-3.

Hoeger, W.W.K., D.R. Hopkins, S.L. Barette, and D.F. Hale. 1990. "Relationship Between Repetitions and Selected Percentages of One Repetition Maximum: A Comparison Between Untrained and Trained Males and Females." *Journal of Applied Sports Science Research* 4: 47-54.

Hughes, C.J., K. Hurd, A. Jones, and S. Sprigle. 1999. "Resistance Properties of Thera-Band Tubing During Shoulder Abduction Exercise." *Journal of Orthopaedic and Sports Physical Therapy* 29(7): 413-20.

Jackson, A.W., and R.D. Dishman. 2000. "Perceived Submaximal Force Production in Young Adult Males and Females." *Medicine and Science in Sports and Exercise* 32(3): 448-51.

Janda, V., and G. Jull. 1987. "Muscles and Motor Control in Low Back Pain." In *Therapy of the Low Back: Clinics in Physical Therapy,* ed. L. Twomey and J.R. Taylor. New York: Churchill Livingstone.

Jette, A.M., B.A. Harris, L. Sleeper, M.E. Lachman, D. Heislein, M. Giorgetti, and C. Levenson. 1996. "A Home-Based Exercise Program for Nondisabled Older Adults." *Journal of the American Geriatric Society* 44(6): 644-9.

Jette, A.M., M. Lachman, M.M. Giorgetti, S.F. Assmann, B.A. Harris, C. Levenson, M. Wernick, and D. Krebs. 1999. "Exercise—It's Never Too Late: The Strong for Life Program." *American Journal of Public Health* 89(1): 66-72.

Klippel, S., N. Olivier, C. Augste, and A. Lowis. 1999. "Mechanical Properties of Thera-Band Resistive Exercisers." Pp. 101-106 in *Proceedings of the First European Congress of OASIS.* Palaiseau, France: OASIS.

Krebs, D.E., A.M. Jette, and S.F. Assmann. 1998. "Moderate Exercise Improves Gait Stability in Disabled Elders." *Archives of Physical Medicine and Rehabilitation* 79(12): 1489-95.

Leiby, K.W., P.J. Neece, S.H. Phipps, and C.J. Hughes. 1995. "A Comparison of Two Methods of Resistance Training on Ipsilateral/Contralateral Hip Abduction Strength" (Abstract). *Journal of Orthopaedic and Sports Physical Therapy* 21(1): 52.

Mayhew, J.L., T.E. Ball, and M.D. Arnold. 1989. "Prediction of 1RM Bench Press From Submaximal Bench Press Performance in College Males and Females." *Journal of Applied Sports Science* 3 (Suppl.): S73.

McDonagh, M.J.N., and C.T.M. Davies. 1984. "Adaptive Responses of Mammalian Skeletal Muscle to Exercise With High Loads." *European Journal of Applied Physiology* 52: 139-55.

Mikesky, A., R. Topp, A. Meyer, and K. Thompson. 1996. "Reliability of Ten Tests for Assessing Functional Performance and Strength in Older Adults" (Abstract). *Medicine and Science in Sports and Exercise* 28(5) (Suppl.): S11.

Mikesky, A.E., R. Topp, J.K. Wigglesworth, D.M. Harsha, and J.E. Edwards. 1994. "Efficacy of a Home-Based Training

Program for Older Adults Using Elastic Tubing." *European Journal of Applied Physiology* 69: 316-20.

Page, P., A. Labbe, and R. Topp. 2000. "Clinical Force Production of Thera-Band Elastic Bands" (Abstract). *Journal of Orthopaedic and Sports Physical Therapy* 30(1): A47-8.

Page, P., M. McNeil, and A. Labbe. 2000. "Torque Characteristics of Two Types of Resistive Exercise" (Abstract). *Physical Therapy* 80(5) (Suppl.): S69.

Page, P.A., J. Lamberth, B. Abadie, R. Boling, R. Collins, and R. Linton. 1993. "Posterior Rotator Cuff Strengthening Using Thera-Band in a Functional Diagonal Pattern in Collegiate Baseball Pitchers." *Journal of Athletic Training* 28(4): 346-54.

Ramsey, R.W., and S.F. Street. 1940. "Isometric Length-Tension Diagram of Isolated Skeletal Muscle Fibers of Frog." *Journal of Cell Composition and Physiology* 15: 11.

Sale, D.B. 1988. "Neural Adaptation to Resistance Training." *Medicine and Science in Sports and Exercise* 20(5) (Suppl.): S135-45.

Simoneau, G.G., S.M. Bereda, D.C. Sobush, and A.J. Starsky. 2001. "Biomechanics of Elastic Resistance in Therapeutic Exercise Programs." *Journal of Orthopaedic and Sports Physical Therapy* 31(1): 16-24.

Skelton, D.A., and A.W. McLaughlin. 1996. "Training Functional Ability in Old Age." *Physiotherapy* 82(3): 159-67.

Skelton, D.A., A. Young, C.A. Greig, and K.E. Malbut. 1995. "Effects of Resistance Training on Strength, Power, and Selected Functional Abilities of Women Aged 75 and Older." *Journal of the American Geriatric Society* 43(10): 1081-7.

Tinetti, M.E., D.I. Baker, G. McAvay, E.B. Claus, P. Garrett, M. Gottschalk, M.L. Koch, K. Trainor, and R.I. Horwitz. 1994. "A Multifactorial Intervention to Reduce the Risk of Falling Among Elderly People Living in the Community." *New England Journal of Medicine* 331(13): 821-7.

Topp, R.A., A. Mikesky, and K. Thompson. 1998. "Determinants of Four Functional Tasks Among Older Adults: An Exploratory Regression Analysis." *Journal of Orthopaedic and Sports Physical Therapy* 27(2): 144-53.

Topp, R.A., A. Mikesky, J. Wigglesworth, W. Holt, and J.E. Edwards. 1993. "The Effect of a 12-Week Dynamic Resistance Strength Training Program on Gait Velocity and Balance of Older Adults." *Gerontologist* 33(4): 501-6.

Treiber, F.A., J. Lott, J. Duncan, G. Slavens, and H. Davis. 1998. "Effects of Thera-Band and Lightweight Dumbbell Training on Shoulder Rotation Torque and Serve Performance in College Tennis Players." *American Journal of Sports Medicine* 26(4): 510-5.

EXERCISE APPLICATIONS

Elastic devices provide a popular means of resistance exercise. They are convenient, portable, inexpensive, and easy to use. Elastic resistance exercises are used in both fitness and rehabilitation settings to strengthen muscle. Although elastic resistive devices are used mostly for extremity exercises, they also can be used for trunk and spine exercise. This section describes the clinical uses of elastic resistance for the upper and lower body as well as for the spine. Each chapter reviews the clinically relevant and functional anatomy and describes the core exercises for each body part including the clinical rationale behind each. In addition, each chapter discusses specific elastic resistance exercises for common injuries.

CHAPTER 4

Upper Extremity Exercises With Elastic Resistance

• • • • •

Todd S. Ellenbecker, MS, PT, SCS, OCS, CSCS
Physiotherapy Associates, Scottsdale Sports Clinic, Scottsdale, Arizona

The challenges presented by the highly mobile and often unstable glenohumeral joint, the extreme osseous congruency of the ulnohumeral joint, and the overuse injuries of the wrist and forearm make the upper extremity an excellent candidate for the application of elastic resistance for both injury rehabilitation and performance enhancement. Exercises aimed at improving scapulothoracic dynamic stabilization form the critical base for all upper extremity rehabilitation and conditioning programs (Kibler 1998). The purpose of this chapter is to review the pertinent functional anatomy of the scapulothoracic, glenohumeral, and elbow joints as well as to review common upper extremity overuse injuries and specific strategies for treatment with elastic resistance. Specific exercises for the upper extremity with elastic resistance are presented, along with a review of the available training literature, which demonstrates the potential efficacy of elastic resistance for the upper extremity.

Scapulothoracic Joint

The scapula consists of a flat blade lying along the thoracic wall that has muscular attachments to provide both stability and movement. The scapula is attached via a strut of the clavicle to the axial skeleton and is stabilized via muscular attachments to the humerus, spinous processes, and ribs (Kibler 1998). The scapulothoracic joint is most noted for the upward rotation it contributes during human arm elevation. The relationship of scapulothoracic motion to glenohumeral motion was termed *scapulohumeral rhythm* by Codman (1934). According to Codman, during arm elevation, for every 2° of glenohumeral motion there is 1° of scapulothoracic motion (Codman 1934; Kibler 1998). Although this ratio between glenohumeral and scapulothoracic movement is not constant during arm elevation (Bagg and Forest 1986; Doody, Freeman, and Waterland 1970), the overall ratio over an 180° arc of elevation is approximately 2:1 (Codman 1934; Kibler

1998). In addition to upward rotation, the scapula also translates forward and backward. These movements are termed protraction and retraction respectively and, depending on the person's size, can account for movement of 15 to 18 cm (Kibler 1991).

Muscular Relationships of the Scapulothoracic Joint

The primary muscular attachments of the scapulothoracic joint include the trapezius, rhomboids, serratus anterior, and levator scapulae. These muscles are responsible for scapular stabilization and rotation (Kibler 1998). Two muscles in this group (trapezius and serratus anterior) work together in a force couple to produce upward rotation. A force couple is technically defined as two or more forces acting on an object that produce rotation, even though the forces may act in opposing directions (Dillman 1995). The trapezius/serratus anterior force couple is an excellent example of how muscular forces working in opposing directions produce upward rotation of the scapulothoracic joint. Of particular importance is the role of the lower trapezius as an upward rotator (Daniels and Worthingham 1980). Using electromyography, Digiovine et al. (1992) investigated the important role of the lower trapezius muscle as a decelerator and stabilizer of the scapulothoracic joint during the follow-through phase of throwing.

The second group of muscles with attachment to the scapula are the deltoid, biceps, and triceps, which are extrinsic shoulder muscles. Finally, the intrinsic muscles of the glenohumeral joint include the rotator cuff (subscapularis, supraspinatus, infraspinatus, and teres minor). Although these later two groups of muscle primarily affect glenohumeral joint motion, the importance of their anatomical origin on the scapula cannot be overlooked.

Measurement of Scapular Position and Scapular Dysfunction

Measurement of scapular position was described by Kibler (1998) using the Kibler lateral scapular slide test. This test involves using a tape measure to measure the distance (in centimeters) between the inferior angle of the scapula and the corresponding spinous process at the level of inferior angle of the scapula (Kibler 1991, 1998). Three positions are used to measure and compare the distance between the inferior angle and the spinous process bilaterally.

These positions are standing with the arms at sides, standing with hands placed on hips with thumbs facing posterior, and standing with 90° of coronal plane abduction with full internal rotation. According to Kibler (1991, 1998), a bilateral difference of greater than 1 to 1.5 cm is considered pathological. This would indicate the need for greater muscular stabilization of the scapulothoracic joint and emphasis during rehabilitation. The validity of the Kibler lateral scapular slide test has been studied. Litchfield, Jeno, and Mabey (1998) found positive lateral scapular slide tests (bilateral difference >1 cm) in a population of patients with unilateral glenohumeral joint impingement, compared with normal subjects with Kibler position 1 (arms resting at sides).

Evaluation of scapular winging (protrusion of the scapula posteriorly off the thoracic wall) is also an important part of the examination process. Placement of the hands at the sides in a resting posture or in the "hands on hips" position often identifies abnormal prominence of the scapula bilaterally or unilaterally. Scapular winging traditionally has been described in clinical situations with long thoracic nerve involvement and extreme weakness of the serratus anterior. Severe upper extremity movement dysfunction and gross dissociation of the scapulothoracic joint are clinical signs of this condition (Zeier 1973).

Additional research has identified the important role that abnormal scapular mechanics play in glenohumeral joint pathology. Warner et al. (1992) used Moire topography to study scapular position in normal shoulders and in patients with impingement and glenohumeral joint instability. Abnormal scapular patterns were measured in 18% of normal subjects but in 32% and 57% in the instability and impingement groups, respectively. Ludewig and Cook (2000) reported similar findings in patients with glenohumeral impingement. A total of 52 male construction workers, 26 diagnosed with unilateral impingement, were measured during elevation of the shoulder in the scapular plane. Subjects with impingement had decreased upward rotation, increased anterior tipping, and medial rotation of the scapula on the involved side. Additionally, impingement subjects had an increase in trapezius electromyographic activity but a decrease in serratus anterior electromyographic activity.

Kibler (1998) attempted to provide a classification system to describe more subtle forms of scapular dysfunction. He described three main types of scapular dysfunction, which are classified based on the location of scapular prominence observed during clinical evaluation and which are relevant to treatment. These three classifications of scapular dysfunction are inferior, medial, and superior. Table 4.01 outlines the specifics of these three types of scapular dysfunction. Additionally, careful inspection of the scapula during active movements often identifies scapular dyskinesis and abnormal prominence of the medial and inferior borders of the scapula, particularly during eccentric lowering from overhead elevation. These important evaluation findings guide the clinician in exercise prescription as he or she designs a resistance exercise treatment plan.

Application of Resistance Exercise for the Scapulothoracic Joint

One of the primary studies that provided a rationale for the use of specific exercise patterns to strengthen and stabilize the scapulothoracic joint was published by Moseley et al. (1992). Their electromyographic study identified exercises that specifically increased serratus anterior activation by placing the shoulder in an exaggerated position of scapular protraction. This protracted position was termed the *plus position* and has been adapted in many scapular strengthen-

ing exercise programs (Ellenbecker and Cappel 2000). Additional exercise patterns studied by Moseley et al. (1992) were the shoulder shrug, which elicited high levels of upper trapezius activity, and the seated row, which highly activated all three portions of the trapezius, levator scapulae, and rhomboids.

Recent research by Decker et al. (1999) confirmed that the plus position elicits high levels of serratus anterior recruitment when elastic resistance is used. Additionally, Decker et al. (1999) introduced an exercise termed the *dynamic hug* (figure 4.01), which also produces high levels of serratus anterior activation and keeps the shoulders below the potential impingement position of 90° of elevation.

Exercise that emphasizes the serratus anterior is indicated to stabilize the scapula and optimize scapular rotation during glenohumeral joint movement patterns. Support for this recommendation comes from electromyographic research by McMahon et al. (1996). They studied subjects with glenohumeral joint instability and normal subjects during planar motions (flexion, abduction, and scaption) of the shoulder in 30° increments. Subjects with glenohumeral joint instability showed significantly less serratus anterior activation in all three planar motions compared with

Table 4.01   Kibler Scapular Dysfunction Classification

Inferior angle dysfunction

Scapula inferior angle tilts posteriorly in the sagittal plane.

Increased anterior tilting of the scapula.

Tenderness often over the coracoid anteriorly attributable to tightness of the pectoralis minor and biceps short head.

Inferior angle prominence often is increased in the hands on hips position or during eccentric lowering of the arms from overhead elevation.

Medial border dysfunction

Entire medial border protruding off the thoracic wall.

Transverse plane dysfunction with internal rotation of the scapula.

Medial border dysfunction often is increased in the hands on hips position or during eccentric lowering of the arms from overhead elevation.

Superior scapular dysfunction

Excessive elevation of the superior border of the scapula with arm elevation.

Occurs primarily with dynamic elevation in the sagittal, frontal, and scapular planes.

Data from W.B. Kibler, 1998, "The role of the scapula in the overhead throwing motion," *American Journal of Sports Medicine* 26(2): 325-337.

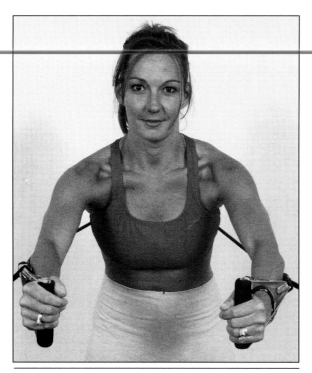

Figure 4.01   Dynamic hug exercise.

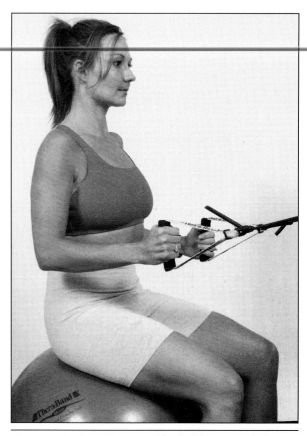

Figure 4.02   Seated rows on Physio ball.

normal subjects. This study clearly shows the importance of scapular muscle training to provide dynamic stabilization during rehabilitation.

McCabe et al. (2001) measured the activation of scapular muscles during several rehabilitation exercises. They found lower trapezius muscular activity to be higher than upper trapezius activity during standing scapular retraction exercise with bilateral resistance of external rotation with elastic resistance. This produced lower trapezius activity 3.3 times that of the upper trapezius. Another exercise, standing scapular retraction with bilateral scapular depression with elastic resistance, also produced high levels of lower trapezius muscular activity. Further research delineating muscular activity patterns during resistance exercise patterns is needed to advance clinicians' understanding and ability to devise optimal exercise programs for patients and individuals who need selected muscle development.

Specific Scapulothoracic Strengthening Exercises

Clinically, several exercises that use elastic resistance can be used to strengthen the musculature that stabilizes and moves the scapulothoracic joint. These exercises are shown in figures 4.01 to 4.10.

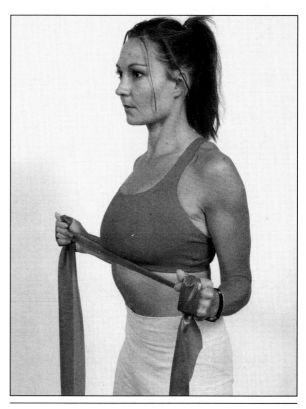

Figure 4.03   Bilateral shoulder external rotation with scapular retraction and depression.

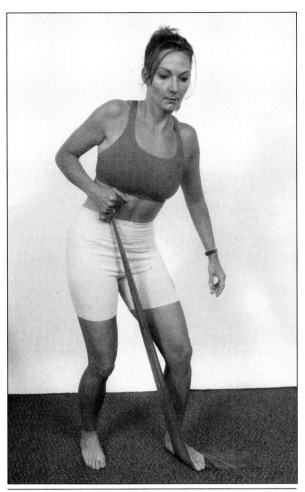

Figure 4.04 Lawn boy exercise.

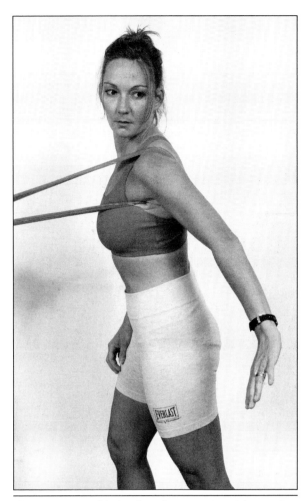

Figure 4.05 Modified unilateral D1 extension with retraction.

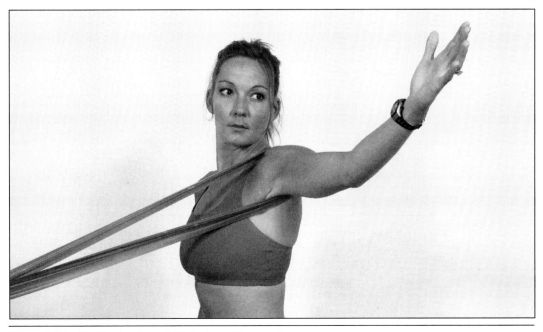

Figure 4.06 Modified unilateral D2 flexion with retraction.

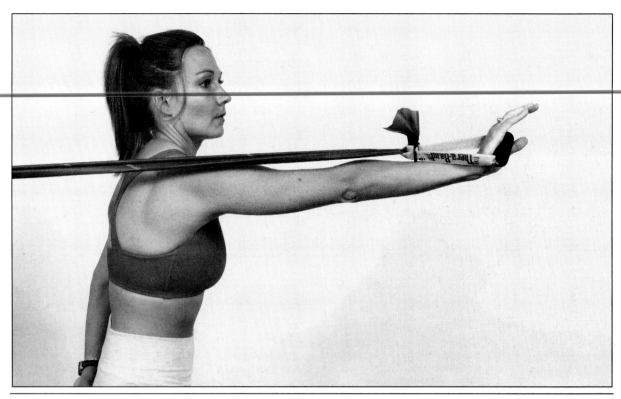

Figure 4.07　Shoulder "serratus" punches.

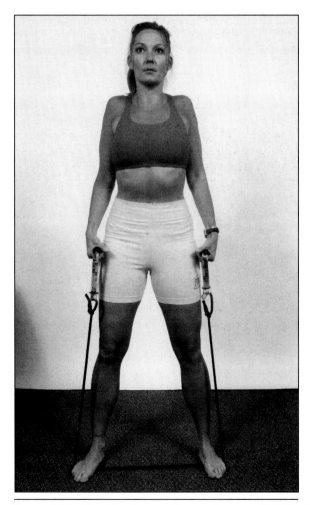

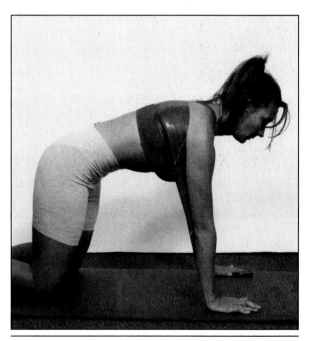

Figure 4.09　Closed chain "plus" exercise (end position).

Figure 4.08　Shoulder shrugs with scapular retraction.

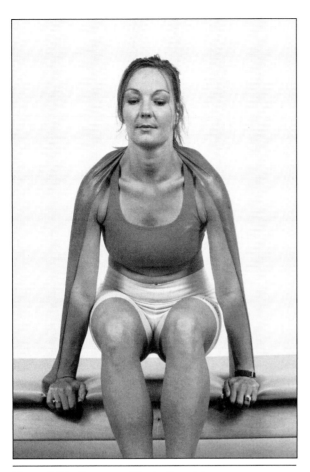

Figure 4.10   Press up with elastic resistance.

Glenohumeral Joint

The osseous relationships of the glenohumeral joint afford little stability, and hence the glenohumeral articulation relies on several additional factors for stability. To enhance resistance exercise prescription for glenohumeral joint pathology, several anatomical and biomechanical concepts must be considered. The neck shaft angle of the humeral head is 135°, which creates an upward orientation to the articulating portion of the humeral head relative to the shaft of the humerus. This angular relationship is coupled with a 30° retrotorsion angle of the humeral head (Saha 1983). The anterior version of the glenoid is between 30 and 40° (Saha 1983). This articular relationship of humeral retrotorsion and anterior facing glenoid results in the "scapular plane" position, which is 30 to 40° anterior to the coronal or frontal plane of the body. The scapular plane position is characterized by optimal osseous congruity and enhanced length-tension relationships of the posterior rotator cuff (Saha, 1983). Use of the

scapular plane position during exercise has been advocated to enhance glenohumeral joint stability and protect the anterior capsule after injury or surgical procedures (Ellenbecker 1995, 1997).

In addition to osseous congruity, several other static stabilizing elements are responsible for glenohumeral joint stability. These include the glenoid labrum, negative intra-articular pressure, joint geometry, and capsular ligaments (Jobe and Kivitne 1989). The glenohumeral joint capsular ligaments attach to the periphery of the labrum and help prevent anterior glenohumeral joint translation (Karduna et al. 1996). O'Brien et al. (1990) studied the specific functional roles of the glenohumeral ligaments and particularly identified the inferior glenohumeral ligament as being the primary stabilizer against anterior and posterior humeral head translation with the shoulder in the functional position of 90° of abduction. Bigliani et al. (1992) measured the tensile strength of the inferior glenohumeral ligament and reported it to have only 15% the tensile strength of the human anterior cruciate ligament. The important interplay between the static restraints and the dynamic stabilization provided by the musculature is required to allow for large arcs of stabilized glenohumeral motion.

Muscular Relationships of the Glenohumeral Joint

One of the most important muscular relationships of the glenohumeral joint is the deltoid/rotator cuff force couple described originally by Inman (1944). The major components of the deltoid/rotator cuff force couple are outlined in figure 4.11. The superior component formed by the deltoid has been shown to pull the humeral head superiorly when contracting unopposed, based on the line of pull of the muscle fiber orientation (Weiner and McNab 1970). The supraspinatus has an approximating or compressing function with muscle contraction and pulls the humeral head into the glenoid (Inman 1944). The infraspinatus, teres minor, and subscapularis muscle tendon units form the inferior component of the deltoid/rotator cuff force couple. These muscles work to oppose the superior pull of the deltoid and control the humeral head during movement (Inman 1944; Kronberg, Nemeth, and Brostrom 1990). Using electromyography, Kronberg Nemeth, and Brostrom (1990) demonstrated how the coordinated muscular activity between the deltoid and rotator cuff musculature occurs during arm elevation. Cocontraction of the deltoid with the rotator cuff is necessary to prevent superior migration and abnormal glenohumeral kinematics. Reddy et al. (2000) compared muscular activity during arm elevation in the scapular plane among subjects with shoulder impingement and normal controls. These researchers found significantly decreased muscular activity in the infraspinatus, subscapularis, and middle deltoid in the arc between 30 and 60° of elevation in the subjects with subacromial impingement. Decreased muscular activity in the infraspinatus also was measured in the impingement subjects with the arm between 60 and 90° of elevation. These findings demonstrate a decrease in the function of the inferior force vector (subscapularis and infraspinatus) in patients with subacromial impingement. Thus, humeral head depression during the critical first portion of elevation may be insufficient in patients with subacromial impingement. Application of exercises to enhance the strength and endurance of the inferior force vectors of the human shoulder appears to be warranted based on the results of this experiment.

In addition to the rotator cuff and deltoid musculature, several additional muscles cross the glenohumeral joint and affect function. Of particular importance is the biceps muscle. The biceps long head tendon inserts on the supraglenoid tubercle

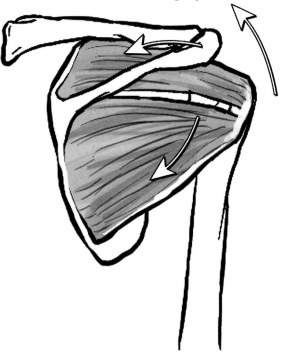

Figure 4.11   Deltoid rotator cuff force couple with solid black lines depicting approximate lines of force of the deltoid (superior arrow), supraspinatus (horizontal arrow), and infraspinatus/teres minor/subscapularis (inferomedially directed arrow).

Adapted, by permission, from T.S. Ellenbecker. 1997. "Etiology and Evaluation of Rotator Cuff Pathology and Rehabilitation." In *Physical Therapy of the Shoulder,* ed. R.A. Donatelli. Philadelphia: Churchill Livingstone.

and blends with the superior labrum. The stabilizing influence of the biceps long head was reported by Itoi et al. (1993) and Rodosky, Harner, and Fu (1994). These authors demonstrated the effect of tension in the biceps long head tendon and its effect on stabilizing against anterior humeral head translation. Inclusion of exercises to increase the strength and endurance of the biceps is indicated, particularly in patients with anterior glenohumeral joint instability (Ellenbecker 1995, 1997).

Additional muscles directly affecting glenohumeral motion are the triceps, teres major, latissimus dorsi, and pectoralis major. Research outlining the specific role of these muscles with regard to glenohumeral joint stability is not available; however, these muscles do play a role in the primary movements of the glenohumeral joint.

Rotator Cuff Dysfunction: Impingement and Instability

It is beyond the scope of this chapter to completely cover glenohumeral joint injuries; however, a brief discussion of two common injuries is clearly warranted. Neer (1972) introduced the concept of shoulder impingement or compressive disease in a classic article outlining three stages. Each of these stages was the direct result of primary mechanical impingement or compression of the rotator cuff tendons between the humeral head and the acromion. The subacromial space is only 6 to 14 mm in normal subjects (Cotton and Rideout 1964), and with muscular imbalance or fatigue, capsular range of motion restriction, and repeated overuse in overhead positions, rotator cuff impingement occurs producing a progression of disability. This progression, according to Neer (1972), starts with edema and hemorrhage initially and, with continued overuse, could result in partial and full thickness tears from the mechanical stresses of compression and impingement. Bigliani et al. (1991) showed the relationship between rotator cuff disease and the shape of the overlying acromion. Acromial shapes that are curved (Type 2) or have a downward spur (Type 3) have an increased likelihood of producing impingement or compressive lesions in the rotator cuff.

Most recently, medical professionals and scientists have understood the important role that glenohumeral joint instability plays in rotator cuff disease. Impingement of the rotator cuff against the acromion may occur secondary to glenohumeral joint instability from attenuation of the static stabilizers such as capsular laxity, labral pathology, and abnormal work or sport biomechanics (Burkhart, Morgan, and Kibler 2000; Jobe and Kivitne 1989; Walch et al. 1992). Additionally, impingement of the undersurface of the rotator cuff tendons on the posterior superior glenoid has been identified as an important cause of rotator cuff dysfunction and shoulder pain (Paley et al. 2000; Walch et al. 1992; figure 4.12). This phenomenon has been termed *posterior impingement* or *internal impingement* and is caused by glenohumeral joint instability, abnormal joint kinematics, and inappropriate overhead movement patterns, such as hyperangulation of the humerus relative to the scapula during throwing (Hammer, Pink, and Jobe 2000; Jobe and Pink 1994).

Application of Resistance Exercise for the Glenohumeral Joint

The anatomical and biomechanical concepts outlined earlier in this chapter provide a framework for the clinician to choose exercise positions and movement patterns to increase both strength and muscular endurance of patients and individuals with shoulder injury or weakness. In addition to concepts such as scapular plane position, avoidance of impingement positions, and the important role that force couples play in producing controlled glenohumeral joint motion, electromyographic studies are available that specifically measure individual muscular activity patterns with traditionally used exercise patterns. Most of the electromyographic studies addressing upper extremity movement patterns use isotonic exercises; however, similar exercise movement patterns can be used with elastic resistance.

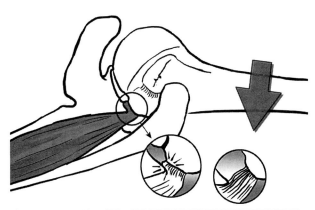

Figure 4.12 Schematic representation of posterosuperior glenoid impingement between the posterior edge of the glenoid and the deep surface of the supraspinatus and infraspinatus tendons.

Adapted by permission from G. Walch, P. Boileau, E. Noel, and S.T. Donell. 1992. "Impingement of the Deep Surface of the Supraspinatus Tendon on the Posterosuperior Glenoid Rim. An Arthroscopic Study." *Journal of Shoulder and Elbow Surgery* 1: 238-45.

Blackburn et al. (1990) used electromyography to measure muscular activity in the posterior rotator cuff during traditional shoulder exercise using isotonic weights. The authors identified a position that has been referred to as the *Blackburn position*, which consists of prone horizontal abduction with 100° of abduction and an externally rotated humeral position (figure 4.13). This position has been reported to involve high levels of muscular activity in the supraspinatus muscle, infraspinatus, teres minor, and scapular stabilizers (Blackburn et al. 1990; Malanga et al. 1996; Townsend et al. 1991). This prone position has become a classic exercise in many rehabilitation programs for both glenohumeral joint impingement and instability (Blackburn et al. 1990). Modifying this exercise to use only 90° of abduction to decrease potential subacromial contact and compression has been recommended (Ellenbecker 1995, 1997).

In addition to the Blackburn et al. (1990) study, Townsend et al. (1991) provided the most comprehensive analysis of shoulder muscle activity during traditional exercises used during rehabilitation programs. Table 4.02 outlines the findings of the Townsend et al. (1991) research, listing the relative activity levels of the rotator cuff and scapular musculature expressed as the percentage of maximal voluntary contraction during common exercise movement patterns. Of particular emphasis in this study is the identification of the *empty can* or *Jobe position* (Townsend et al. 1991). This position and exercise also have been termed *scaption* or scapular plane elevation. The elevation of the shoulder in the scapular plane (30° anterior to the coronal plane) with full internal rotation was found to produce the highest levels of supraspinatus muscle activation of the many exercises studied in this investigation. Additionally, Townsend et al. (1991) found the prone shoulder exercises such as prone horizontal abduction (with external humeral rotation), prone extension (with external humeral rotation), and prone external rotation at 90° of abduction to produce high levels of posterior rotator cuff activity.

Malanga et al. (1996) also used electromyography to compare the muscular activity patterns of the Blackburn and Jobe exercise movement patterns. The results of their study showed no significant difference statistically in the muscular activity between the two positions, and they concluded that "both positions activate the supraspinatus, but neither isolate the supraspinatus." This information can be applied clinically by using both positions during rehabilitation or by using the position of maximal comfort for the patient with rotator cuff dysfunction.

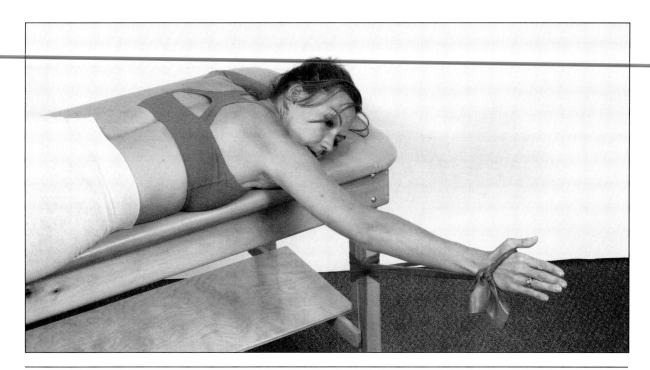

Figure 4.13   Blackburn position. (Prone horizontal abduction with 100° of abduction and external rotation.)

Table 4.02   Rotator Cuff Muscular Activity Patterns During Shoulder Exercises

Movement pattern	Muscle	%MMT
Empty can (scaption with internal rotation)	Supraspinatus	74
	Subscapularis	62
Side-lying external rotation	Infraspinatus	85
	Teres minor	80
Prone horizontal abduction with external rotation	Infraspinatus	88
	Teres minor	74

Note: %MMT is the percentage of maximal manual muscle test activity used to normalize muscular activity in this research. IR = internal rotation.

The combined motion of elevation with internal rotation often exacerbates the impingement process because of the position of the greater tuberosity under the acromion (Neer 1972) and hence may be contraindicated during early stages or even during all stages of rehabilitation for some patients. Using the objective research presented in this section of the chapter would lead the clinician to substitute the Blackburn exercise to recruit the supraspinatus muscle.

Ballantyne et al. (1993) studied three exercises (scaption, side-lying external rotation, and prone external rotation with 90° of abduction) using elec-tromyography. They found that scaption elicited the highest levels of supraspinatus activity, with both side-lying external rotation and prone external rotation being more optimal for both infraspinatus and teres minor activation. Additionally, prone external rotation produced the highest lower trapezius activity of the three exercises studied by Ballantyne et al. (1993).

Hintermeister et al. (1998) also studied traditional elastic resistance exercises for the shoulder by using electromyography. They monitored the rotator cuff, pectoralis major, trapezius, and serratus anterior by using surface and indwelling electrodes. Exercises tested were internal and external rotation, seated rowing in multiple grips, forward punching, and the shoulder shrug. The authors measured loads from 21 to 54 N (approximately 4.5-12 lb) during the exercises using the elastic resistance. Table 4.03 shows the average electromyographic activity of the muscles during each of the five exercises. Of particular importance clinically was the level of posterior rotator cuff (infraspinatus) activity during external rotation exercise and the level of subscapularis activity during internal rotation exercise with elastic resistance. Additionally, the subscapularis and trapezius were both active during the rowing exercises, with the serratus anterior being the predominant muscle activity during the forward punch exercise. Additional electromyographic research that uses elastic resistance is currently not available in the literature, but the available studies (Decker et al. 1999; Hintermeister et al. 1998) clearly demonstrate the muscular activity patterns of commonly used therapeutic exercises with elastic resistance.

Additional Research on the Use of Elastic Resistance in the Shoulder

Treiber et al. (1998) studied the effects of a training program that used elastic resistance and dumbbells in a population of elite tennis players. Players trained for 4 weeks, 3 times per week, using both the Thera-Band for internal and external rotation at the side and dumbbells for the empty can exercise. Two sets of 20 repetitions were performed over the 4-week training program. Pre- and posttesting was conducted with the Cybex 6000 (Cybex Inc, Ronkonkoma, NY) isokinetic dynamometer. Results of testing showed statistically significant improvements in internal rotation at both slow and fast isokinetic testing speeds. External rotation improvements in the training group were exhibited only at the fast isokinetic testing speed. Subjects in the training group also exhibited improvement in a functional performance measurement. The maximal ball speed on a serve was measured before and after the training program, with subjects in the experimental group exhibiting a 6% increase in serving speed. This study supports the use of elastic resistance training to increase both internal and external rotation strength as well as functional performance in tennis players.

Page et al. (1993) studied the effects of elastic resistance training in collegiate baseball pitchers. Subjects trained the posterior rotator cuff 3 times a week for 6 weeks by using the diagonal 2 (D2) flexion proprioceptive neuromuscular facilitation (PNF) pattern with

Table 4.03   Rotator Cuff and Scapular Muscle Activity During Rehabilitative Shoulder Exercises With Elastic Resistance

Movement pattern	Muscle	%MMT
Internal rotation, arm at side	Subscapularis	52
External rotation, arm at side	Infraspinatus	47
Seated rowing	Supraspinatus	32
	Subscapularis	87
	Infraspinatus	30
	Trapezius	33
Forward punch	Serratus anterior	48
	Subscapularis	27
	Supraspinatus	48
Shoulder shrug, retraction phase	Supraspinatus	44
	Subscapularis	98
	Infraspinatus	24
	Trapezius	54
	Serratus anterior	31

Note: %MMT is the percentage of maximal manual muscle test activity used to normalize muscular activity in this research.

elastic resistance. The authors found a 19.8% increase in eccentric strength of the posterior rotator cuff, measured isokinetically, when using a diagonal testing pattern. This study clearly shows the important benefit of elastic resistance in a functional (D2) training and testing pattern in collegiate baseball pitchers.

Another training study that used elastic resistance was performed by Bleacher and Roush (1999), who studied healthy female subjects. Subjects trained using the D2 flexion PNF pattern with elastic resistance, with 3 sets of 15 repetitions. Training occurred 3 times a week for 6 weeks. Before and immediately after the training, subjects were tested on a NORM isokinetic dynamometer (Henley HealthCare, Austin, TX) to measure shoulder internal and external rotation strength at 45° of glenohumeral joint abduction in the seated position. No significant differences pre- and posttraining were measured in shoulder internal and external rotation strength, indicating no significant increase in rotator cuff strength from the D2 flexion pattern used in the experimental group. This finding supports the specificity principle, in that using a D2 pattern may not provide an adequate strength training stimulus for the rotator cuff. Therefore, more specific patterns of training similar to the one used by Treiber et al. (1998) that use internal and external rotation should be emphasized to increase rotator cuff strength.

Similar specificity of training responses was demonstrated by Anderson et al. (1992). Twenty-eight subjects trained 3 times per week using elastic resistance in the pattern of glenohumeral joint internal rotation. Concentric and eccentric pre- and posttesting of shoulder internal rotation identified mean increases of 10% in the training group, particularly eccentrically, over the 6-week training program. A similar study was performed by Macko et al. (1999) using the shoulder external rotators. Female subjects age 18 to 30 trained 3 times a week, performing external shoulder rotation with elastic resistance. Three sets of 4 to 6 repetitions were used with isometric and isokinetic pre- and posttesting of external rotation strength. Results showed significant increases in both isometric and isokinetic external rotation strength from the 6-week training program.

These studies support the clinical use of elastic resistance. Most of these studies included healthy, uninjured subjects or athletes (Anderson et al. 1992; Bleacher and Rousch 1999; Macko et al. 1999; Page et al. 1993). Burkhead and Rockwood (1992) studied patients with glenohumeral joint instability, who performed elastic resistance exercises consisting of internal and external humeral rotation, seated rowing, front rowing, and 45° limited arc abduction. The authors reported 80% good or excellent results with nonoperative management with elastic resistance exercises in patients with a traumatic instability. Additional research on the interaction and effects of elastic resistance on injured patients will further assist clinicians in applying elastic resistance in rehabilitation.

Finally, Simoneau et al. (2001) reviewed the biomechanics of elastic resistance for shoulder rehabilitation. The authors demonstrated the differences in performing a standard external rotation exercise in neutral abduction under two conditions (securing the elastic in a doorway and securing the elastic resistance with the contralateral extremity). The condition where the elastic material was supported in a door began with a starting length of the elastic material of 0.6 m. During a standard external rotation exercise where the exercising extremity coursed through an arc of 90°, the elastic material elongated to a final length from the door of 1 m. This ultimately changed the length by 0.4 m, for a relative deformation of the band of 67%.

In the second example by these authors, the band was secured in the contralateral extremity while the ipsilateral extremity did the 90° arc of external rotation. The elastic material moved from a resting length of 0.3 to 0.7 m. This also resulted in a total elongation of 0.4 m but instead resulted in a relative elongation of 133%. This example highlights specific issues regarding load, percentage elongation, and consistent start and end positioning when elastic resistance is used during rehabilitation and exercise. Simply changing the length or distance from the point of attachment to the point of application can greatly change the level of resistance and may alter a patient's perception of strength level during a change from one method to another, as shown in the previous example.

Additional Factors for Implementing Humeral Rotation Exercise

Several additional factors are important when implementing glenohumeral joint internal and external rotation exercise with elastic resistance. Rathburn and McNab (1970) identified a region of hypovascularity in the rotator cuff tendons (specifically the supraspinatus) near its insertion on the greater tuberosity of the humerus. This region of hypovascularity was greatest when the arm was placed in neutral abduction/adduction (arm at side), attributable to the wrapping of the suprapinatus tendon over the top of the humeral head. Rathburn and McNab (1970) termed this the *wringing-out* phenomenon, because of the apparent decrease in vascularity with the shoulder held in the neutral adducted position. Placing the shoulder in a more abducted position reduced the wringing-out phenomenon and improved the vascularity of the supraspinatus tendon in that area. This finding led clinicians (Davies 1992; Ellenbecker 1997) to advocate using a towel roll or pillow during exercises such as humeral internal and external rotation with elastic resistance. Exercises in this text include the addition of the towel roll to encourage positioning in slight abduction and slight forward flexion, to place the shoulder in a theoretically advantaged vascular position during exercise.

Another study that supported the use of multiple positions of rotational exercise was published by Bassett et al. (1990). They studied glenohumeral muscle force and moment mechanics with the shoulder in a position of 90° of abduction with 90° of external rotation. The findings of their complex biomechanical investigation showed an alteration of muscle function in the 90/90 position, which is inherent in many sport activities such as throwing and tennis (Elliot, Marsh, and Blanksby 1986). The findings of this study showed that the infraspinatus functions more as an extensor than an external rotator in this position, with the supraspinatus also serving as an extensor, adductor, and external rotator. These functions differ from the traditional functions of these muscle tendon units, and this finding supports the use of the 90° abducted positions for training, to ensure that specific muscular functions are enhanced with training. Listed in this chapter are several exercises that place the shoulder into the 90/90 (abduction/external rotation) position for advanced activity or sport-specific training. Care must be taken, however, to ensure proper scapular control and humeral head control before the glenohumeral joint is placed in this more advanced position, to reduce the risk of exercise-induced irritation (Ellenbecker 1995, 1997; Davies 1992).

Specific Exercises for the Glenohumeral Joint With Elastic Resistance

Specific exercises to improve muscular strength and endurance of the glenohumeral joint are listed in figures 4.14 to 4.30.

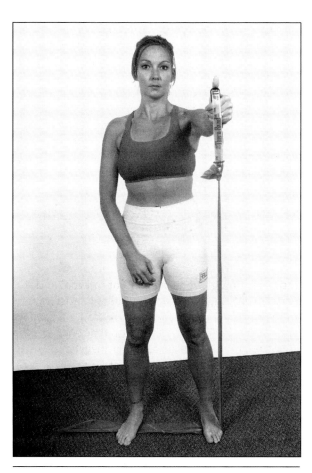

Figure 4.14   Shoulder flexion to 90°.

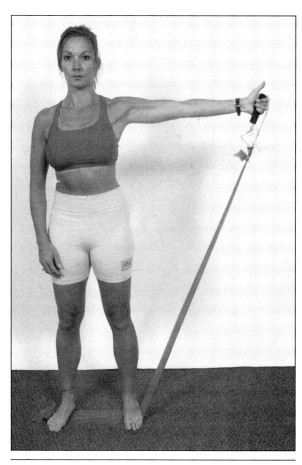

Figure 4.15   Shoulder abduction to 90°.

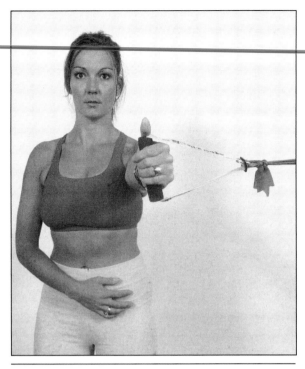

Figure 4.16 Shoulder horizontal adduction to 90° of elevation.

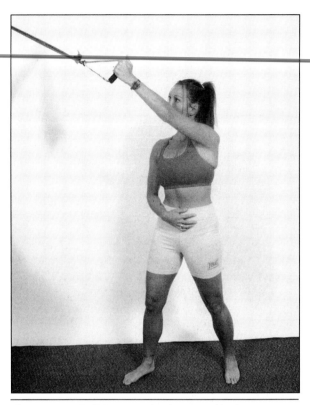

Figure 4.17 PNF D1 extension (start position).

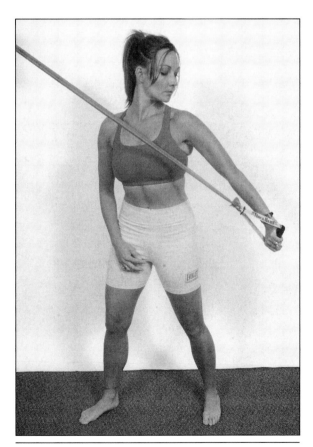

Figure 4.18 PNF D1 extension (end position).

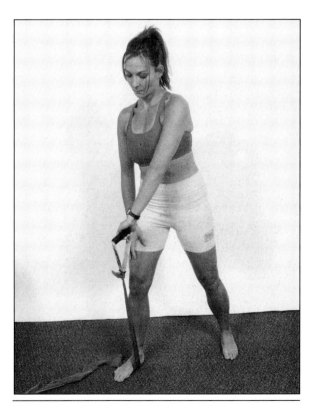

Figure 4.19 PNF D2 flexion (start position).

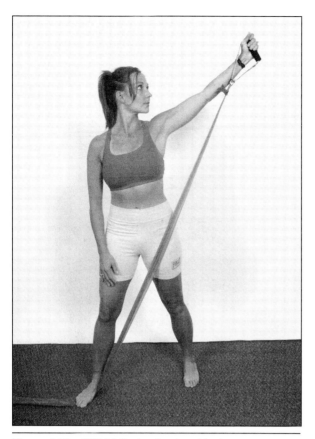

Figure 4.20   PNF D2 flexion (end position).

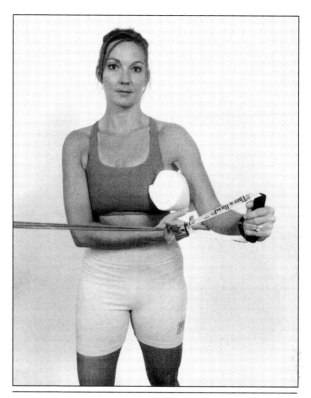

Figure 4.21   Shoulder external rotation in neutral.

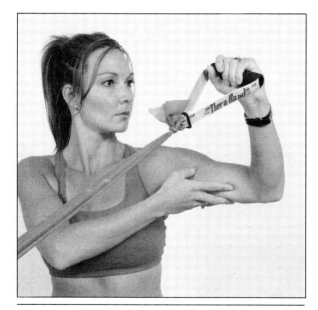

Figure 4.22   Shoulder external rotation with 90° of elevation in the scapular plane.

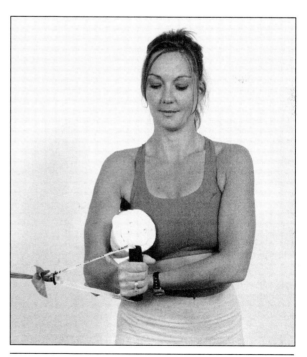

Figure 4.23   Shoulder internal rotation in neutral.

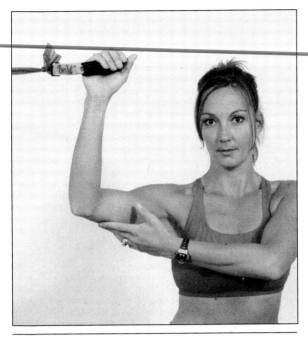

Figure 4.24 Shoulder internal rotation with 90° of elevation in the scapular plane.

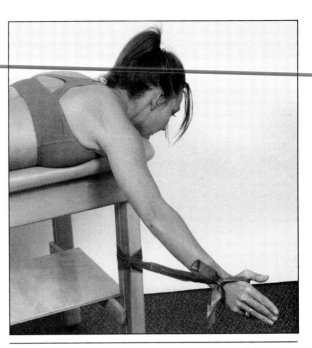

Figure 4.25 Prone horizontal abduction with 90° of abduction.

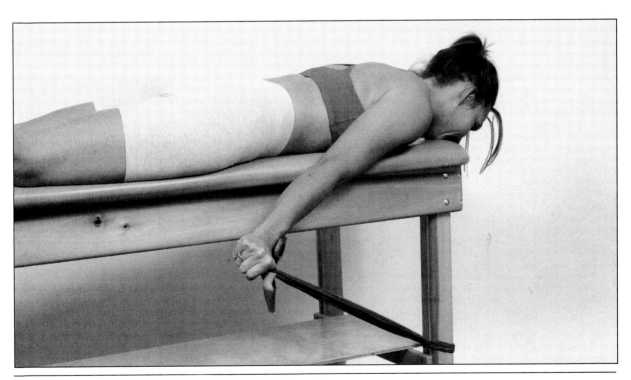

Figure 4.26 Prone extension with externally rotated arm position.

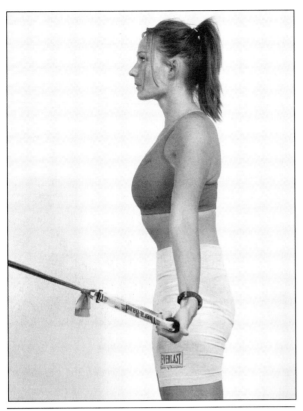

Figure 4.27 Standing shoulder extension with externally rotated arm position.

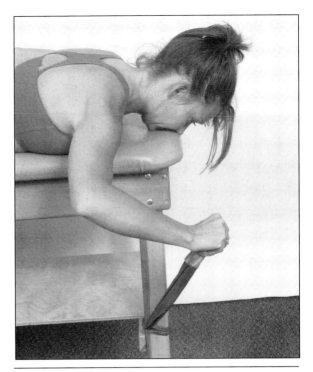

Figure 4.28 Prone external rotation with 90° of abduction.

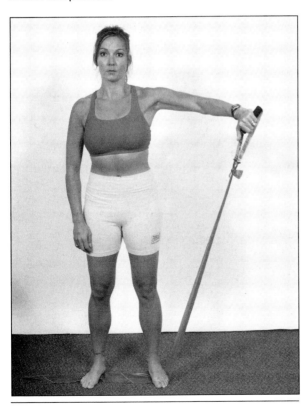

Figure 4.29 Shoulder empty can exercise.

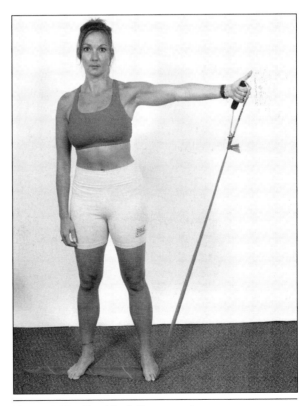

Figure 4.30 Shoulder full can exercise.

Elbow Joint

The elbow is a trochoginglymoid joint and consists of the ulnohumeral, radiocapitellar, and proximal radioulnar joints in one common capsule (Morrey 1993). Unlike the glenohumeral joint, the ulnohumeral joint has a high degree of osseous congruency and is a very stable joint that primarily functions in the sagittal plane, performing flexion and extension. Several articular relationships are important for clinicians to design resistance training programs that use elastic resistance. The medial aspect of the distal humerus, the trochlea, projects further distally compared with the distal lateral aspect of the humerus, the capitellum. This bony relationship results in the formation of the carrying angle that is a normally occurring valgus angulation of the elbow. Normal carrying angle in males is 10°, with 13° being the average for females. Increases in carrying angle after injury or in throwing athletes of up to 10 to 15° have been reported (King, Brelsford, and Tullos 1969).

Another important articular relationship in the human elbow is the relationship between the distal humerus and ulna. The distal aspect of the humerus is angulated 30° anterior, with the sigmoid notch (proximal ulna that receives the trochlea of the humerus) of the ulna being angulated 30° posteriorly (Morrey 1993). This articular relationship allows the elbow to extend fully and flex to 140 or 150° without bony impingement.

In addition to the capsule, the static stabilizers of the elbow joint consist mainly of the ligaments. The primary restraint against valgus stress is the medial ulnar collateral ligament (Morrey and An 1983). This ligament consists of three bands, with the anterior band being the primary restraint against valgus stress with the elbow at or near extension. The anterior band is taut during the final 30° of extension of the elbow. The posterior band of the ulnar collateral ligament becomes taut after 60° of elbow flexion. Table 4.04 shows the relative contribution of the ligament, capsule, and bone to stability of the human elbow in both extended and flexed positions. Of particular importance is the increased relative contribution of the ulnar collateral ligament with the elbow in flexion, compared with a more equal distribution of stress with the elbow in extension. This has significant clinical ramifications, because many patients lose valuable elbow extension range of motion after injury, surgery, or fracture of the elbow. This leads to increased demands on the ligamentous structure (ulnar collateral ligament) during activities of daily living or sport-specific overhead movement patterns (Ellenbecker and Mattalino 1996; Morrey 1993; Morrey and An 1983).

The primary restraint against varus stress is the lateral ulnar collateral ligament. This structure, not the radial collateral ligament, is primarily responsible for limiting varus stress at the human elbow. O'Driscoll, Bell, and Morrey (1991) showed that release of the lateral ulnar collateral ligament leads to posterolateral rotary instability of the elbow and is an important structure for normal elbow function. Although several other ligaments around the elbow are important, they are beyond the scope of this chapter. The final ligament to mention is the

Table 4.04   Percent Contribution of Restraining Force During Displacement (Rotational or Distractional)

Position	Stabilizing element	Distraction	Varus	Valgus
Extension	MCL	12	—	31
	LCL	10	14	—
	Capsule	70	32	38
	Articulation	—	55	31
Flexion	MCL	78	—	54
	LCL	10	9	—
	Capsule	8	13	10
	Articulation	—	75	33

MCL = Medial collateral ligament complex; LCL = Lateral collateral ligament complex.
Reprinted, by permission, from T.S. Ellenbecker and A.J. Mattalino, 1996, *The Elbow in Sport*, Champaign, IL: Human Kinetics, 8.
Data from B.F. Morrey, 1993, *The Elbow and Its Disorders*, 2nd ed., Philadelphia: Saunders.

annular ligament. This broad ligament surrounds the radial head, allowing 180° of rotation of the radial head while stabilizing the proximal radioulnar joint. With supination, the anterior aspect of the annular ligament becomes taut, and in pronation, the posterior portion of the annular ligament becomes taut.

Muscular Forces Around the Elbow Joint

Functionally, the muscles around the elbow joint can be grouped as elbow flexors and extensors, wrist flexors and extensors, and forearm pronators and supinators. An and colleagues (1981) studied the muscular structures around the elbow extensively and, through moment arm analysis, found that most muscles have one primary function. These authors found that the muscles which contribute most to elbow flexion were the brachioradialis, biceps, brachialis, and extensor carpi radialis. The muscles with the greatest moment arms for elbow extension were the triceps, flexor carpi ulnaris, and anconeus. The flexor carpi radialis was found to have an extension moment with the elbow in extension and a flexion moment with the elbow in a flexed position. Muscles creating a valgus moment that would resist varus stress at the elbow were the anconeus, brachioradialis, extensor carpi radialis, and extensor carpi ulnaris. The pronator teres, flexor carpi radialis, and flexor carpi ulnaris all created varus moments about the elbow and would resist valgus stress.

Knowledge of the muscular activity patterns during common sport activities can assist clinicians in understanding injury patterns and prioritizing muscular development programs for performance enhancement. Morris et al. (1989) studied the elbow and forearm muscles during tennis strokes and found extremely high activity of the wrist extensors, particularly the extensor carpi radialis brevis, during groundstrokes and serving. High levels of wrist flexor and forearm pronator activity present during the acceleration phase of the throwing motion or in tennis stabilize the medial aspect of the elbow (Sisto et al. 1987). Changes in the muscular activity patterns surrounding the elbow have been measured in tennis players with tennis elbow (Kelley et al. 1994) and in throwing athletes with ulnar collateral ligament injury (Glousman et al. 1992). These studies clearly demonstrate that alterations in optimal dynamic muscular stabilization and increased activation and subsequent muscular fatigue have deleterious effects on the human elbow.

Common Injuries to the Elbow Joint

By far, one of the most common injuries seen in most orthopedic and sports medicine clinics is humeral epicondylitis. Although humeral epicondylitis initially was thought to be an inflammatory condition or tendinitis (Nirschl and Sobel 1981), recent research has clearly shown an absence of inflammatory cells in the tissue in elbows with humeral epicondylitis (Kraushaar and Nirschl 1999). In fact, histopathological studies have shown that specimens taken from areas of chronic tendon overuse injury do not contain macrophages, lymphocytes, or neutrophils. This has led to the development of the term *tendinosis*, a condition characterized by the presence of primarily degenerative tissue, disorganized collagen, dense populations of fibroblasts, and vascular hyperplasia (Kraushaar and Nirschl 1999).

The primary tendons involved in lateral humeral epicondylitis include the extensor carpi radialis brevis, extensor carpi radialis longus, and extensor digitorum communis. In athletics, lateral humeral epicondylitis occurs most often in tennis and golf. It occurs in tennis because of overload of the extensor muscles on the backhand groundstroke. In golf, the condition affects the left hand of a right-handed golfer. The primary tendon sites of overuse injury in medial epicondylitis are the flexor carpi radialis and pronator teres. This injury occurs in tennis players from overload on the forehand groundstroke and serve, and it occurs in the right arm in a right-handed golfer and in the throwing athlete (Ellenbecker and Mattalino 1996). In addition to initially decreasing pain and optimizing range of motion, progressive resistance exercise has been a primary treatment for individuals with humeral epicondylitis (Ellenbecker and Mattalino, 1996; Kraushaar and Nirschl 1999). Elastic resistance is an important adjunct in the treatment of humeral epicondylitis and can be used to provide both strength and endurance stimuli to the injured extremity.

Additional injuries common in the active elbow can be grouped or classified as valgus extension overload injuries. This type of injury specifically refers to the valgus stress imparted to the elbow during the acceleration phase of throwing, serving, spiking, or golfing while the elbow is also extending (Fleisig, Dillman, and Andrews 1989; Indelicato et al. 1979). Injuries caused by valgus stress to the elbow include ulnar collateral ligament sprains, ulnar nerve irritation, and osteophyte development in the posterior medial aspect of the olecranon (Ellenbecker and Mattalino 1996). In addition to the injuries mentioned on the medial aspect of the elbow from tension or tensile loading, the lateral aspect of the elbow suffers compression at the radiocapitellar joint during the valgus extension overload. This can lead to osteochondritis dissecans of the radial head or capitellum as well as osteophyte development.

Strengthening of the elbow is also an important aspect of treating the elbow, and elastic resistance can play a part in resistance exercise programming as well. Several important concepts provide a rationale for the inclusion of specific exercises to target muscular strength in the distal upper extremity. Davidson et al. (1995) showed the close approximation of the flexor carpi ulnaris tendon and medial ulnar collateral ligament in the human elbow. The important role that dynamic stabilization plays in the active elbow cannot be overlooked.

Research Using Elastic Resistance for the Elbow

Ellenbecker, Kingma, and Kim (1994) studied the effects of a 6-week training program that used elastic resistance in healthy high school students. Subjects trained 3 times per week, using 3 sets of 15 repetitions of wrist flexion and extension unilaterally, with the contralateral extremity serving as a control group. Before and immediately after the 6 weeks of training, isokinetic wrist flexion and extension strength were measured on a Cybex 6000 isokinetic dynamometer. Results of the study showed no significant improvement in wrist flexion or extension strength over the 6-week training program in healthy uninjured subjects. Clearly, further research is needed to determine optimal training intensities and training volumes to increase muscular strength around the elbow and wrist. No further research is currently available in the literature that involves elastic resistance for the elbow or wrist.

Specific Patterns of Exercise for the Elbow With Elastic Resistance

Specific exercises to improve strength and endurance of the muscles that cross and ultimately affect function at the elbow, forearm, and wrist are shown in figures 4.31 through 4.44.

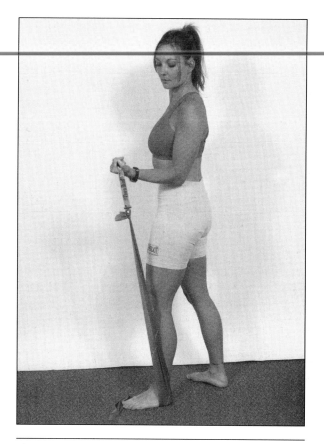

Figure 4.31   Elbow flexion (neutral at side).

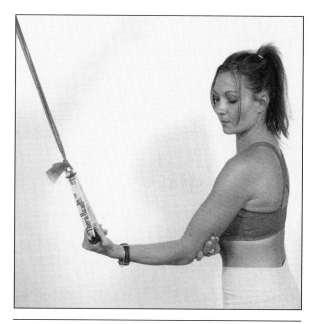

Figure 4.32   Elbow extension (neutral at side).

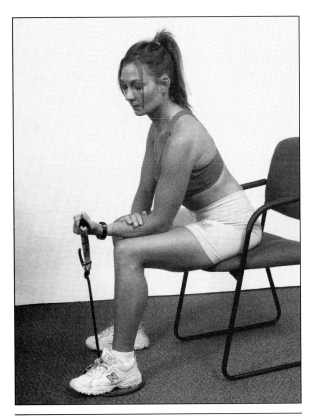

Figure 4.33 Wrist flexion.

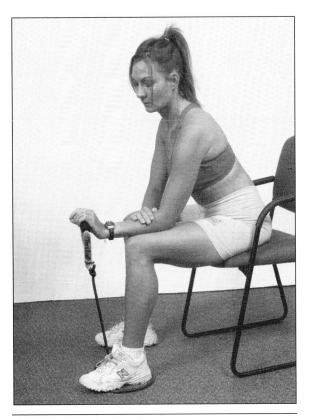

Figure 4.34 Wrist extension.

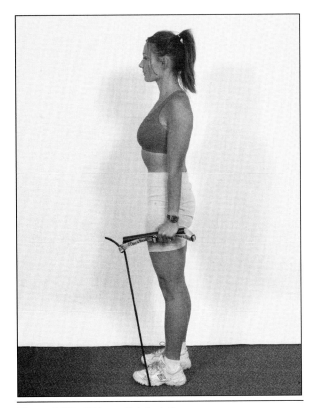

Figure 4.35 Wrist radial deviation.

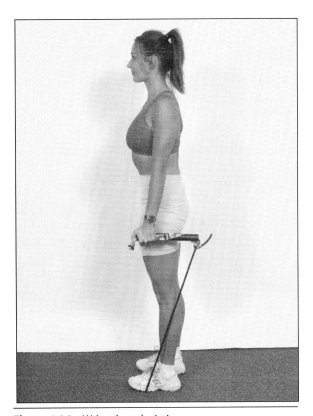

Figure 4.36 Wrist ulnar deviation.

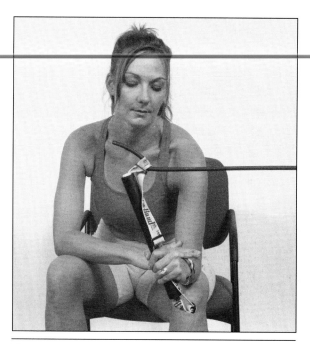

Figure 4.37   Forearm pronation.

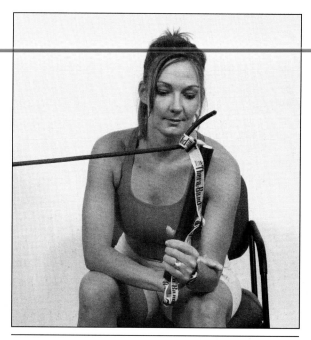

Figure 4.38   Forearm supination.

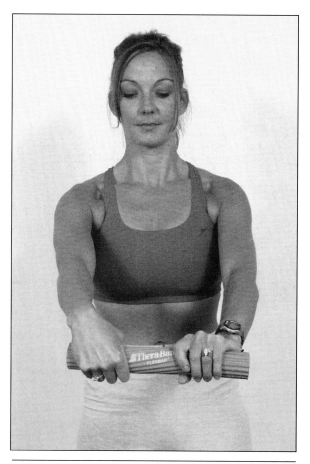

Figure 4.39   FlexBar flexion.

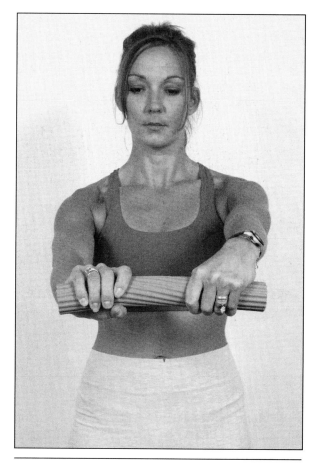

Figure 4.40   FlexBar extension.

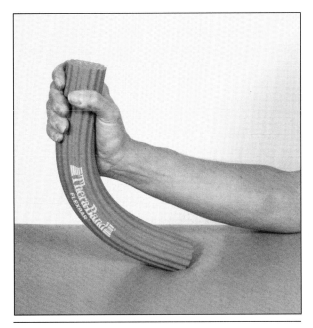

Figure 4.41 FlexBar radial deviation.

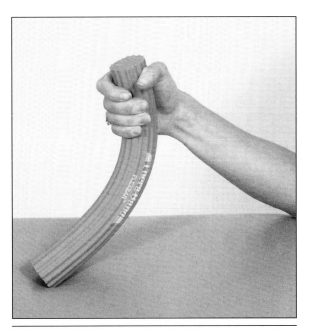

Figure 4.42 FlexBar ulnar deviation.

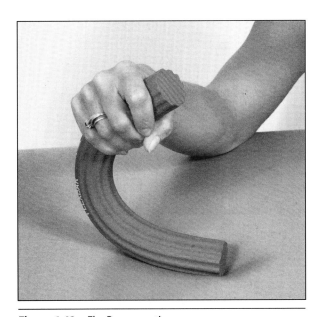

Figure 4.43 FlexBar pronation.

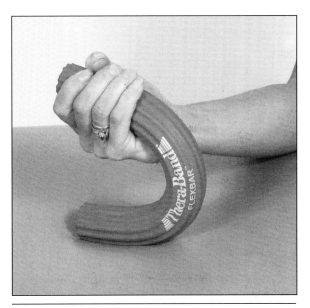

Figure 4.44 FlexBar supination.

Additional Uses of Elastic Resistance in Elbow Rehabilitation

Another frequent complication after fracture, surgery, or extensive injury to the elbow is range of motion loss. Morrey (1993) called the elbow the most "unforgiving" joint in the human body. Specific anatomical factors often limit range of motion in the human elbow. One of these factors is the presence of actual muscle coursing anteriorly to the elbow joint, rather than tendon. This is very unique to the elbow, with the brachialis muscle, not tendon, passing over the anterior capsule. Therefore, overly aggressive attempts at stretching the elbow into extension may lead to bleeding of the anterior capsule of the elbow and subsequently may lead to capsular thickening and contracture and possibly myositis ossificans (Morrey 1992). This unique response of the anterior capsule of the elbow, coupled with the high degree of joint congruity in the ulnohumeral joint, often makes regaining range of motion in the human elbow a rehabilitative challenge.

The clinical application of elastic resistance to assist in regaining range of motion during rehabilitation can be demonstrated by the use of the low-load prolonged stretch (LLPS) concept (Hepburn and Cirvelli 1984). Figure 4.45 shows the placement and application of elastic resistance to gently move the elbow into extension, to facilitate elbow extension range of motion. Placing the

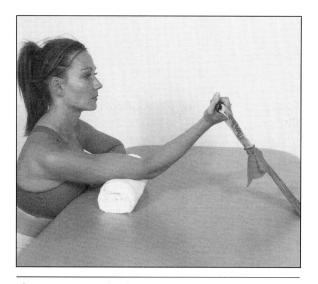

Figure 4.45   Low load prolonged stretch technique for increasing elastic resistance.

elastic in the hand or distal to the wrist may increase the muscular activity of the wrist and finger flexors and can prohibit maximal relaxation of the musculature around the elbow during stretching (Ellenbecker and Mattalino 1996). This technique is used for longer durations with very light resistance (such as yellow or red level Thera-Band) to apply the LLPS concept. Additionally, a towel roll is placed just proximal to the olecranon to position the humerus in a more optimal position during the stretch.

Wrist Joint

The wrist and hand contain 27 bones. The distal radius has a broad concave articular surface where it articulates with the scaphoid and lunate bones. The radial styloid process projects further distally, allowing approximately 15 to 20° of radial deviation. Medially, the distal radius contains the ulnar notch, providing a concave articular surface for articulation with the distal ulna and formation of the distal radioulnar joint (Wadsworth 1997). In conjunction with the proximal radioulnar joint, the distal radioulnar joint allows for 170 to 180° of pronation/supination of the forearm. A mobile radius rotates around a relatively stable ulna. During pronation, the ulna moves in a posterolateral and distal direction (Palmer and Werner 1984).

The ulnar styloid process is shorter than the radial styloid process and allows for 30 to 40° of ulnar deviation. At the distal end of the ulna, the articular disk only attaches to the distal ulna but also has radial attachments at the medial margin and attaches the radius to the ulna. This biconcave disk articulates proximally with the ulna and distally with the proximal carpal row, primarily the triquetrum, preventing direct contact between the distal ulna and carpals (Wadsworth 1997). This articulation is technically referred to as the ulnomeniscaltriquetral articulation and the triangular fibrocartilage complex. Finally, the bones of the carpus lie in two transverse rows. The approximate range of motion of the wrist is 80° of extension and 85° of flexion.

Specific exercises with elastic resistance for the wrist are presented in the elbow section of this chapter. Because of the common muscle tendon unit arrangement shared by the elbow, forearm, and wrist, movement patterns for resistance exercise used in elbow rehabilitation also involve the wrist and, specifically, the muscle/tendon units that cross and stabilize the wrist joint. Exercise patterns such as forearm pronation and supination, wrist flexion and extension, and wrist radial and ulnar deviation are important parts of a wrist rehabilitation program (Wadsworth 1997). Additionally, strips of elastic resistance can be used to provide resistance for finger flexion and extension during rehabilitation of the wrist and hand.

Conclusion

This chapter reviewed anatomical and biomechanical principles to provide a detailed rationale for the use of elastic resistance in rehabilitation and resistance training for the upper extremity. The exercises contained in this chapter can provide a framework for the development of resistance exercise programs for the upper extremity, for both rehabilitation and performance enhancement. The specific positions described, along with the electromyographic research, will provide the necessary guidance for clinical application of elastic resistance. Further research is needed to better understand the unique benefits of elastic resistance training and specific parameters for its direct application for the upper extremity.

CASE STUDY

Lindsay is a 14-year-old right-handed female elite junior tennis player with a 2-week history of posterior shoulder pain. The pain initiated during heavy serving at a tournament and initially bothered her only with overhead activities but now is present at low levels with any exertion. Pain is 8/10 with overhead serving, 2/10 with other activities, and 0/10 at rest and at night. She denies any significant history of shoulder problems and has not changed her equipment or playing technique recently.

Physical examination reveals a prominent medial border of the right scapula and mild atrophy in the infraspinous fossa of the right scapula as compared to the left. Protrusion of the medial border of the scapula is present with pressure taken via the upper extremities and during eccentric lowering of the right arm from full flexion and abduction. Lindsay shows a 1+ sulcus sign and 2+ anterior posterior humeral head translation at 90° of abduction in the right shoulder. Positive Neer and Hawkins impingement tests are present, as well as a positive subluxation/relocation test in the right shoulder. Gross manual muscle testing of the right shoulder reveals 4/5 external rotation and supraspinatus strength with reproduction of posterior pain in the right shoulder. All other muscle tests are 5/5 and unremarkable. Right shoulder external rotation is 120° with 90° of abduction and 100° on the contralateral left extremity. Internal rotation is 20° with 90° of abduction on the right and 55° on the left.

Lindsay presents with signs and symptoms consistent with impingement secondary to instability and concomitant scapular dysfunction.

Lindsay's treatment consists of modality care to decrease pain and inflammation in the right shoulder coupled with posterior capsule and stretching to gently improve internal rotation range of motion in the right shoulder. She is started on elastic resistance exercises to address the focused weakness in the external rotators and scapular stabilizers. These scapular exercises, which include the seated row (figure 4.02), bilateral ER with scapular retraction (figure 4.03), the serratus punch (figure 4.07), and push-up with a plus (figure 4.09) address the important force couple between the serratus anterior and lower trapezius. Additionally, Lindsay is instructed to perform external rotation in neutral (figure 4.21), prone shoulder extension (figure 4.26), and prone horizontal abduction with external rotation (figure 4.25). These exercises are used with 3 sets of 15 repetitions using red level Thera-Band.

After 2 weeks of strengthening, Lindsay is progressed to 90° abducted exercise for external rotation (figure 4.22), prone external rotation with 90° of abduction (figure 4.28), lawnboys (figure 4.04), and the diagonal 2 modified scapular retraction exercise (figure 4.06).

Isokinetic testing performed on Lindsay shows only 10% deficits in right shoulder external rotation, and external/internal rotation ratios from 62% to 66% after three weeks of rehabilitation. Additionally, she now has 30° of internal rotation with 90° of abduction. She is started on an interval tennis program with groundstrokes initially, and after 2 additional weeks begins light serving. She is given the above-mentioned exercises as a home program to continue to increase posterior rotator cuff strength and scapular stabilization. She returns to unrestricted tennis play.

References

An, K.N., F.C. Hui, B.F. Morrey, R.L. Linscheid, and E.Y. Chao. 1981. "Muscles Across the Elbow Joint: A Biomechanical Analysis." *Journal of Biomechanics* 14: 659-69.

Anderson, L., R. Rush, L. Shearer, and C.J. Hughes. 1992. "The Effects of a Thera-Band Exercise Program on Shoulder Internal Rotation Strength" (Abstract). *Physical Therapy* 72(6): S40.

Bagg, S.D., and W.J. Forrest. 1986. "Electromyographic Study of the Scapular Rotators During Arm Abduction in the Scapular Plane." *American Journal of Physical Medicine* 65: 111-24.

Ballantyne, B.T., S.J. O'Hare, J.L. Paschall, M.M. Pavia-Smith, A.M. Pitz, J.F. Gillon, and G.L. Soderberg. 1993. "Electromyographic Activity of Selected Shoulder Muscles in Commonly Used Therapeutic Exercises." *Physical Therapy* 73: 668-82.

Bassett, R.W., A.O. Browne, B.F. Morrey, and K.N. An. 1990. "Glenohumeral Muscle Force and Moment Mechanics in a Position of Shoulder Instability." *Journal of Biomechanics* 23: 405- 415.

Bigliani, L.U., R.G. Pollock, L.J. Soslowsky, E.L. Flatow, R.J. Pawluk, and V.C. Mow. 1992. "Tensile Properties of the Inferior Glenohumeral Ligament." *Journal of Orthopedic Research* 10: 187-97.

Bigliani, L.U., J.B. Ticker, E.L. Flatow, L.J. Soslowsky, and V.C. Mow. 1991. "The Relationship of the Acromial Architecture to Rotator Cuff Disease." *Clinics in Sports Medicine* 10: 823-838.

Blackburn, T.A., W.E. McLeod, B. White, and L. Wofford. 1990. "EMG Analysis of Posterior Rotator Cuff Exercises." *Athletic Training* 25: 40-5.

Bleacher, J., and J. Roush. 1999. "The Effects of a Six-Week Home Exercise Program Using Elastic Resistance on Shoulder External Rotator Peak Torque" (Abstract). *Physical Therapy* (Suppl) 79(5): S31.

Burkhart, S.S., C.D. Morgan, and W.B. Kibler. 2000. "Shoulder Injuries in Overhead Athletes: The 'Dead Arm' Revisited." *Clinics in Sports Medicine* 19(1): 125-58.

Burkhead, W.Z., and C.A. Rockwood. 1992. "Treatment of Instability of the Shoulder With an Exercise Program." *Journal of Bone and Joint Surgery* 74-A(6): 890-6.

Codman, E.A. 1934. *The Shoulder.* 2nd ed. Boston: Thomas Todd.

Cotton, R.E., and D.F. Rideout. 1964. "Tears of the Humeral Rotator Cuff: A Radiological and Pathological Necropsy Survey." *Journal of Bone and Joint Surgery* 46B:314.

Daniels, L., and C. Worthingham. 1980. *Muscle Testing: Techniques of Manual Examination.* Philadelphia: Saunders.

Davidson, P.A., M.M. Pink, J. Perry, and F.W. Jobe. 1995. "Functional Anatomy of the Flexor Pronator Muscle Group in Relation to the Medial Collateral Ligament of the Elbow." *American Journal of Sports Medicine* 23(2): 245-50.

Davies, G.J. 1992. *A Compendium of Isokinetics in Clinical Usage.* 2nd ed. LaCrosse, WI: S&S Publishers.

Decker, M.J., R.A. Hintermeister, K.J. Faber, and R.J. Hawkins. 1999. "Serratus Anterior Muscle Activity During Selected Rehabilitation Exercises." *American Journal of Sports Medicine* 27(6): 784-91.

Digiovine, N.M., F.W. Jobe, M. Pink, and J. Perry. 1992. "An Electromyographic Analysis of the Upper Extremity in Pitching." *Journal of Shoulder and Elbow Surgery* 1: 15-5.

Dillman, C.J. 1995. "Biomechanics of the Rotator Cuff." *Sports Medicine and Arthroscopy Review* 3: 2.

Doody, S.G., L. Freeman, and J.C. Waterland. 1970. "Shoulder Movements During Abduction in the Scapular Plane." *Archives of Physical Medicine and Rehabilitation* 51: 595-604.

Ellenbecker, T.S. 1995. "Rehabilitation of Shoulder and Elbow Injuries in Tennis Players." *Clinics in Sports Medicine* 14(1): 87-110.

Ellenbecker, T.S. 1997. "Etiology and Evaluation of Rotator Cuff Pathology and Rehabilitation." In *Physical Therapy of the Shoulder*, ed. R.A. Donatelli. Philadelphia: Churchill Livingstone.

Ellenbecker, T.S., and K. Cappel. 2000. "Clinical Application of Closed Kinetic Chain Exercises in the Upper Extremities." *Orthopaedic Physical Therapy Clinics in North America* 9(2): 231-45.

Ellenbecker, T.S., J. Kingma, and A. Kim. 1994. "A Six-Week Isotonic Training Study of the Forearm Flexors and Extensors in Healthy Subjects." Unpublished research.

Ellenbecker, T.S., and A.J. Mattalino. 1996. *The Elbow in Sport.* Champaign, IL: Human Kinetics.

Elliot, B., T. Marsh, and B. Blanksby. 1986. "A Three Dimensional Cinematographic Analysis of the Tennis Serve." *International Journal of Sport Biomechanics* 2: 260-71.

Fleisig, G.S., C.J. Dillman, and J.R. Andrews. 1989. "Proper Mechanics for Baseball Pitching." *Clinics in Sports Medicine* 1: 151-70.

Glousman, R.E., J. Barron, F.W. Jobe, J. Perry, and M.M. Pink. 1992. "An Electromyographic Analysis of the Elbow in Normal and Injured Pitchers With Medial Collateral Ligament Insufficiency." *American Journal of Sports Medicine* 20(3): 311-7.

Hammer, D.L., M.M. Pink, and F.W. Jobe. 2000. "A Modification of the Relocation Test: Arthroscopic Findings Associated With a Positive Test." *Journal of Shoulder and Elbow Surgery* 9: 263-7.

Hepburn G.R., and K.J. Cirvelli. 1984. "Use of Elbow Dynasplint for Reduction of Elbow Flexion Contractures: A Case Study." *Journal of Orthopaedic and Sports Physical Therapy.* 5: 269-274.

Hintermeister, R.A., G.W. Lange, J.M. Schultheis, M.J. Bey, and R.J. Hawkins. 1998. "Electromyographic Activity and Applied Load During Shoulder Rehabilitation Exercises Using Elastic Resistance." *American Journal of Sports Medicine* 26(2): 210-20.

Indelicato, P.A., F.W. Jobe, R.K. Kerlan, V.S. Carter, C.L. Sheilds, and S.J. Lombardo. 1979. "Correctable Elbow Lesions in Professional Baseball Players. A Review of 25 Cases." *American Journal of Sports Medicine* 7: 72-5.

Inman, V.T., J.B. Saunders, and L.C. Abbot. 1944. "Observations on the function of the Shoulder Joint. *Journal of Bone Joint Surgery*, A26: 1-30.

Itoi, E., D.K. Kuenchle, S.R. Newman, B.F. Morrey, and K.N. An. 1993. "Stablising Function of the Biceps in Stable and Unstable Shoulders." *Journal of Bone and Joint Surgery* 75BR: 546-50.

Jobe, F.W., and R.S. Kivitne. 1989. "Shoulder Pain in the Overhand or Throwing Athlete. The Relationship of Anterior

Instability and Rotator Cuff Impingement." *Orthopaedic Review* 18: 963-75.

Jobe, F.W., and M. Pink. 1994. "The Athlete's Shoulder." *Journal of Hand Therapy*, p. 107.

Karduna, A.R., G.R. Williams, J.L. Williams, and J.P. Iannotti. 1996. "Kinematics of the Glenohumeral Joint: Influences of Muscle Forces, Ligamentous Constraints, and Articular Geometry." *Journal of Bone and Joint Surgery* 14: 986-93.

Kelley, J.D., S.J. Lombardo, M.M. Pink, and J. Perry. 1994. "Electromyographic and Cinematographic Analysis of Elbow Function in Tennis Players With Lateral Epicondylitis." *American Journal of Sports Medicine* 22: 359-63.

Kibler, W.B. 1991. "The Role of the Scapula in the Overhead Throwing Motion." *Contemporary Orthopaedics* 22: 525-32.

Kibler, W.B. 1998. "The Role of the Scapula in Athletic Shoulder Function." *American Journal of Sports Medicine* 26(2): 325-37.

King, J.W., H.J. Brelsford, and H.S. Tullos. 1969. "Analysis of the pitching arm of the professional baseball pitcher." *Clinical Orthopaedics and Related Research* 67:116-23.

Kraushaar, B.S., and R.P. Nirschl. 1999. "Tendinosis of the Elbow (Tennis Elbow)." *Journal of Bone and Joint Surgery* 81-A: 259-78.

Kronberg, M., F. Nemeth, and L.A. Brostrom. 1990. "Muscle Activity and Coordination in the Normal Shoulder: An Electromyographic Study." *Clinical Orthopaedics and Related Research* 257: 76-85.

Litchfield, D.G., S. Jeno, and R. Mabey 1998. "The Lateral Scapular Slide Test: Is It Valid in Detecting Glenohumeral Impingement?" (Abstract). *Physical Therapy* 78(5): S29.

Ludewig, P.M., and T.M. Cook. 2000. "Alterations in Shoulder Kinematics and Associated Muscle Activity in People With Symptoms of Shoulder Impingement." *Physical Therapy* 80(3): 276-91.

Macko, S.D., M.L. Manley, C.A. Maul, B.E. Roth, and M.A. Sakalas. 1999. "Effectiveness of Theraband on Strengthening the Shoulder External Rotators" (Abstract). *Physical Therapy* 79(5) (Suppl.): S82-3.

Malanga, G.A., Y.N. Jenp, E.S. Growney, and K.N. An. 1996. "EMG Analysis of Shoulder Positioning in Testing and Strengthening the Supraspinatus." *Medicine and Science in Sports and Exercise* 28: 661-4.

McCabe, R.A., T.F. Tyler, S.J. Nicholas, and M.P. McHugh. 2001. "Selective Activation of the Lower Trapezius Muscle in Patients With Shoulder Impingement." *Journal of Orthopaedics and Sports Physical Therapy* 31(1): (Abstract) 45.

McMahon, P.J., F.W. Jobe, M.M. Pink, et al. 1996. "Comparative Electromyographic Analysis of Shoulder Muscles During Planar Motions. Anterior Glenohumeral Instability Versus Normal." *Journal of Shoulder and Elbow Surgery* 5: 118-23.

Morrey, B.F. 1992. "Postraumatic Stiffness: Distraction Arthroplasty." *Orthopaedics* 15: 863-9.

Morrey, B.F. 1993. *The Elbow and Its Disorders*. 2nd ed. Philadelphia: Saunders.

Morrey, B.F., and K.N. An. 1983. "Articular and Ligamentous Contributions to the Stability of the Elbow Joint." *American Journal of Sports Medicine* 11: 315-319.

Morris, M., F.W. Jobe, J. Perry, M.M. Pink, and B.S. Healy. 1989. "Electromyographic Analysis of Elbow Function in Tennis Players." *American Journal of Sports Medicine* 17: 241-7.

Moseley, J.B., F.W. Jobe, M. Pink, J. Perry, and J. Tibone. 1992. "EMG Analysis of the Scapular Muscles During a Shoulder Rehabilitation Program." *American Journal of Sports Medicine* 20(2): 128-34.

Neer, C.J. 1972. "Anterior Acromioplasty for the Chronic Impingement Syndrome in the Shoulder." *Journal of Bone and Joint Surgery* 54A: 41-50.

Nirschl, R.P., and J. Sobel. 1981. "Conservative Treatment of Tennis Elbow." *The Physician and Sportsmedicine* 9(6): 43-54.

O'Brien, S.J., M.C. Neves, S.P. Arnoczky, S.R. Rozbruck, E.F. DiCarlo, R.F. Warren, R. Schwartz, and T.L. Wickiewicz. 1990. "The Anatomy and Histology of the Inferior Glenohumeral Ligament Complex of the Shoulder." *American Journal of Sports Medicine* 18: 449-56.

O'Driscoll, S.W., D.F. Bell, and B.F. Morrey. 1991. "Posterolateral Rotary Instability of the Elbow." *Journal of Bone and Joint Surgery* 74A: 440-6.

Page, P.A., J. Lamberth, B. Abadie, R. Boling, R. Collins, and R. Linton. 1993. "Posterior Rotator Cuff Strengthening Using Thera-Band in a Functional Diagonal Pattern in Collegiate Baseball Pitchers." *Journal of Athletic Training* 28(4): 346-54.

Paley, K.J., F.W. Jobe, M.M. Pink, R.S. Kvitne, and N.S. Elattrache NS. 2000. "Arthroscopic Findings in the Overhand Throwing Athlete: Evidence for Posterior Internal Impingement of the Rotator Cuff." *Arthroscopy* 16(1): 35-40.

Palmer, A.K., and F.M. Werner. 1984. "Biomechanics of the Distal Radioulnar Joint." *Clinical Orthopaedics and Related Research* 187: 26-35.

Rathbun, J.B., and I. McNab. 1970. "The Microvascular Pattern of the Rotator Cuff." *Journal of Bone and Joint Surgery* 52B: 540-53.

Reddy, A.S., K.J. Mohr, M.M. Pink, and F.W. Jobe. 2000. "Electromyographic Analysis of the Deltoid and Rotator Cuff Muscles in Persons With Subacromial Impingement." *Journal of Shoulder and Elbow Surgery* 9: 519-23.

Rodosky, M.W., C.D. Harner, and F.F. Fu. 1994. "The Role of the Long Head of the Biceps Muscle and Superior Glenoid Labrum in Anterior Stability of the Shoulder." *American Journal of Sports Medicine* 22: 121-30.

Saha, A.K. 1983. "Mechanism of Shoulder Movements and a Plea for the Recognition of 'Zero-Position' of Glenohumeral Joint." *Clinical Orthopaedics and Related Research* 173: 3-10.

Simoneau, G.G., S.M. Bereda, D.C. Sobush, and A.J. Starsky 2001. "Biomechanics of Elastic Resistance in Therapeutic Exercise Programs." *Journal of Orthopaedic and Sports Physical Therapy*. 31:16-24.

Sisto, D., F.W. Jobe, D. R. Moynes, and D.J. Antonelli. 1987. "An Electromyographic Analysis of the Elbow in Pitching." *American Journal of Sports Medicine* 15(3): 260-3.

Townsend, H., F.W. Jobe, M. Pink, J. Perry. 1991. "Electromyographic Analysis of the Glenohumeral Muscles During a Baseball Rehabilitation Program." *American Journal of Sports Medicine* 19: 264-72.

Treiber, F.A., J. Lott, J. Duncan, F. Slavens, and H. Davis. 1998. "Effects of Theraband and Lightweight Dumbbell

Training on Shoulder Rotation Torque and Serve Performance in College Tennis Players." *American Journal of Sports Medicine* 26: 510-515.

Wadsworth, C. 1997. "The Wrist and Hand." In *Orthopaedic and Sports Physical Therapy*, ed. T.R. Malone, T. McPoil, and A.J. Nitz. St. Louis: Mosby.

Walch, G., P. Boileau, E. Noel, and S.T. Donell. 1992. "Impingement of the Deep Surface of the Supraspinatus Tendon on the Posterosuperior Glenoid Rim. An Arthroscopic Study." *Journal of Shoulder and Elbow Surgery* 1: 238-45.

Warner, J.J.P., L.J. Micheli, L.E. Arslanian, J. Kennedy, and R. Kennedy. 1992. "Scapulothoracic Motion in Normal Shoulders and Shoulders With Glenohumeral Joint Instability and Impingement Syndrome." *Clinical Orthopaedics and Related Research* 285: 191-9.

Weiner, D.S., and I. McNab. 1970. "Superior Migration of the Humeral Head." *Journal of Bone and Joint Surgery* 52B: 524-7.

Zeier, F.G. 1973. "The Treatment of Winged-Scapula." *Clinical Orthopaedics and Related Research* 91: 128-33.

CHAPTER 5

Lower Extremity Exercises With Elastic Resistance

• • • • •

Jill Thein-Nissenbaum, MPT, SCS, ATC
University of Wisconsin at Madison

Jill C. Orzehoskie, MPT, ATC
Sheboygan Memorial Hospital, Sheboygan, Wisconsin

Rehabilitation of the lower extremities—the hip, knee, lower leg, ankle, and foot—is a common reason for referral to the health care professional. Factors that necessitate intervention and rehabilitation include pain, impaired strength and range of motion, and decreased balance and proprioception. These impairments commonly are seen in persons with orthopedic concerns such as trochanteric bursitis, degenerative joint disease, knee ligament reconstruction, patellofemoral stress syndrome, ankle sprains, and plantar fasciitis.

With the advent of managed care and dwindling health care benefits, patients may find themselves with a decreased number of rehabilitation visits. Thus, an effective home exercise program is crucial. Because many patients do not have access to health clubs or exercise facilities, clinicians and patients alike are seeking alternative rehabilitation programs that can be performed without expensive equipment. Consequently, the use of elastic resistance has become popular, because of its low cost, simplicity, portability, and nonreliance on gravity

(Hughes et al. 1999). Elastic resistive devices, such as bands and tubing, come in varying degrees of tension and can be cut to the length required by the patient. Because they are portable, they can be transported by the patient to any location, which can enhance compliance.

In this chapter we discuss the use of elastic resistance in hip, knee, ankle, and foot rehabilitation. We briefly review anatomy and discuss pathologies and impairments commonly seen at each joint. This is followed by exercise prescription for each joint, in which the exercise is correlated to the pathologies previously described. Last, we discuss balance and proprioception for the lower extremity with the use of elastic resistance.

The Hip

The diarthrodial hip joint is comprised of the acetabulum and femur. It is capable of performing flexion/extension in the sagittal plane, adduction/

abduction in the frontal plane, and internal/external rotation in the transverse plane. Normal active range of motion (ROM) for hip motions is 120° of flexion, 15° of extension, 50° of abduction, 30° of adduction, 60° of external rotation, and 40° of internal rotation (Magee 1992).

The primary flexors of the hip joint include the psoas and the iliacus. Secondary hip flexors include rectus femoris, sartorius, and adductors. The primary extensors are the gluteus maximus, hamstrings, adductor magnus, and the posterior portion of the gluteus medius. The adductors, gracilis, and pectineus accomplish adduction, whereas abduction is achieved by the gluteus medius and minimus, tensor fascia latae, and piriformis. Internal rotation is performed by the adductors, the anterior portion of gluteus medius and minimus, and tensor fascia latae. Last, external rotation is performed by gluteus maximus, piriformis, obturator internus and externus, gemellus inferior and superior, and quadratus femoris (Magee 1992; Soderberg 1996). Ligamentous stability is accomplished by the iliofemoral ligament (also termed the *Y ligament of Bigelow*), the ischiofemoral ligament, and the pubofemoral ligament (Norkin and Levangie 1990).

Elastic Resistance Exercises for the Hip

A variety of pathologies, diseases, diagnoses, and subsequent impairments involving the hip affect people of all ages. A few common diagnoses in the adult population include degenerative joint disease (Soderberg 1996), greater trochanteric bursitis, osteitis pubis, tendinitis, and hamstring and adductor muscle strains (Sanders and Nemeth 1996). Hip pathology in the prepubescent child includes slipped capital femoral epiphysis and Legg-Calvé-Perthes disease (Thein 1996).

An impairment commonly seen with hip pathologies is loss of strength. Elastic resistance exercises have demonstrated muscle activation via electromyography in various lower extremity rehabilitation exercises (Hintermeister et al. 1998; Hopkins et al. 1999; Schulthies et al. 1998). Thus, elastic resistance exercises commonly are used to address weakness.

Much of the musculature of the lower extremity is diarthrodial, which means that it functions at two joints. Consequently, many muscles that function at the hip also function at the knee. Subsequently, we explain and demonstrate exercises that isolate the hip musculature as well as multijoint exercises incorporating muscles that cross the knee joint.

Sagittal plane movements at the hip include flexion and extension. The hip flexors typically demonstrate a loss of flexibility rather than a loss of strength, because of the prolonged sitting dictated by our society. Hip flexors can be strengthened, when necessary, with knee extension to bias the iliacus and psoas. This will decrease the mechanical advantage of the rectus femoris (figure 5.01). When combined with knee flexion, the rectus femoris contributes to hip flexion (figure 5.02).

The hip extensors are often weak, an impairment frequently addressed in rehabilitation. Hip extensor strength—both concentric and eccentric—is necessary for activities of daily living (ADLs), such as stair climbing, squatting, and lowering oneself to a chair. With many of these activities, hip extension (from a flexed position to neutral) and knee extension occur simultaneously, as do hip and knee flexion. Elastic resistance activities may be performed to isolate hip movement, or in combination with knee movement, making the exercise more functional. Hip extension with the knee flexed will isolate the gluteals (figure 5.03), whereas hip extension with the knee extended will incorporate the hamstrings. Combined hip and knee flexion and extension movements can be executed in open (figures 5.04 and 5.05) or closed (figures 5.06-5.08) chain

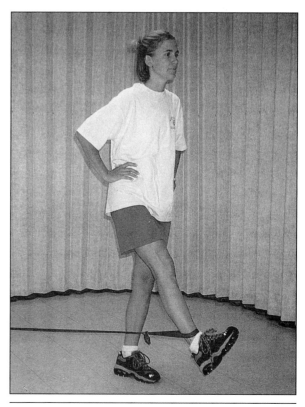

Figure 5.01   Standing hip flexion with knee extended.

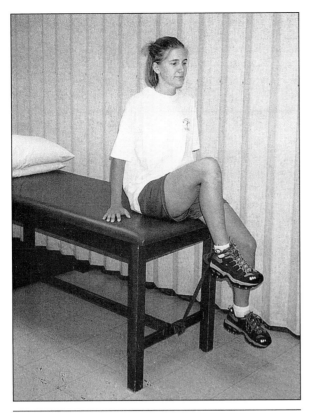

Figure 5.02 Seated hip flexion with knee flexed.

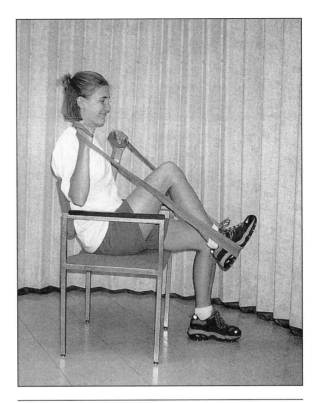

Figure 5.04 Leg press: Seated hip and knee extension (start position).

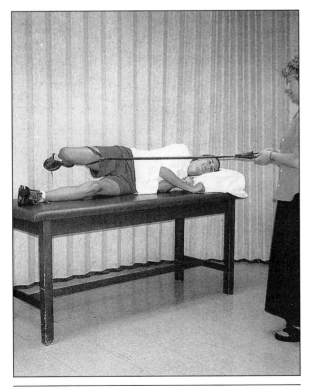

Figure 5.03 Sidelying hip extension with knee flexed.

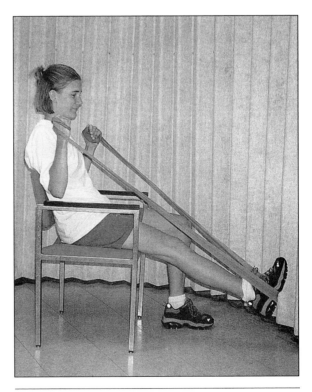

Figure 5.05 Leg press: Seated hip and knee extension (end position)

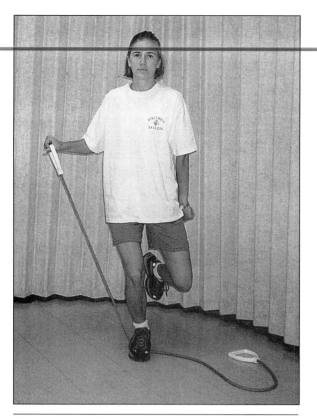

Figure 5.06   Unilateral mini-squat: standing hip and knee extension.

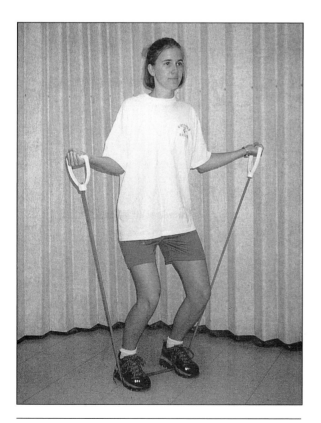

Figure 5.07   Bilateral mini-squat.

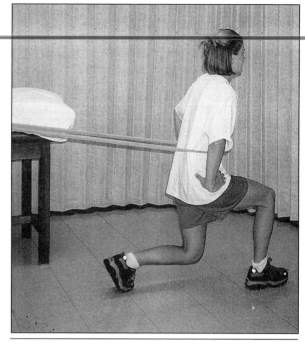

Figure 5.08   Lunges. Elastic resistance can be placed anterior or posterior to the patient and secured at waist height.

with elastic resistance. Single-leg squats, double-leg squats, and lunges all incorporate hip and knee movements and may be a functional progression in rehabilitation for patients with either hip or knee impairments. The cocontraction of the flexors and extensors offers lower extremity stability and carries over to sports that involve running, jumping, and landing. In the elderly, this exercise proves to be functional in ADLs such as raising and lowering from a chair and ascending and descending stairs.

Frontal plane hip motions (adduction and abduction) are performed primarily by one-joint muscles; as such, knee position is not as significant with frontal plane hip movement compared with sagittal plane hip movement (Kendall, Kendall, and Wadsworth 1972; Magee 1992; Soderberg 1996). However, increasing the length of the lever will make the exercise more challenging. Resisted hip motions are more difficult with the elastic resistance around the ankle than the distal thigh, if the resistance remains unchanged. Attaching the elastic resistance distal to the knee joint will cause a valgus or varus stress on the knee joint, which may provoke symptoms, especially if the patient has ligamentous instability at the knee. Resisted hip adduction and abduction may be completed in supine (figure 5.09), side-lying, or standing positions (figure 5.10). If the patient is elderly or has bilateral hip abduction weakness, or if balance is an issue, the supine or side-lying position may be the best position

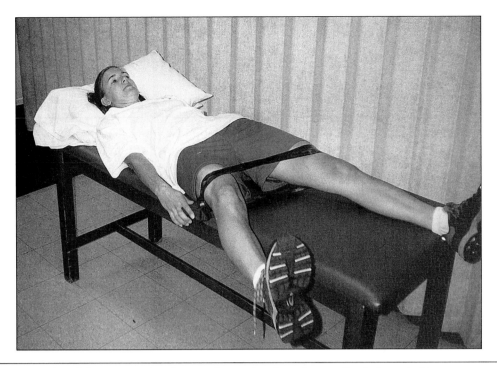

Figure 5.09 Supine hip abduction exercises. Progress by moving the resistance distally from the hip.

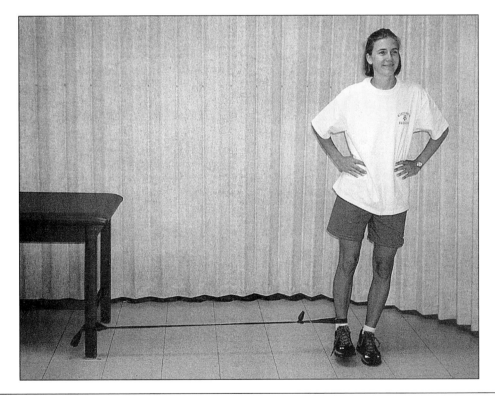

Figure 5.10 Standing hip adduction with knee extended.

initially. When exercises are executed in standing position, the hip abductors of the standing leg also must contract to stabilize the pelvis. Leiby et al. (1995) found an increase in strength of the stance leg compared with the kicking leg after 6 weeks of standing hip abduction strength training with elastic bands. The author suggested that clinicians should have the patient stand on the injured leg when performing this rehabilitation exercise. Incorporating hip extension and external rotation with abduction will isolate the posterior fibers of the gluteus medius in the moving leg, which may benefit the patient with patellofemoral stress syndrome (discussed in the knee section; figure 5.11).

Patients with degenerative joint disease at the hip often demonstrate pain, loss of motion, and weakness. They may benefit from joint unloading (via an assistive device), gentle stretching, and strengthening of the hip extensors and abductors (Lewis and Bottomley 1994). The patient who has undergone a total hip arthroplasty with a lateral surgical incision often demonstrates weakness in hip abduction, which may effect ambulation and cause a Trendelenburg gait. For these patients, the aforementioned strengthening exercises may be an important component of their exercise prescription.

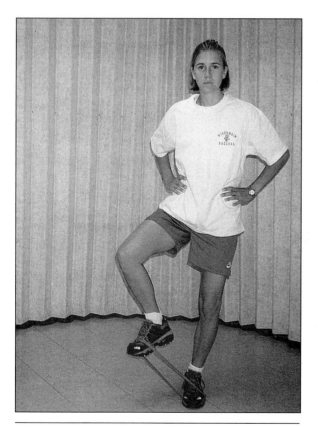

Figure 5.11　Standing hip abduction and extension with external rotation.

Strengthening exercises with elastic resistance also may be beneficial in patients who have had a hip fracture. Tinetti et al. (1997) created a systematic multicomponent rehabilitation program and then implemented it with elderly patients who had incurred a hip fracture. The program was performed at the patient's home, after the hospital stay. The rehabilitation strategy addressed many issues, including lower extremity strength loss, balance, bed mobility, and gait. Elastic bands were used to address impairments, and patients were progressed by using color-coded resistive bands. The results of the study showed that patients progressed to higher levels of resistive bands and balance exercises in 6 months of exercise. In a follow-up study by the same authors, the systematic multicomponent rehabilitation program was compared with "usual care" in the same population (Tinetti et al. 1999). The results showed that both groups showed improvements, with little differences between the groups. The authors noted that their "usual care" group received more rehabilitative services than typical, which possibly could explain their higher rate of recovery. The authors concluded that interventions after hip fracture, including strengthening exercises for the extremities with elastic resistance, are beneficial for return to function.

Internal and external rotation of the hip may be best performed seated, with the hip and knee in 90° of flexion (figures 5.12 and 5.13). Johnston, Lindsay, and Wiley (1999) found these exercises beneficial when treating patients with iliopsoas syndrome. This position requires the elastic resistance to be placed distal to the knee; the clinician is encouraged to monitor for symptoms of knee pain or discomfort.

Rotation of the hip also can be combined with other hip motions, as commonly performed in proprioceptive neuromuscular facilitation (PNF) techniques. PNF techniques are methods of promoting or hastening the response of the neuromuscular mechanism through stimulation of the proprioceptors (Vos, Ionta, and Myers 1985). PNF often is used when a patient has inefficient motor patterns or posture. The specific patterns may be used to improve timing or firing of certain musculature, to enhance range of motion, and to improve strength, because the specific patterns follow a diagonal and incorporate all planes of movement (Hanson 1999). With such training, the patient learns multiplanar movements, which are similar to movements found in ADLs, hobbies, and sports. The lower extremity intermediate segment (the knee) can be either flexed or extended during the pattern, specific to the patient's needs. Although isolated elastic resistance

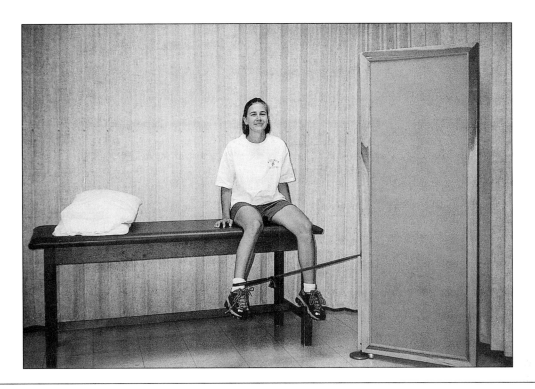

Figure 5.12 Seated hip internal rotation.

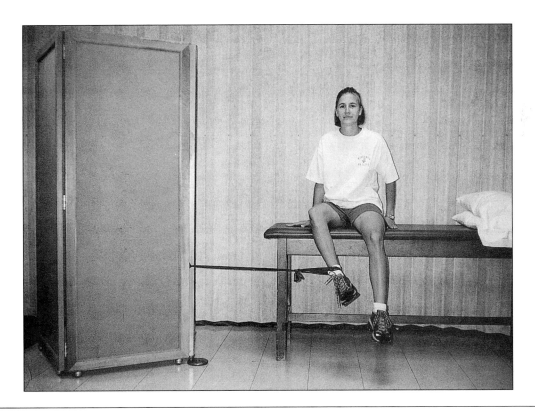

Figure 5.13 Seated hip external rotation.

can only provide resistance in one plane—typically in the diagonal plane of the PNF pattern—the patient may learn to move, cocontract, and stabilize while performing the diagonal against resistance. PNF diagonal 1 flexion incorporates hip flexion, adduction, and external rotation. Diagonal 1 extension involves hip extension, abduction, and internal rotation (figures 5.14 and 5.15). Diagonal 2 flexion is combined hip flexion, abduction, and internal rotation, whereas diagonal 2 extension is hip extension, adduction, and external rotation (figures 5.16 and 5.17; Vos, Ionta, and Myers 1985). PNF patterns are functional for the patient and offer strength and balance challenges to the standing leg. Other sport-specific drills can be found in subsequent chapters.

The Knee

The knee joint is very susceptible to injury, because it is located at the end of long lever arms—the femur

and the tibia. It provides mobility, as during ambulation, and stability during support of body weight (Magee 1992; Norkin and Levangie 1990). The joint relies on both bony configuration and soft tissue for support.

Normal sagittal plane active ROM is 0° to 135° (Magee 1992). The hamstrings (semitendinosus, semimembranosus, and biceps femoris) primarily perform knee flexion, whereas knee extension is achieved by the quadriceps femoris (rectus femoris, vasti intermedius, lateralis, and medialis). Knee flexion causes the patella to engage in the intercondylar notch, and with increased knee flexion the compressive forces of the patella and the femur are altered. A larger surface area of contact allows forces to be dissipated, and any alterations in the mechanics of the patellofemoral joint may cause increased forces on a decreased area of contact, threatening the health of the articular cartilage of the patella (McConnell and Fulkerson 1996). Various contributing factors (both intrinsic and extrinsic) may cause

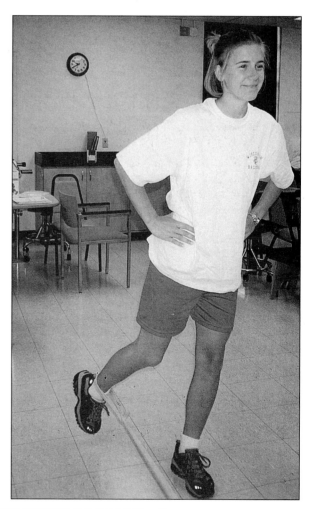

Figure 5.14-5.15   PNF D1 extension: start position (5.14); end position (5.15).

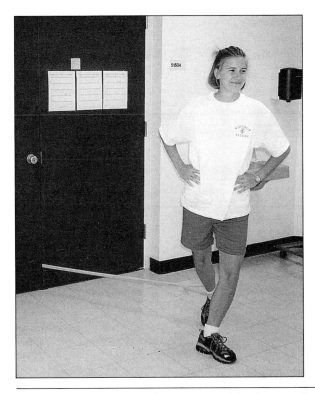 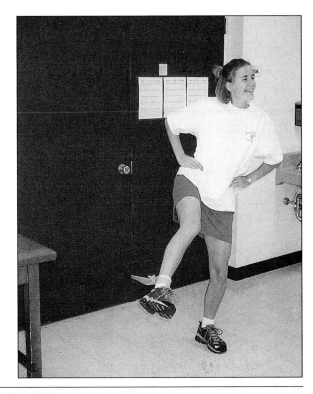

Figure 5.16-5.17   PNF D2 flexion: start position (5.16); end position (5.17).

patellofemoral pain. Several authors provide comprehensive discussion of patellofemoral pain (Brody and Thein 1998; Grelsamer and Klein 1998; Holmes and Clancy 1998; McConnell 2000; McConnell and Fulkerson 1996; Wilk et al. 1998).

Elastic Resistance Exercises for the Knee

Numerous injuries occur around the knee, including ligamentous injuries, meniscal injuries, patellofemoral pain, and tendinitis. The most common ligamentous injuries are tears of the anterior cruciate ligament (ACL) or medial collateral ligament (MCL), with the ACL often requiring surgical reconstruction (Brody and Tremain 1999). The medial meniscus is injured more frequently than the lateral meniscus, possibly because of its secure attachment and small displacement. Patellofemoral pain commonly is seen in women as well as in many athletes who play sports requiring flexion and extension, such as running and cycling. Patellar tendinitis is commonly seen in young athletes participating in jumping sports, whereas quadriceps tendinitis is commonly seen in the recreational athlete over the age of 40. Degenerative joint changes

and arthritis are seen at both the tibiofemoral and patellofemoral joints. Strengthening exercises are often imperative for patients with these pathologies.

Exercises to address deficits in quadriceps and hamstring strength frequently are prescribed in the clinical environment. The clinician must consider the cause of the weakness—such as lack of use, pain, or reflex inhibition. Knee joint effusion immediately postoperatively may contribute to decreased quadriceps activity. Spencer, Hayes, and Alexander (1984) found that 20 to 30 ml of saline injected into the knee joint was enough to cause reflex inhibition of the vastus medialis. These authors found that 59 to 60 ml of saline caused inhibition in the vastus lateralis and rectus femoris. These results demonstrate that if edema is present, it needs to be treated concurrently with the decreased quadriceps activity.

Isolated quadriceps exercises can be performed in the open chain with elastic resistance. Sitting or side-lying knee extension exercises can be performed that use the entire range of motion if the patient is asymptomatic and the exercise is not contraindicated (figures 5.18 and 5.19). The open-chain terminal knee extension position, from 0° to 30°, often is used sparingly with patients who are ACL-deficient or who have recently had an ACL reconstruction. It is commonly believed that the knee joint

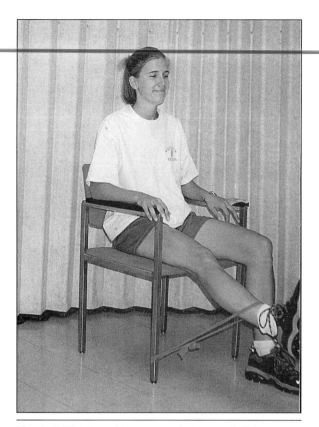

Figure 5.18   Seated knee extension (open chain).

experiences increased anterior tibial translation between approximately 30° of flexion and full extension in the open kinetic chain, which increases stress on the graft. Beynnon et al. (1997), however, found no differences in ACL strain behavior in vivo in patients with normal ligaments. The authors compared open-chain knee flexion-extension to the closed-chain squat, both with and without elastic resistance. The results demonstrated no difference in ACL strain behavior at 10° and 20° of knee flexion for all three exercises. The authors concluded that there is no difference between the strain on a normal ACL when a patient performs open-chain knee flexion-extension, squats, and squats with elastic resistance (figure 5.07). However, this study did not determine the strain on the ACL when open-chain knee flexion-extension exercises are performed against elastic resistance. Further research in this area is needed. To avoid any potential stress on a healing graft, terminal extension may be addressed in the closed chain (figure 5.20).

Steinkamp et al. (1993) found patellofemoral joint reaction force and patellofemoral joint stress to be greater in leg extension exercise between 0° and 30°

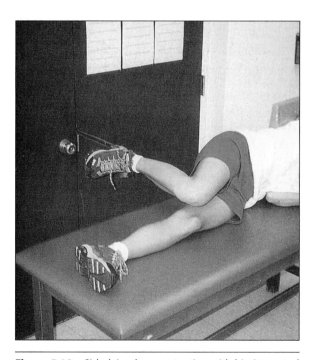

Figure 5.19   Side-lying knee extension with hip in neutral (start position).

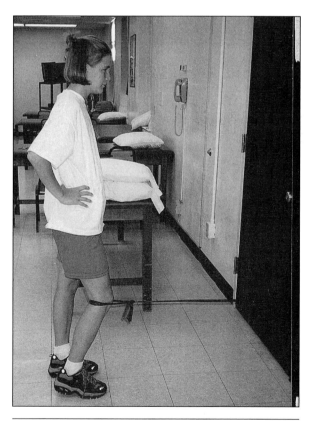

Figure 5.20   Standing terminal knee extension (30° to 0°).

than with the closed-chain leg press. The authors also found increased patellofemoral joint reaction force and patellofemoral joint stress at 60° and 90° in the leg press when compared with the open-chain leg extension exercise. These findings indicate that the clinician should use open-chain leg extension exercise through the full ROM with scrutiny in patients with ACL impairments or patellofemoral stress syndrome (PFSS). Terminal extension can be achieved in the closed chain with the aid of elastic resistance (figure 5.20).

Patients with PFSS frequently experience a lateral glide of the patella with quadriceps contraction because of a multitude of factors, including a tight lateral retinaculum and a weak vastus medialis oblique (VMO; Brody and Thein 1998). Strengthening exercises designed to specifically isolate the VMO remain controversial. Several studies of subjects performing a variety of exercises found no difference in VMO versus vastus lateralis (VL) activity (Cerny 1995; Dunleavy and McNeven 1997; Karst and Willett 1995; Powers, Landel, and Perry 1996). Other authors found that selective training of the VMO can affect an individual's activation pattern (King et al. 1984; LeVeau and Rogers 1980; McConnell 1986). Other authors have theorized that if VMO force is essential to proper tracking, general quadriceps strengthening may bring the VMO up to the "threshold" needed for adequate patellar tracking, without selectively training the VMO (Grabiner, Koh, and Draganich 1994).

Strengthening exercises for patients with PFSS include both open- and closed-chain exercises that limit patellofemoral joint reaction forces. Closed-chain exercises should be performed near terminal extension (0-30°; figure 5.20), whereas the remainder of the range of motion can be strengthened in the open-chain position. In a study by Willett et al. (1998), 16 subjects without knee pathology performed weight-bearing terminal knee extension through 0° to 30° four different ways—with and without elastic bands in neutral hip rotation, and with the bands in 30° of both external and internal hip rotation. The elastic band was set at a tension equivalent to a force of 4.5 kg, and electromyographic activity of the VMO and VL was assessed via surface electrodes. The results showed significantly increased VMO and VL activity in the three exercises that used elastic resistance compared with the exercise without elastic resistance. The ratio of VMO/VL activity was not different in any of the groups. The authors concluded that elastic resis-

tance exercises increase electromyographic activity of the VMO and VL but do not enhance VMO activity relative to the VL.

Other authors believe that concurrent adductor contraction with knee extension may enhance VMO firing, because of its close relation to the adductor muscles (Brody and Tremain 1999). As such, mini-squats with elastic resistance for adduction may be beneficial in VMO recruitment (figure 5.21).

Strengthening the hip external rotators, specifically the gluteus medius, also may benefit the patient with PFSS. If the gluteus medius is working well, there is less activity in the tensor fascia lata. Ultimately, this decreases the lateral pull of the patella via the lateral retinaculum and fibrous slips from the iliotibial band. Combined hip abduction, extension, and external rotation can strengthen the posterior fibers of the gluteus medius, affecting the iliotibial band via the tensor fascia lata, and ultimately will affect the patellofemoral joint (figure 5.11; McConnell and Fulkerson 1996).

The strength of the hamstrings often is overlooked in lower extremity rehabilitation, because rehabilitation tends to focus primarily on quadriceps strength. The hamstrings play a vital role in controlling anterior tibial translation, which is of

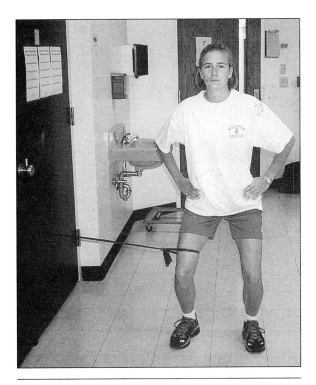

Figure 5.21 Mini-squats with concurrent resisted adduction (start position).

utmost importance in the newly reconstructed or ACL-deficient knee (Blair and Wills 1991). Eccentric strength of the hamstrings is necessary for controlled deceleration of the tibia during activities such as running and should be a component of the postoperative ACL rehabilitation program. Blair and Wills (1991) recommended hamstring strengthening with elastic resistance as early as 5 to 7 days postoperatively.

Isolated strengthening of the hamstrings can be performed seated with both concentric and eccentric muscular contractions (figure 5.22). The same exercise can be performed in prone position (figure 5.23). To focus on the eccentric portion of the exercise, the patient should use both lower extremities to flex the knee and then slowly extend the involved knee in a controlled fashion (figure 5.24). Resisted knee flexion increases stress on the posterior cruciate ligament (PCL) attributable to the posterior movement of the tibia on the femur. As such, this exercise should be used cautiously in patients with PCL deficiencies or reconstructions (Irrgang, Safran, and Fu 1996).

The ratio of hamstrings to quadriceps strength is a parameter often reviewed in isokinetic studies. It has been well established in the literature that this ratio is velocity dependent for concentric contractions. As the speed of testing increases, the ratio approaches 1.0 (Noyes, Barber, and Mangine 1991; Sapega 1990; Wojtys and Huston 1994). Eccentric

muscular contractions also have been studied, and the eccentric hamstrings/concentric quadriceps ratio has been studied in ACL-deficient knees. These ratios in the ACL-deficient limb and normal limbs were similar, leading the authors to suggest that neuromuscular strategies may have been implemented in the ACL-deficient knee (St Clair Gibson et al. 2000). A well-devised rehabilitation program may play a key role in the development of this neuromuscular adaptation.

The hamstrings/quadriceps strength ratio is an important consideration in rehabilitation. Because muscular activity serves as a major shock-absorbing mechanism for joints, adequate muscular balance of agonists and antagonists can help maintain overall joint health (Lewis and Bottomley 1994). Consequently, most patients with knee impairments benefit from isolated quadriceps and hamstrings strengthening. Once isolated strength is adequate, a functional strengthening program that uses co-contractions of the agonists and antagonists is implemented. Closed-chain exercises encourage co-contractions and potentially decrease the anterior shear of the tibia and stress on the newly reconstructed ACL. As such, they are beneficial in the early stages of ACL rehabilitation (Graham, Gehlsen, and Edwards 1993; Hopkins et al. 1999). In a prospective study by Bynum, Barrack, and Alexander (1995), 100 patients who underwent ACL reconstruction with a patellar-tendon graft were

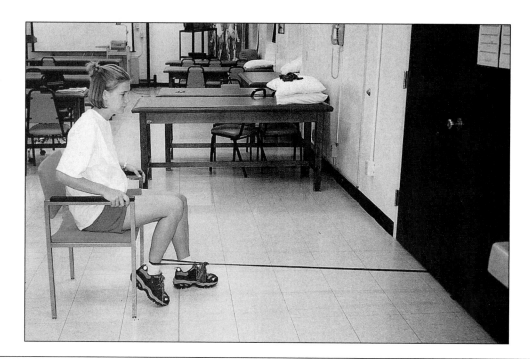

Figure 5.22   Seated knee flexion (hamstring curl).

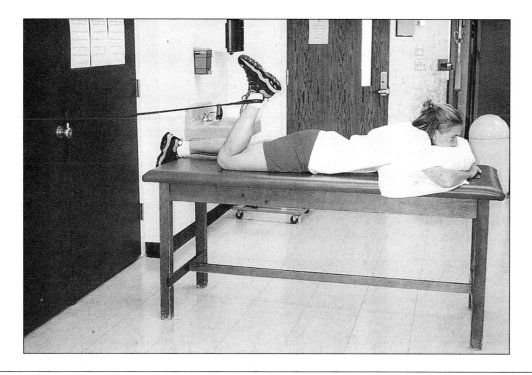

Figure 5.23   Prone knee flexion (hamstring curl).

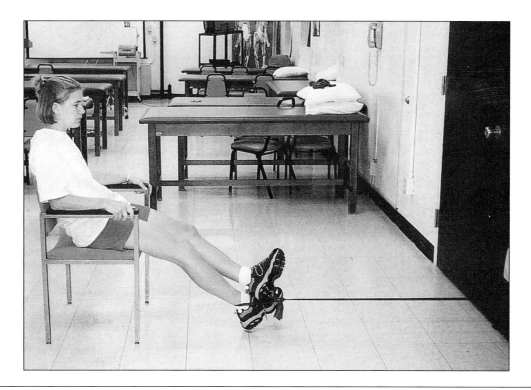

Figure 5.24   Seated knee flexion with emphasis on the eccentric phase. The uninvolved leg assists with the flexion portion of the movement, then is removed to allow the beginning of the eccentric phase of the hamstring contraction on the involved leg from a flexed position.

assigned randomly to a closed-chain or open-chain exercise group. The subjects in the open-chain exercise group performed activities such as isotonic and isokinetic quadriceps and hamstrings strengthening and treadmill jogging. Subjects in the closed-chain group performed activities using elastic resistance, such as squats, resisted walking, and seated leg press. At 1-year follow-up, the subjects in the closed-chain group demonstrated lower mean scores via a KT-1000 knee ligament arthrometer, less patellofemoral pain, and a perceived return to ADLs sooner than expected. The authors concluded that closed-chain exercises using elastic resistance were safe and effective in ACL postoperative rehabilitation.

Closed-chain exercises (figures 5.06-5.08) can be progressed to meet the patient's rehabilitative needs. Lunges also can be progressed by applying elastic resistance at various angles to the plane of movement, thereby challenging lower extremity and trunk control (figure 5.25). To make the exercise more challenging, lunges can be performed on an unstable surface (figure 5.26).

Cook, Burton, and Fields (1999) used elastic resistance when performing neuromuscular retraining in a collegiate female basketball player who was ACL-deficient. Daily, she performed activities such as alternate upper extremity movements against elastic resistance while standing on the affected leg, resisted running, and resisted scissors running using elastic resistance. The athlete had significant strength gains in 1 week, which the authors attributed to neuromuscular changes. The authors concluded that neuromuscular retraining may be performed effectively by using elastic resistance, ultimately enhancing performance.

In another study of ACL insufficiency, Lephart et al. (1991) devised norms for three functional performance tests to be used when the clinician assessed the ACL-insufficient athlete for return to sport. The authors included the cocontraction test, which uses elastic tubing secured to a Velcro belt around the patient's waist and to a hook on a wall. The athlete then shuffles in a semicircle with continuous tension on the tubing. The authors believed that this test would reproduce rotational forces at the knee. The results of the study demonstrated that athletes who perform sports that require lateral running performed better on this functional performance test. The results of each test were listed by sport, for the clinician to use as reference when assessing the ACL-insufficient athlete.

Hopkins et al. (1999) studied electromyographic activity in the VL, vastus medialis, and biceps femo-

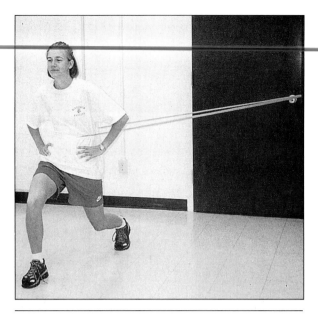

Figure 5.25   Lunge with weight shift.

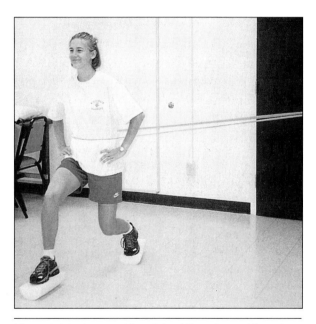

Figure 5.26   Lunge with weight shift and unstable surface.

ris during four closed-chain exercises. The unilateral one-quarter squat, lateral step-up, elastic-resisted front-pull (figure 5.27), and elastic-resisted back-pull (figure 5.28) were performed by 38 active healthy female college students without knee pathology. The subjects maintained closed-chain knee active ROM of 5° to 30° on their standing (involved) leg, which is similar to the active ROM used in postoperative ACL rehabilitation. The results of the

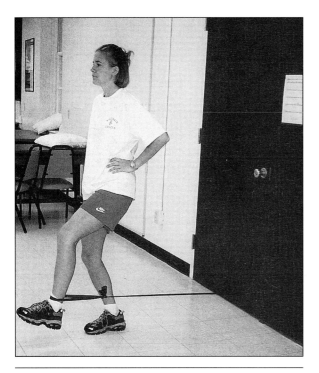

Figure 5.27 Standing hip flexion ("front pull").

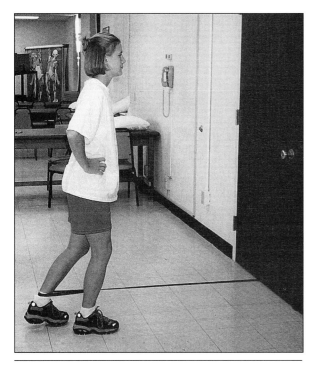

Figure 5.28 Standing hip extension ("back pull").

standing leg muscle activity demonstrated that the biceps femoris had higher levels of activity during the front-pull and back-pull than during the extension phase of the lateral step-up. During the flexion phase, the front-pull and back-pull demonstrated higher levels of biceps femoris activity than

during the unilateral one-quarter squat and the lateral step-up exercise. The front-pull also produced higher levels of vastus medialis activity than any other exercise. The authors concluded that the elastic-resisted exercises produced as much electromyographic activity in the quadriceps as traditional exercises, including the unilateral one-quarter squat and the lateral step-up, and that they also produced a strong biceps femoris contraction. Because of the high degree of hamstring activity during the front-pull exercise, the authors suggested that this exercise might, in fact, be safer than the traditional one-quarter squat and the lateral step-up (Hopkins et al. 1999). Although the electromyographic activity during each exercise was presented in the study, the maximum electromyographic readings or ratios were not provided. Consequently, one cannot determine the maximal percentage of electromyographic activity during each exercise. All subjects in the study were healthy; therefore, the results cannot be applied to subjects with pathology. Nonetheless, the authors concluded that the front-pull (figure 5.27) and back-pull (figure 5.28) are good rehabilitation exercises for general knee rehabilitation.

Schulthies et al. (1998) studied the electromyographic activity of the vastus medialis, vastus lateralis, semimembranosus, semitendinosus, and biceps femoris during four elastic tubing closed-chain exercises in patients 5 to 24 weeks after ACL reconstruction. Resistance was applied to the uninvolved lower extremity (LE) during four exercises—front-pull (figure 5.27), back-pull (figure 5.28), crossover (figure 5.29), and reverse-crossover (figure 5.30)—while the involved LE stabilized body weight. Electromyographic data gathered on muscle activity in the involved LE during the four exercises revealed significantly greater hamstrings/quadriceps (H/Q) ratios during the front-pull exercise (137%) than all other conditions and significantly greater H/Q ratio during the crossover exercise (115%) than the back-pull (70%) and reverse-crossover exercises (60%; table 5.01). The hamstrings contraction generates a posterior shear force on the tibia, which decreases ACL stress, suggesting that patients can activate the quadriceps with a co-contraction of the hamstrings with a reduced risk of stressing the ACL graft. This study suggested that the front-pull and crossover exercises can be safely performed early in the rehabilitation process to promote normal proprioceptive and functional patterns in musculature, balance, and coordination. This study also suggests that these four exercises produce myoelectric activity in excess of 30% of maximal

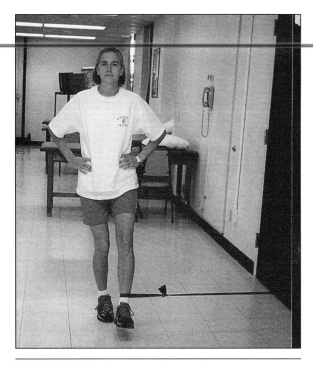

Figure 5.29 Standing hip adduction ("crossover").

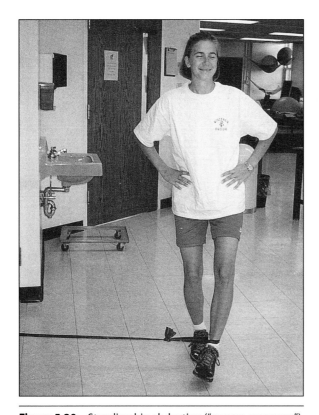

Figure 5.30 Standing hip abduction ("reverse crossover").

Table 5.01   Hamstring/Quadriceps Ratio of Electromyographic Activity for Various Exercises

Exercise	Hamstring/quadriceps ratio per electromyography (%)
Front-pull	137
Back-pull	70
Crossover	115
Reverse crossover	60

Reprinted by permission, from S.S. Schulthies, M.D. Ricard, K.J. Alexander, and J.W. Myer, 1998, "An Electromyographic Investigation of 4 Elastic-Tubing Closed Kinetic Chain Exercises After Anterior Cruciate Ligament Reconstruction," *Journal of Athletic Training* 33(4): 333.

voluntary isometric contraction, higher than that produced by squats, stair stepping, or step-ups, suggesting that these exercises may result in greater strength gains.

Hintermeister et al. (1998) studied muscle activation levels, knee joint angles, and applied force during five rehabilitation exercise with an elastic resistance device in 12 healthy subjects. The five exercises were the double-knee dip, leg press, hamstring pull, single-knee dip, and side-to-side jump. The double-knee dip was characterized by notable quadriceps activity, with peak electromyographic amplitude of 74.0% maximal voluntary contraction (MVC) for the vastus medialis (Table 5.02). Peak activity occurred as the subject ended the flexion phase and began the extension phase (figure 5.07). The leg press resulted in substantial rectus femoris activity with average amplitude of 25.5% MVC (figures 5.04 and 5.05). The hamstring pull was characterized by pronounced activity in the medial hamstrings and biceps femoris with peak amplitudes of 54.2% and 35.3% MVC, respectively (figure 5.22). The single-knee dip was similar to the double-knee dip but resulted in more pronounced quadriceps activity. The vastus medialis, vastus lateralis, and rectus femoris muscles had peak amplitudes of 102.6%, 82.6%, and 73.2% MVC, respectively (figure 5.6). The side-to-side jump required the greatest muscle activity with 113.4% and 93.8% MVC of vastus medialis and vastus lateralis, respectively (figure 5.31). The authors offered suggestions about when to implement these exercises in a rehabilitation program,

Table 5.02   Notable Percentages of Maximal Voluntary Contractions (MVC) During Five Lower Extremity Exercises

Exercise	Notable %MVC of various muscles during exercise				
	VM	VL	RF	MH	BF
Double-knee dip	74.0%	56.4%	48.7%	—	—
Leg press	—	—	25.5%	—	—
Hamstring pull	—	—	—	54.2%	35.3%
Single-knee dip	102.6%	82.6%	73.2%	—	—
Side-to-side jump	113.4%	93.8%	87.9%	—	—

VM = vastus medialis; VL = vastus lateralis; RF = rectus femoris; MH = medial hamstrings; BF = biceps femoris.
Data from R.A. Hintermeister, M.J. Bey, G.W. Lange, J.R. Steadman, and C.J. Dillman, 1998, "Quantification of Elastic Resistance Knee Rehabilitation Exercises," *Journal of Orthopaedic and Sports Physical Therapy* 28(1): 40-50.

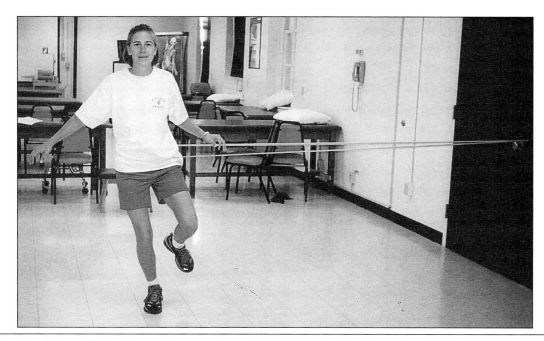

Figure 5.31   Side-to-side jump.

suggesting that a continuum of elastic resistance exercises be performed for a variety of knee impairments, including non-operative injury, debridement/menisectomy, and ACL reconstruction. Time frames are dependent on the severity of the initial injury and the patients pre-existing fitness level. Three exercises, the double-knee dip, hamstring pull, and leg press should be instituted as soon as possible. The single-knee dip can be introduced at 4 to 6 weeks, while the side-to-side jump can be introduced at 6 to 8 weeks. For ACL reconstruction, however, the authors recommend waiting 12 weeks before introducing the side-to-side jump (Hintermeister et al. 1998).

The Ankle and Foot

The ankle and foot complex consists of 28 bones and 25 joints, which provide both stability and mobility. Numerous ligaments and musculature support the ankle and foot. The normal active ROM for the talocrural joint is considered to be 0 to 20° of dorsiflexion and 0 to 30° or 0 to 50° of plantar flexion from neutral (Norkin and Levangie 1990). The major dorsiflexors are the tibialis anterior, extensor hallucis longus, and extensor digitorum longus. The gastrocnemius, soleus, posterior tibialis, and plantaris primarily perform plantar flexion (Kendall, Kendall, and Wadsworth 1972).

The talocalcaneal, or subtalar, joint consists of three articulations between the talus and the calcaneus and is supported by ligaments. The motions that occur about an oblique axis at the subtalar joint include inversion (combined motions of foot adduction, foot supination, and foot plantar flexion) and eversion (combined motions of foot abduction, foot pronation, and foot dorsiflexion; Soderberg 1996).

Normal active ROM at the subtalar joint is difficult to assess but generally is accepted as 10° of pronation and 20° of supination (Norkin and Levangie 1990). The muscles responsible for inversion at the subtalar joint include tibialis anterior and posterior. The peroneus brevis and peroneus longus function as the major evertors of the ankle (Kendall, Kendall, and Wadsworth 1972; Soderberg 1996).

The talonavicular and the calcaneocuboid joints comprise the compound joint known as the midtarsal joint. This joint allows for motions of pronation/supination and eversion/inversion. The tarsometatarsal joints are plane synovial joints reinforced by numerous ligaments. Motions of the tarsometatarsal joints function to allow supination/pronation twists of the forefoot. The metatarsophalangeal joints primarily function to allow the hind foot to pass over the toes during weight bearing, allowing movements of flexion/extension and abduction/adduction. The interphalangeal joints are synovial hinge joints, allowing flexion and extension (Norkin and Levangie 1990). Numerous foot intrinsic muscles perform movement at the metatarsophalangeal and interphalangeal joints (Kendall, Kendall, and Wadsworth 1972).

The bony architecture of the foot forms longitudinal and transverse arches, which are designed to facilitate absorption and distribution of body weight during weight bearing. Several ligaments support the arches, with active muscle contraction also contributing to the dynamic stability of the arches.

Elastic Resistance Exercises for the Ankle and Foot

Patients with a variety of ankle and foot impairments are commonly referred for rehabilitation. Nonoperative diagnoses include ankle sprains, tendinitis (Achilles or posterior tibialis), stress fractures, and plantar fasciitis. Strengthening exercises are often necessary in postoperative cases, as with a repaired Achilles tendon, repair of a navicular nonunion fracture, compartment release, or calcaneal osteotomy. The clinician must use sound clinical decision making to prescribe an exercise program that will enhance the strength of the patient's lower extremity without exacerbating symptoms. Pain and fatigue in the ankle and foot may produce an antalgic gait, which can irritate surrounding structures. For this reason, the clinician must exercise good judgment when designing an exercise program for the ankle and foot.

The primary dorsiflexor of the ankle is the tibialis anterior, whereas the extensor hallucis longus, extensor digitorum longus, and peroneus tertius assist in the movement. Weakness is often present after periods of immobilization and with decreased weight bearing. Open-chain strengthening of the dorsiflexors can be achieved with the use of elastic resistance in supine, long-sitting, side-lying, or seated positions (figures 5.32 and 5.33). Knee extension combined with dorsiflexion puts the gastrocnemius on maximal stretch. If there is tightness in the gastrocnemius, knee flexion will increase the amount of dorsiflexion available. The joint also will experience a mild load when the exercise is performed in a seated position. The exercise is progressed by increasing the resistance, frequency, and duration of the exercise.

Strengthening of the plantar flexors (gastrocnemius, soleus, posterior tibialis, and plantaris) is often required for patients after immobilization, Achilles tendon repair, or bouts of Achilles tendinitis or retrocalcaneal bursitis. The plantar flexors also play a vital role in explosive movements, such as jumping. Strengthening with elastic resistance can be achieved in the open chain in long-sitting, supine, or side-lying positions (figure 5.34). To decrease the mechanical advantage of the gastrocnemius and increase the use of the soleus, the exercise is performed with the knee flexed (figure 5.35). Eccentric contractions play an important role in shock absorption, as when an athlete lands from a jump. Consequently, plantar flexion exercises with a focus on the eccentric phase play an important role in the comprehensive rehabilitation program.

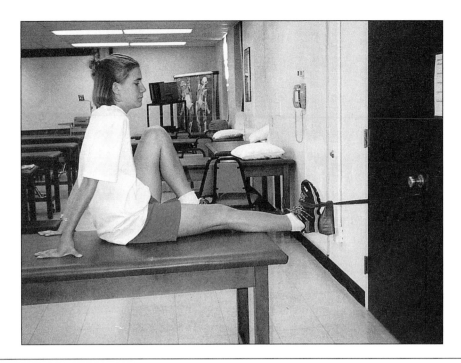

Figure 5.32 Long-sitting ankle dorsiflexion.

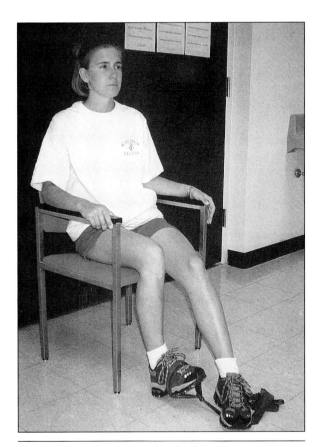

Figure 5.33 Seated ankle dorsiflexion.

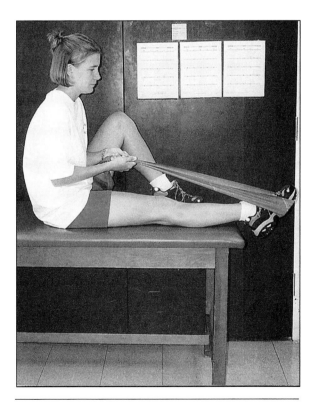

Figure 5.34 Long-sitting ankle plantar flexion.

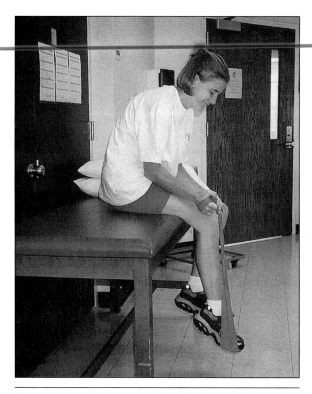

Figure 5.35 Seated ankle plantar flexion (emphasis on soleus muscle).

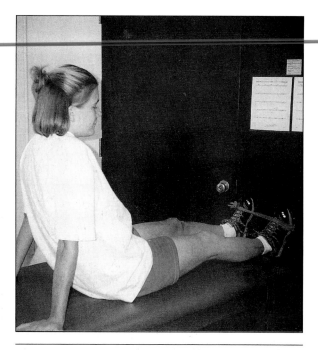

Figure 5.36 Long-sitting ankle eversion.

Inversion ankle sprains are the most common types of ankle sprain, accounting for more than 85% of all ankle sprains (Docherty, Moore, and Arnold 1998). The frequency of inversion ankle sprains is most likely attributable to the poor ligamentous stability and bony structure of the lateral aspect of the ankle joint. Strengthening of the evertor muscles (peroneus longus and brevis) is often necessary after an inversion ankle sprain. Elastic resistance strengthening exercises for the peroneal musculature can be performed in long-sitting, supine, or sitting positions. The patient can secure the elastic resistance to the opposite foot, if necessary (figure 5.36).

Although the medial aspect of the ankle joint provides stability via bony congruence and the deltoid ligament, strengthening of the invertor muscles (anterior and posterior tibialis) may be necessary. As with all joints, muscle balance of the agonists and antagonists offers stability and increased shock absorption. Consequently, inversion ankle strengthening should be included in the comprehensive ankle rehabilitation program. As with eversion strengthening, inversion exercises may be completed in long-sitting, supine, or seated positions (figure 5.37).

Strength training programs that use elastic resistance also enhance joint position sense in the functionally unstable ankle. In a study by Docherty, Moore, and Arnold (1998), 20 subjects with functionally unstable ankles were divided into a control and exercise group. The exercise group performed sets of 10 repetitions of dorsiflexion, plantar flexion, inversion, and eversion with elastic bands 3 times a week for 6 weeks, as outlined by a resistance tubing training protocol established by the authors (table 5.04). The tubing was stretched to what was calculated to be 70% of its maximal stretch before the exercise began. Pre- and posttest assessments included dorsiflexion and eversion strength and plantar flexion/dorsiflexion and inversion/eversion joint position sense (JPS). Results showed an increase in strength, as well as JPS for inversion, plantar flexion, and dorsiflexion. The authors suggested that strength training may play a role in increasing JPS as well as increasing strength. They attributed the increase in JPS to increased muscle spindle activity.

In a similar study, Hawke et al. (1998) determined the acute proprioceptive benefits of open-chain elastic resistance ankle exercises. Twenty-six high school athletes with functional instability in one or both ankles performed 30 repetitions of dorsiflexion, plantar flexion, inversion, and eversion using elastic resistance stretched to 50% of its maximum length. Balance testing via the Biodex Stability System was performed before treatment, immediately after treatment, and 30 min after treatment (while

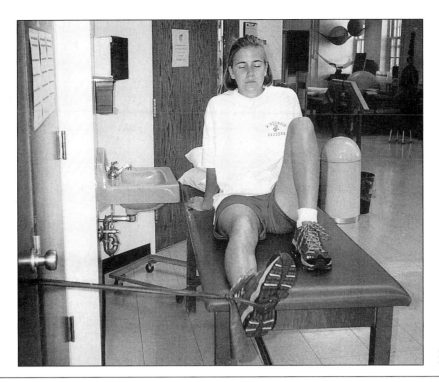

Figure 5.37   Long-sitting ankle inversion.

Table 5.03   Thera-Band Resistive Tubing Training Protocol

Week	Tubing	Sets	Repetitions
1	Blue—extra heavy	3	10
2	Blue—extra heavy	4	10
3	Black—special heavy	3	10
4	Black—special heavy	4	10
5	Silver—super heavy	3	10
6	Silver—super heavy	4	10

Reprinted, with permission, from C.L. Docherty, J.H. Moore, and B.L. Arnold,1998,"Effects of Strength Training on Strength Development and Joint Position Sense in Functionally Unstable Ankles," *Journal of Athletic Training* 33(4): 312.

participants maintained a non-weight-bearing status). Results showed no difference between the pre- and posttest data. The authors concluded that open-chain resistance exercises with an elastic band had no effect on postural stability as measured by the Biodex Stability System. However, the subjects performed only one bout of exercise, and the study did not indicate whether the subjects were allowed visual input. As such, data from this study should be interpreted cautiously.

Many movements at the ankle joint are combined movements of the planar movements (dorsiflexion/ plantar flexion, inversion/eversion) previously described. Therefore, the clinician may consider adding PNF patterns to the rehabilitation program once strength in planar motions is adequate. The movement of dorsiflexion, inversion, and supination from the position of plantar flexion, eversion, and pronation is similar to PNF diagonal 1 (figures 5.38 and 5.39). PNF diagonal 2 consists of the movement of dorsiflexion, eversion, and pronation, from plantar flexion, inversion, and supination (figures 5.40 and 5.41). Resistance can be applied to the diagonal plane of movement.

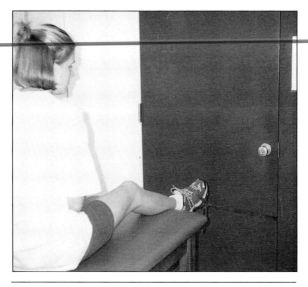

Figure 5.38 Ankle PNF D1 diagonal flexion (start position).

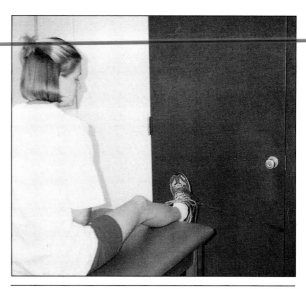

Figure 5.39 Ankle PNF D1 diagonal flexion (end position of dorsiflexion, inversion, and supination).

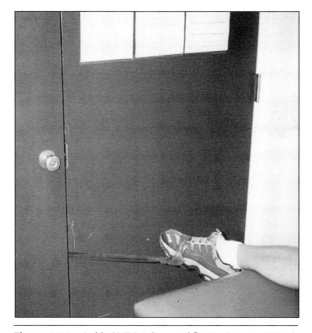

Figure 5.40 Ankle PNF D2 diagonal flexion (start position).

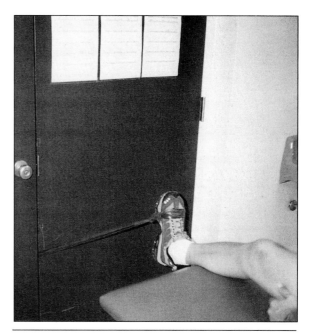

Figure 5.41 Ankle PNF D1 diagonal flexion (end position of dorsiflexion, eversion, and pronation).

Closed-chain exercises for the ankle and foot are also important, because they can enhance strength, balance, and proprioception. Cordova, Jutte, and Hopkins (1999) compared the electromyographic activity of the tibialis anterior, medial gastrocnemius, and peroneus longus muscles in four closed-chain activities. The activities consisted of single-leg stance, single-leg stance on a trampoline, Thera-Band kicks (kicking against elastic resistance with the unaffected leg while standing on the affected leg), and single-leg stance with perturbations. The authors found that the elastic-resisted kicks that involved hip flexion, as well as kicks at a 45° angle laterally and medially to hip flexion, induced greater electromyographic activity in all three muscles. The authors concluded that the elastic resistance exercises in a closed chain produced the greatest challenge, as evidenced by the heightened muscle activity, and they recommended this activity in the late stages of rehabilitation.

Tomaszewski (1991) suggested that athletes perform small, quick, elastic-resisted kicks with rapid oscillations in both the sagittal and frontal planes while standing on the involved foot (figures 5.27-5.30). The author believed that the proprioceptors around the ankle joint would be constantly stimulated with this type of activity. Although this activity may not directly affect strength, it might enhance proprioceptive input. Lower extremity balance and proprioception are discussed in detail in the next section.

Balance and Proprioception

Balance is necessary for all static and dynamic ADLs, such as standing, walking, running, and stair climbing. Balance is defined as the ability to maintain the center of gravity over the base of support and is achieved through the interaction of several systems, including the visual, vestibular, and somatosensory systems (Crutchfield, Shumway-Cook, and Horak 1989). Several physical impairments (such as decreased motion, strength, and mobility) can negatively affect balance. Other factors, including vestibular dysfunction, visual impairment, or diminished proprioception, can also negatively affect balance (Lewis and Bottomley 1994).

The risk for falls increases dramatically with age because of an interaction of underlying physical dysfunctions, medications, and environmental hazards (Blake et al. 1988; Christiansen and Huhl 1987; Hornbrook et al. 1994; Tinetti et al. 1994). Falls are the leading cause of death for people over the age of 65, and approximately 25% to 35% of people over the age of 65 experience one or more falls each year (Hornbrook et al. 1994; Nevitt et al. 1989; Sattin 1992; Tinetti and Ginter 1988).

Almost 70% of emergency room visits by people 75 years or over are related to falls (Sattin 1992).

Several researchers have found that strengthening programs prevent falls by improving overall strength, coordination, balance responses, and reaction time (Brown and Holloszy 1991; Lewis and Bottomley 1994; Roberts 1989; Shumway-Cook et al. 1997). Krebs, Jette, and Assmann (1998) found that a home exercise program that included elastic resistance improved gait stability in people age 60 or older, and the authors concluded that this improvement could, in turn, confer a degree of protection from falls among disabled community-dwelling seniors. The older adults in a study completed by Taaffe et al. (1999) improved in both strength and neuromuscular performance after participating in a weekly resistance exercise program. The improvements in neuromuscular function suggest a decreased risk for falls in the elderly as well as enhancement of daily functional activities.

Elastic Resistance Exercises to Improve Balance and Proprioception

Injury or trauma to a joint and surrounding structures may cause a loss of proprioceptive feedback from mechanoreceptors, which subsequently may interfere with balance. Thus, it is imperative to address balance as part of a comprehensive rehabilitation program. Balance exercises should be specific to each patient and should emphasize the control necessary for functional tasks. Balance training activities have many benefits, including improved trunk stability, biomechanical alignment, and weight distribution as well as increased awareness of center of mass and limits of stability. Other benefits include heightened awareness of musculoskeletal responses to perturbation, improved balance strategies and synergies, and use of all systems responsible for balance (O'Sullivan and Schmitz 1999). Balance training teaches safety awareness and compensation when necessary. Patients should receive education, in addition to functional training, about the ways that medication, postural hypotension, and environmental risks affect balance.

Balance training should focus on the different systems responsible for balance. Removing input from one system will force the patient to rely on other systems to maintain balance. Visual input can be removed by having the patient close his or her eyes, thus forcing the patient to rely on somatosensory and vestibular input to maintain equilibrium. Altering the surface on which the exercise is performed, such as changing from tile floor to foam, will alter proprioceptive input (figure 5.26). Vestibular inputs can be varied by having the patient move his or her head in several directions during the exercise or by transitioning from a moving surface to a stationary one. A clinical progression might combine several strategies, such as having the patient perform the exercise on an unstable surface, then closing the eyes (figure 5.42).

Many balance exercises can be enhanced or progressed with elastic resistance. Single-leg stance, a common balance challenge, can be progressed by placing elastic resistance around the LE at various angles. This exercise can be progressed further in a variety of ways, including increasing the amount of resistance by using bands of different tension. Narrowing the patient's base of support or progressing to single-limb support also will make the balance exercise more challenging (figure 5.43). The activity can be progressed further by changing the surface. Progressing the environment from a closed (stable) to an open (variable) one is often an appropriate clinical progression. Internal perturbations, such as adding arm movements during the exercise (figure 5.42), as well as external perturbations, such as nudges by a therapist, can increase the difficulty of balance activities (figure 5.44). Balls of varying size and weight can be thrown to the patient during exercises to add to the complexity of the exercise (figure 5.45). Because balance activities

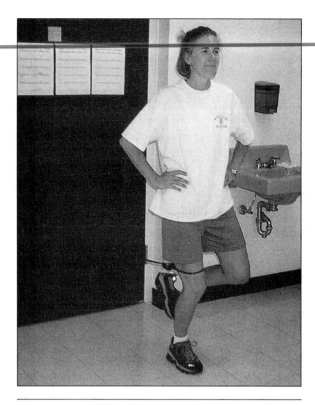

Figure 5.43 Unilateral balance with elastic resistance around involved extremity.

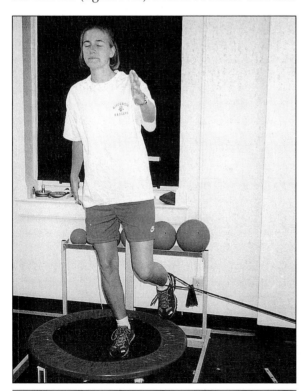

Figure 5.42 Unilateral balance on minitrampoline with elastic resistance around uninvolved extremity (eyes closed).

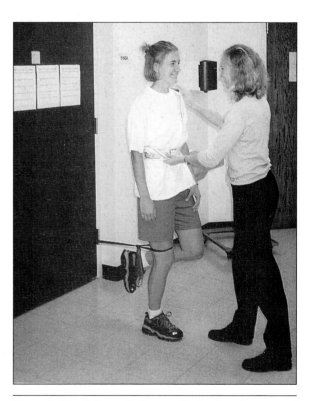

Figure 5.44 Unilateral balance with elastic resistance and perturbations.

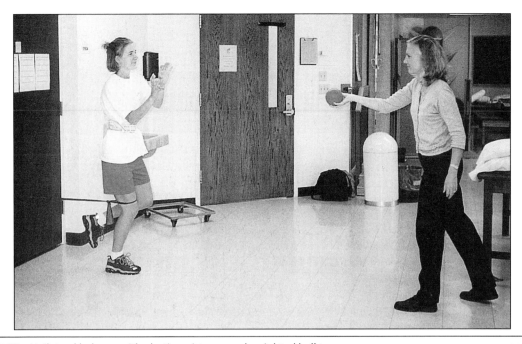

Figure 5.45   Unilateral balance with elastic resistance and weighted ball toss.

can be very challenging for patients and can cause a temporary loss of balance, the clinician must determine the appropriateness of the activities for each patient and must always take proper safety precautions when patients perform these exercises.

Mini-lunges or full lunges with elastic resistance were mentioned previously as closed-chain exercises that benefit both the hip and knee. These exercises also are appropriate for challenging balance and increasing joint awareness for the LE (figure 5.08). These exercises challenge the knee extensors, hip extensors, and ankle dorsiflexors. Exercises that were described for knee rehabilitation that are also appropriate balance challenges are the front-pull (figure 5.27), back-pull (figure 5.28), crossover (figure 5.29), and reverse crossover (figure 5.30). The stabilizing musculature that will maintain balance during these four exercises will vary depending on where the center of mass is at a given point during the exercise. For example, during the front pull, the uninvolved LE and center of mass begin posterior to the body, and, therefore, contraction of the anterior musculature on the involved LE will maintain upright posture. As the uninvolved hip is flexed beyond neutral, the center of mass moves anterior to the body, and posterior musculature on the involved LE will contract to maintain posture.

Dynamic balance can be improved by performing multiplanar double-leg hops, progressing to single-leg hops, with elastic resistance. Elastic resistance can be applied around the trunk while the patient performs hops in a pattern (figure 5.46). The patient also

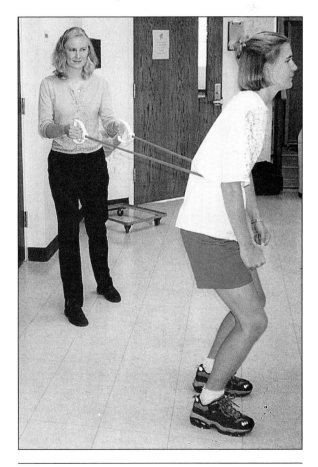

Figure 5.46   Double leg hops. Weight shifting can be performed in different directions with resistance applied in various angles

can perform double- and single-leg hops on and off a platform to further challenge balance (figure 5.47).

Dynamic gait balance can be improved by adding resistance to the trunk or LE during gait activities. Resistance can be applied to specific body segments during portions of gait in which an abnormality is noted. Resistance also can be applied in a lateral direction during gait to challenge lateral stability (figure 5.48).

Other common clinical balance tools include the balance board, trampoline, therapeutic exercise ball, and slide board. Elastic resistance can be added to such equipment to further challenge the patient. A patient can perform multidirectional weight shifting on a balance board with resistance applied to the body at various angles (figure 5.49). Resistance also can be applied to the body during exercises on the trampoline including single-leg stance, multidirectional single-leg hops, and mini-squats. Sitting weight shifts on a therapeutic exercise ball with lower extremity weight bearing or loading is another balance activity to which resistance can be applied. As previously mentioned, these exercises can be made more challenging by having the patients close their eyes, decreasing their base of support, and adding internal or external perturbations. Other chapters provide information on neuromuscular retraining and sport-specific proprioception drills.

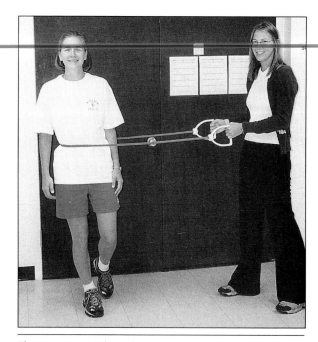

Figure 5.48 Unilateral stance with weight shift in frontal plane. Weight shifting can be performed in different directions with resistance applied in various angles.

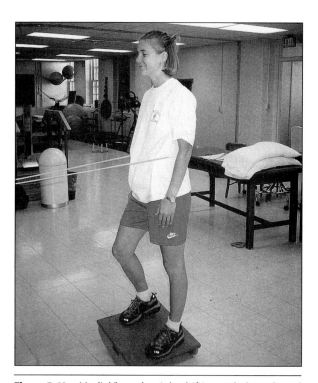

Figure 5.49 Medial/lateral weight shifting on balance board with weight shift in sagittal plane. Weight shifting can be performed in different directions with resistance applied in various angles.

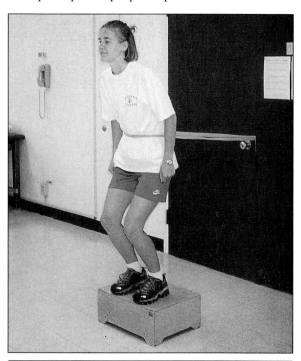

Figure 5.47 Box jumps with elastic resistance in sagittal plane.

Conclusion

Exercises to increase strength, balance, and proprioception are key components of a comprehensive lower extremity rehabilitation program, and elastic resistance is a useful tool to achieve rehabilitation goals. All strength deficits may be addressed with elastic resistance, and progression is achieved easily by increasing the length of the lever arm or the thickness of the elastic band. Balance and proprioception exercises are important in lower extremity rehabilitation, not only to return the athlete to high-level sport but also to reduce the risk of falls in the elderly patient. This chapter discussed lower extremity rehabilitation of the hip, knee, ankle, and foot. Sample exercises, including their relation to common pathologies, were explained, and progression of exercise was reviewed. Elastic resistance is an essential rehabilitation tool for lower extremity weakness and balance impairments. Because of its low cost and portability, the use of elastic resistance in lower extremity rehabilitation may increase compliance, thereby decreasing the number of visits with the health care provider. Ultimately, elastic resistance may become a major comprehensive cost-saving tool in today's health care environment.

CASE STUDY 1

Herbert is a 72-year-old widowed male with a history of bilateral degenerative joint disease of the hips. He underwent a total arthroplasty of the left hip via a lateral incision 14 days ago with cement fixation. His hospital course of 5 days was uneventful, and he was discharged to his daughter's home for assistance with ADLs of dressing and grooming. He was discharged with a standard walker for ambulation and was instructed to use weight bearing as tolerated. The patient's goals are to return to living at home independently, to drive independently, and to ambulate without an assistive device. His home environment consists of a one-story home, with three steps to enter the home, railing on the L during ascension. He would also like to return to walking for exercise (20-min walk 3 times per week) and recreational dancing once per week at the senior citizens center.

His medical history is significant for angioplasty (3 years ago), history of smoking, and hypertension. His current medications include atenolol, Advil as needed, and a multivitamin.

Physical exam reveals a mildly obese male who can ambulate independently with a standard walker independently. He requires minimal assistance with sitting down from a standing position, rising from a sitting position, sitting up from a supine position, and lying down from a sitting position. He follows all precautions for total hip arthroplasty. His active and passive ROMs are symmetrical to his right side (within precautions for total hip arthroplasty).

Strength tests are as follows:

Gluteus medius = 3+/5	Iliopsoas = 4/5
Gluteus maximus = 3+/5	Adductors = 4+/5
Quadriceps = 4–/5	Hamstrings = 4/5

A lateral surgical incision appears to be healing, with no signs of infection; staples were removed 2 days ago. The patient requests to do as many activities at his daughter's home as possible, because he cannot drive and his daughter lives approximately 45 min from therapy.

His treatment is a home program consisting of lateral weight shifting near a table or counter for support. He is prescribed elastic resistance exercises consisting of hip flexion (in supine, to 90° of flexion), hip extension (with a pillow between the knees to maintain abduction; figure 5.03), hip abduction (with pillow between the legs to avoid adduction; figure 5.09), leg press (similar to figures 5.04 and 5.05, in supine, no greater than 90° of hip flexion), and knee flexion and extension (as in figures 5.22 and 5.18, in a semireclined position in a chair). The patient may starts with 2 sets of 10 repetitions twice a day and progresses to 3 sets of 10 repetitions twice a day.

The patient eventually can progress to standing hip flexion (figure 5.01), extension (figure 5.28), and abduction (figure 5.30; the patient with a total hip arthroplasty will not be allowed to cross midline, however) and resisted movements in all planes while standing on the left leg to increase balance and gluteus medius strength (figures 5.27-5.30).

CASE STUDY 2

Maggie is a 28-year-old female who recently sustained an isolated ACL tear of her right knee while playing soccer. She underwent ACL reconstruction with a patellar tendon graft 10 days ago. She has returned to work part time as a computer software engineer. She is ambulating with a hinged brace, unlocked, and is using one crutch for community ambulation. She will travel to a satellite office for work for the next 2 weeks, will stay in a hotel, and will have no access to exercise equipment. She will have access to ice at the hotel.

Physical exam reveals moderate effusion, a well-healing scar (sutures removed today), active ROM consisting of 0 to 0 to 100°, and passive ROM consisting of 3 to 0 to 105° with a capsular end feel. Strength testing was deferred. There is a visible quadriceps contraction with a quadriceps set and a mild decrease in patellar mobility, especially superior glide.

Her treatment is a home program using elastic resistance consisting of closed-chain terminal knee extension (figure 5.20), double-leg squats (figure 5.07), seated hamstrings curls (figure 5.22), and knee extension (90-45° only; figure 5.18). For balance, Maggie can perform front-pulls, back-pulls, crossover, and reverse crossover, all while standing on the surgical leg (figures 5.27-5.30). Other activities, such as active/passive ROM, quadriceps sets, patellar mobilizations, and straight-leg raises, also can be performed to complete the program.

CASE STUDY 3

Mike is a 44-year-old carpenter and recreational soccer player. He has a history of right lateral ankle instability from numerous inversion sprains sustained while playing club soccer in college. He most recently suffered an inversion ankle sprain 3 weeks ago when he was carrying a load of lumber down a flight of stairs and missed the last step. He was seen at a local urgent care clinic, where X-rays were negative. He was placed in a walking boot and instructed in partial weight bearing with axillary crutches. He is now ambulating without crutches but still uses the boot for ambulation, ADLs, and work. He has returned to work (light duty), with a goal of returning to work full time without restrictions and returning to play recreational soccer 3 times per week.

Physical examination reveals antalgic gait without the walking boot (decreased dorsiflexion and decreased stance time on the right foot), moderate effusion and ecchymosis on the lateral aspect of the ankle, a 10° loss of both active ROM for dorsiflexion and plantar flexion with the knee flexed, a 5° loss of inversion and eversion (when compared with the uninvolved side), and strength assessment as follows: inversion = 4+/5, eversion = 4/5, dorsiflexion = 4/5, and plantar flexion = 4/5. Special tests reveal a Grade II anterior drawer and (+) talar tilt test. Mike is point tender over the anterior talofibular ligament and the calcaneofibular ligament.

Mike currently is working at a job site approximately 75 min away from the closest physical therapy clinic and would like an exercise program that he is able to perform independently.

His treatment is a home program consisting of elastic resistance strengthening for eversion (figure 5.36), inversion (figure 5.37), plantar flexion (figures 5.34 and 5.35), and dorsiflexion (figures 5.32 and 5.33) in the open chain. To increase balance and proprioception, Mike will perform elastic resistance front-pulls, back-pulls, crossovers, and reverse crossovers while standing on the involved leg (figures 5.27-5.30). To progress his balance exercise, Mike can close his eyes, stand on an uneven surface (a pillow from his hotel room), or both. Once cardinal plane strength is adequate, Mike can add PNF diagonals with elastic resistance (figures 5.38-5.41), lunges on an uneven surface (similar to figure 5.26), and various hopping drills with elastic resistance (figures, 5.31, 5.46, and 5.47).

References

Beynnon, B.D., R.J. Johnson, B.C. Fleming, C.J. Stankewich, P.A. Renstrom, and C.E. Nichols. 1997. "The Strain Behavior of the Anterior Cruciate Ligament During Squatting and Active Knee Flexion-Extension. A Comparison of an Open and a Closed Kinetic Chain Exercise." *American Journal of Sports Medicine* 25: 823-9.

Blair, D.F., and R.P. Wills. 1991. "Rapid Rehabilitation Following Anterior Cruciate Reconstruction." *Athletic Training, JNATA* 26: 32-40.

Blake, A.J., K. Morgan, M.J. Bendall, H. Dallosso, S.B. Ebrahim, T.H. Arie, P.H. Fentem, and E.J. Bassey. 1988. "Falls by Elderly People at Home: Prevalence and Associated Factors." *Age and Aging* 17: 365-72.

Brody, L.T., and J.M. Thein. 1998. "Nonoperative Treatment for Patellofemoral Pain." *Journal of Orthopaedic and Sports Physical Therapy* 28(5): 336-44.

Brody, L.T., and L. Tremain. 1999. "The Knee." In *Therapeutic Exercise: Moving Towards Function*, ed. C.M. Hall and L.T. Brody. Philadelphia: Lippincott, Williams & Wilkins.

Brown, M., and J.O. Holloszy. 1991. "Effects of a Low-Intensity Exercise Program on Selected Physical Performance Characteristics of 60- to 70-Year-Olds." *Aging* 3: 129-39.

Bynum, E.B., R.L. Barrack, and A.H. Alexander. 1995. "Open Versus Closed Chain Kinetic Exercises After Anterior Cruciate Ligament Reconstruction." *American Journal of Sports Medicine* 23: 401-6.

Cerny, K. 1995. "Vastus Medialis Oblique/Vastus Lateralis Activity Ratios for Selected Exercises in Persons With and Without Patellofemoral Pain Syndrome." *Physical Therapy* 75(8): 672-83.

Christiansen, J., and E. Huhl, eds. 1987. "The Prevention of Falls in Later Life." *Danish Medical Bulletin* 34 (Suppl.) 4: 1-24.

Cook G., L. Burton, and K. Fields. 1999. "Reactive Neuromuscular Training for the Anterior Cruciate Deficient Ligament-Knee: A Case Report." *Journal of Athletic Training* 34: 194-201.

Cordova, M.L., L.S. Jutte, and J.T. Hopkins. 1999. "EMG Comparison of Selected Ankle Rehabilitation Exercises." *Journal of Sport Rehabilitation* 8: 209-18.

Crutchfield, C.A., A. Shumway-Cook, and F.B. Horak. 1989. "Balance and Coordination Training." In *Physical Therapy*, ed. R. Scully and M. Barnes. Philadelphia: Lippincott.

Docherty, C.L., J.H. Moore, and B.L. Arnold. 1998. "Effects of Strength Training on Strength Development and Joint Position Sense in Functionally Unstable Ankles." *Journal of Athletic Training* 33(4): 310-4.

Dunleavy, K., and N. McNeven. 1997. "Muscle Firing Patterns in a Ballroom Dancer With Patellofemoral Dysfunction Related to Taping, Bracing and Heel Height: A Case Report" (Abstract). *Physical Therapy* 77(5): S39.

Grabiner, M.D., T.J. Koh, and L.F. Draganich. 1994. "Neuromechanics of the Patellofemoral Joint." *Medicine and Science in Sports and Exercise* 26(1): 10-21.

Graham, V.L., G.M. Gehlsen, and J.A. Edwards. 1993. "Electromyographic Evaluation of Closed and Open Kinetic Chain Knee Rehabilitation Exercises." *Journal of Athletic Training* 28(1): 23-30.

Grelsamer, R.P., and J.R. Klein. 1998. "The Biomechanics of the Patellofemoral Joint." *Journal of Orthopaedic and Sports Physical Therapy* 28(5): 286-98.

Hanson, C. 1999. "Proprioceptive Neuromuscular Facilitation." In *Therapeutic Exercise: Moving Towards Function*, ed. C.M. Hall and L.T. Brody. Philadelphia: Lippincott, Williams & Wilkins.

Hawke, R.L., B.L. Van Lunen, B.L. Arnold, and B.M. Gansneder. 1998. "Acute Proprioceptive Measurements Following Resistive Ankle Exercises." *Journal of Athletic Training* 33 (Suppl.): S26.

Hintermeister, R.A., M.J. Bey, G.W. Lange, J.R. Steadman, and C.J. Dillman. 1998. "Quantification of Elastic Resistance Knee Rehabilitation Exercises." *Journal of Orthopaedic and Sports Physical Therapy* 28(1): 40-50.

Holmes, S.W., and W.G. Clancy. 1998. "Clinical Classification of Patellofemoral Pain and Dysfunction." *Journal of Orthopaedic and Sports Physical Therapy* 28(5): 299-306.

Hopkins, J.T., C.D. Ingersoll, M.A. Sandrey, and S.D. Bleggi. 1999. "An Electromyographic Comparison of 4 Closed Chain Exercises." *Journal of Athletic Training* 34(4): 353-7.

Hornbrook, M.C., V.J. Stevens, D.J. Wingfield, J.F. Hollis, M.R. Greenlick, and M.G. Ory. 1994. "Preventing Falls Among Community-Dwelling Older Persons: Results From a Randomized Trial." *Gerontologist* 34: 16-23.

Hughes, C.J., K. Hurd, A. Jones, and S. Sprigle. 1999. "Resistance Properties of Thera-Band Tubing During Shoulder Abduction Exercise." *Journal of Orthopaedic and Sports Physical Therapy* 29(7): 413-20.

Irrgang, J.J., M.R. Safran, and F.H. Fu. 1996. "The Knee: Ligamentous and Meniscal Injuries." In *Athletic Injuries and Rehabilitation*, ed. J.E. Zachazewski, D.J. Magee, and W.S. Quillen. Philadelphia: Saunders.

Johnston, C.A.M, D.M. Lindsay, and J.P. Wiley. 1999. "Treatment of Iliopsoas Syndrome With a Hip Rotation Strengthening Program: A Retrospective Case Series." *Journal of Orthopaedic and Sports Physical Therapy* 29(4): 218-24.

Karst, G.M, and G.M. Willett. 1995. "Onset Timing of Electromyographic Activity in the Vastus Medialis Oblique and Vastus Lateralis Muscles in Subjects With and Without Patellofemoral Pain." *Physical Therapy* 75: 813-23.

Kendall, H.O., F.P. Kendall, and G.E. Wadsworth, eds. 1972. *Muscles: Testing and Function*. Baltimore: Williams & Wilkins.

King, A.C., T.A. Ahles, J.E. Martin, and R. White. 1984. "EMG Biofeedback-Controlled Exercise in Chronic Arthritic Knee Pain." *Archives of Physical Medicine and Rehabilitation* 65: 341-3.

Krebs D.E., A.M. Jette, and S.F. Assmann. 1998. "Moderate Exercise Improved Gait Stability in Disabled Elders." *Archives of Physical Medicine and Rehabilitation* 79: 1489-95.

LeVeau, B.F., and C. Rogers. 1980. "Selective Training of the Vastus Medialis Muscle Using EMG Biofeedback." *Physical Therapy* 60(11): 1410-5.

Leiby, K.W., P.L. Neece, S.H. Phipps, and C.J. Hughes. 1995. "A Comparison of Two Methods of Resistance Training on Ipsilateral/Contralateral Hip Abduction Strength" (Abstract). *Journal of Orthopaedic and Sports Physical Therapy* 21(1): 52.

Lephart, S.M., D.H. Perrin, F.H. Fu, and K. Minger. 1991. "Functional Performance Tests for the Anterior Cruciate Ligament Insufficient Athlete." *Athletic Training, JNATA* 26: 44-50.

Lewis, C.B., and J.M. Bottomley, eds. 1994. *Geriatric Physical Therapy: A Clinical Approach.* Norwalk, CT: Appleton and Lange.

Magee, D.J. 1992. *Orthopedic Physical Assessment.* Philadelphia: Saunders.

McConnell, J. 1986. "The Management of Chondromalacia Patellae: A Long Term Solution." *Australian Journal of Physiotherapy* 32(4): 215-23.

McConnell, J. 2000. "Patellofemoral Joint Complications and Considerations." In *Knee Ligament Rehabilitation*, ed. T.S. Ellenbecker. Philadelphia: Churchill Livingstone.

McConnell, J., and J. Fulkerson. 1996. "The Knee: Patellofemoral and Soft Tissue Injuries." In *Athletic Injuries and Rehabilitation*, ed. J.E. Zachazewski, D.J. Magee, and W.S. Quillen. Philadelphia: Saunders.

Nevitt, M., S.R. Cummings, S. Kidd, and D. Black. 1989. "Risk Factors for Recurrent Non-Syncopal Falls: A Prospective Study." *Journal of the American Medical Association* 261: 2663-8.

Norkin, C.C., and P.K. Levangie, eds. 1990. *Joint Structure and Function: A Comprehensive Analysis.* Philadelphia: Davis.

Noyes, F.R., S.D. Barber, and R.E. Mangine. 1991. "Abnormal Lower Limb Symmetry Determined by Function Hop Tests After Anterior Cruciate Ligament Rupture." *American Journal of Sports Medicine* 19(5): 513-8.

O'Sullivan, S.B., and T.J. Schmitz. 1999. *Physical Rehabilitation Laboratory Manual: Focus on Functional Training.* Philadelphia: Davis.

Powers, C.M., R. Landel, and J. Perry. 1996. "Timing and Intensity of Vastus Muscle Activity During Functional Activities in Subjects With and Without Patellofemoral Pain." *Physical Therapy* 76(9): 946-68.

Roberts, B.L. 1989. "Effects of Walking on Balance Among Elders." *Nursing Research* 38(3): 180-3.

Sanders, B., and W.C. Nemeth. 1996. "Hip and Thigh Injuries." In *Athletic Injuries and Rehabilitation*, ed. J.E. Zachazewski, D.J. Magee, and W.S. Quillen. Philadelphia: Saunders.

Sapega, A.A. 1990. "Muscle Performance Evaluation in Orthopaedic Practice." *Journal of Bone and Joint Surgery* 72(10): 1562-74.

Sattin, R.W. 1992. "Falls Among Older Persons: A Public Health Perspective." *Annual Review of Public Health* 13: 489-508.

Schulthies, S.S., M.D. Ricard, K.J. Alexander, and J.W. Myer. 1998. "An Electromyographic Investigation of 4 Elastic-Tubing Closed Kinetic Chain Exercises After Anterior Cruciate Ligament Reconstruction." *Journal of Athletic Training* 33(4): 328-35.

Shumway-Cook, A., W. Gruber, M. Baldwin, and S. Liao. 1997. "The Effect of Multidimensional Exercises on Balance, Mobility, and Fall Risk in Community-Dwelling Older Adults." *Physical Therapy* 77: 46-57.

Soderberg, G.L., ed. 1996. *Kinesiology: Application to Pathological Motion.* Baltimore: Williams & Wilkins.

Spencer, J.D., K.C. Hayes, and I.J. Alexander. 1984. "Knee Joint Effusion and Quadriceps Reflex Inhibition in Man." *Archives of Physical Medicine and Rehabilitation* 65(4): 171-7.

St. Clair Gibson, A., M.I. Lambert, J.J. Durandt, N. Scales, and T.D. Noakes. 2000. "Quadriceps and Hamstrings Peak Torque Ratio Changes in Persons With Chronic Anterior Cruciate Ligament Deficiency." *Journal of Orthopaedic and Sports Physical Therapy* 30(7): 418-27.

Steinkamp, L.A., M.F. Dillingham, M.D. Markel, J.A. Hill, and K.R. Kaufman. 1993. "Biomechanical Considerations in Patellofemoral Joint Rehabilitation." *American Journal of Sports Medicine* 21(3): 438-44.

Taaffe, D.R, C. Duret, S. Wheeler, and R. Marcus. 1999. "Once-Weekly Resistance Exercise Improves Muscle Strength and Neuromuscular Performance in Older Adults." *Journal of the American Geriatric Society* 47: 1208-14.

Thein, L.A. 1996. "The Child and Adolescent Athlete." In *Athletic Injuries and Rehabilitation*, ed. J.E. Zachazewski, D.J. Magee, and W.S. Quillen. Philadelphia: Saunders.

Tinetti, M.E., D.I. Baker, M. Gottschalk, P. Garrett, S. McGeary, D. Pollack, and P. Charpentier. 1997. "Systematic Home-Based Physical and Functional Therapy for Older Persons After Hip Fracture." *Archives of Physical Medicine and Rehabilitation* 78: 1237-47.

Tinetti, M.E., D.I. Baker, M. Gottschalk, C.S. Williams, D. Pollack, P. Garrett, T.M. Gill, R.A. Marottoli, and D. Acampora. 1999. "Home-Based Multicomponent Rehabilitation Program for Older Persons After Hip Fracture: A Randomized Trial." *Archives of Physical Medicine and Rehabilitation* 80: 916-22.

Tinetti, M.E., D.I. Baker, G. McAvay, E.B. Claus, P. Garrett, M. Gottschalk, M.L. Koch, K. Trainor, and R.I. Horwitz. 1994. "A Multifactorial Intervention to Reduce the Risk of Falling Among Elderly People Living in the Community." *New England Journal of Medicine* 331: 821-7.

Tinetti, M.E., and S.F. Ginter. 1988. "Identifying Mobility Dysfunctions in Elderly Patients: Standard Neuromuscular Examination or Direct Assessment?" *Journal of the American Medical Association* 259: 1190-3.

Tomaszewski, D. 1991. "'T-Band' Kicks Ankle Proprioception Program." *Athletic Training, JNATA* 26: 216-9.

Vos, D.E., M.K. Ionta, and B.J. Myers. 1985. "Proprioceptive Neuromuscular Facilitation: Patterns and Techniques." Philadelphia: Harper and Row.

Wilk, K.E., G.J. Davies, R.E. Mangine, and T.R. Malone. 1998. "Patellofemoral Disorders: A Classification System and Clinical Guidelines for Nonoperative Rehabilitation." *Journal of Orthopaedic and Sports Physical Therapy* 28(5): 307-22.

Willett, G.M, J.B. Paladino, K.M. Barr, J.N. Korta, and G.M. Karst. 1998. "Medial and Lateral Quadriceps Muscle Activity During Weight-Bearing Knee Extension Exercise." *Journal of Sport Rehabilitation* 7: 248-57.

Wojtys, E.M., and L.J. Huston. 1994. "Neuromuscular Performance in Normal and Anterior Cruciate Ligament Deficient Lower Extremities." *American Journal of Sports Medicine* 22(1): 89-104.

CHAPTER 6

Spinal Exercises
With Elastic Resistance

• • • • •

Andre Labbe, PT, MOMT
Advantage Physical Therapy, New Orleans, Louisiana

Rehabilitation of the spine has evolved into a very complicated and diverse specialty within health care. Twenty-five percent to 50% of all patient visits to physical therapy are spine related (Jackson 2000). The treatment of spine-related problems is one of the most common and expensive health care issues in our society. According to the National Safety Council, the total cost of occupational injuries and illnesses amounts to $117 billion, with the majority of these related to low back pain. These issues have forced clinicians to provide more objective and outcome-oriented treatment as well as to focus on cost-effective and scientifically based interventions.

One common thread within the treatment of pathologies is that exercise is a large part of rehabilitation. Exercise is the most powerful intervention that the clinician can use to expedite rehabilitation. Exercise has the following benefits in spinal rehabilitation:

- Increases tissue tolerance to stress
- Promotes healing and nutrition in synovial joints
- Helps restore proper arthro- and osteokinematics (Grimsby 1994)

Exercise also has been shown to decrease the psychosocial stress associated with low back pain (Viru and Smirnova 1995). Unfortunately, many therapists do not know how to prescribe specific exercises for the spine and tend to use very general and nonspecific methods of treatment. In the past, clinicians have relied on very passive methods of treating the spine that focused on pain relief and symptom reduction. This practice has poor outcomes and a high recurrence rate among patients returning for the same pathology (Cherkin et al. 1998). Clinicians must be more active and specific in treating the spine. For example, they must be as aggressive and exercise-oriented with treatment of multifidus in the spine as with treatment of vastus medialis of the knee or supraspinatus of the shoulder. Most clinicians can demonstrate the proper exercise to activate the extremity muscles but not the muscles of the spine.

Elastic resistance provides creativity and specificity with a very inexpensive and adaptable tool that the patient can use in a home program. The home exercise program is arguably the most important aspect of rehabilitation. The time a patient may spend with a clinician is useless if the patient does nothing at home to help the process.

The key is to apply the basic sciences in day-to-day treatment of patients. A clinician must be able to consider anatomy, osteokinematics, arthrokinematics, and tissue tolerance in his or her evaluation and treatment of the spine. In this chapter, functionally and clinically relevant anatomy and physiology are discussed and applied to the treatment of some common pathologies with the use of specific exercises for the cervical, thoracic, and lumbar spine.

General Anatomy of the Spine

The spine can be divided into three basic regions of anatomy and function. The seven cervical, 12 thoracic, and five lumbar spine segments make up the most mobile regions of the spine. General anatomical characteristics of the entire spine are reviewed first, followed by functional anatomy and specific exercises for each region.

Bony Anatomy

The spinal segment is divided into an anterior and a posterior region. The anterior region is dominated by the kidney-shaped body. The posterior section is made of the pedicle, laminae, transverse, and spinous processes. These bony prominences act as attachments for muscles and ligaments throughout the spine and help disperse load over the intervertebral disk.

The Disc

The typical spinal disc is made of two parts: the nucleus pulposus and annulus fibrosus. As a unit, they make up the intervertebral disc. The functions of the intervertebral disc are threefold. First, it transfers weight from one vertebra to the next without collapsing. It then must be able to accommodate the rocking movement of the vertebra above without moving the one below. Third, it also must be strong enough not to be injured during normal motions of rotation, flexion, and side bending (Bogduk and Twomey 1991). The structure of the nucleus pulposus is dominated by Type 2 collagen, which makes up 15 to 20% of its dry weight. The nucleus itself is made of 70 to 90% water (Bogduk and Twomey 1991). This allows it to withstand compressive forces and disperse the force over the area of the vertebral end plate of the disc below. Compression and decompression of the Type 2 collagen fi-

bers will increase the tolerance of the nucleus pulposus to stress and increase synthesis of nutrients through the vertebral end plates.

The annulus fibrosus is made up of 10 to 12 sheets of tightly packed collagen called lamellae, which surround the nucleus pulposus. Like the nucleus, the annulus is made up of 50 to 60% water, with collagen fibers making up 50 to 60% of its dry weight. In contrast to the nucleus, Type 1 collagen dominates the annulus fibrosus. These fibers are aligned at 45 to 60° angles to the horizontal plane as they run from vertebra to vertebra. The direction of inclination changes from lamella to lamella.

To stimulate Type 1 collagen for regeneration, we must use tensile forces along the length of the strand. This increases its ability to resist shear and rotary forces that dominate the function of the intervertebral disc. Because of the alignment of the fibers, left rotation in midrange will create tensile forces in half of the fibers, whereas right rotation will create tensile forces in the other half.

General Ligamentous Structures

Several ligaments support the vertebrae. The anterior longitudinal ligament and posterior longitudinal ligaments lie anterior and posterior, respectively, to the vertebral body. The anterior ligament attaches to the vertebral bodies and the posterior ligament attaches to the vertebral discs. They limit flexion and extension, and the posterior ligament supplies added support to the intervertebral disc (Kapandji and D'Aubigné 1974; Porterfield and Derosa 1998). The ligamentum flavum attaches from the laminae above to the laminae below. This ligament has a high elastic component that allows it to become taut with spinal flexion without buckling during spinal extension. It also becomes one of the posterior borders of the spinal canal. The ligamentum flavum also supports and contributes to the anterior wall of the apophyseal (facet) joint capsule. The ligamentum flavum's thickness and ability to resist shearing forces add to its importance as a spinal stabilizer (Bogduk and Twomey 1991).

The Apophyseal Joint

Each vertebral segment, excluding the upper cervical spine, has four articulations that are used specifically for interaction with the adjacent vertebral body. The superior articular facets of one vertebra articulate with the inferior articular facets of the vertebra above. These articulations form the apophyseal joints. They function as a true synovial joint and provide motion between vertebrae. They are also an important load-bearing structure within the spine. The surfaces of the joints are covered with articular cartilage and withstand compressive forces. The joint capsule has a balloon-type cavity above and below, which houses articular fat that assists in absorbing some of the compressive forces. The capsule is supported superiorly by the deep fibers of the multifidus muscle and inferiorly by the ligamentum flavum (Bogduk and Twomey 1991). In the lumbar spine, the capsule also has a small hole that allows the articular fat to move into the extra-articular space (Bogduk and Twomey 1991).

The apophyseal joint capsule ligaments surround the apophyseal joints to stabilize and retain the integrity of the synovial membrane of the joint. The joint is innervated by the medial branch of the posterior primary rami and may be a source of mechanical pain within the spine. Mechanical stimulation of the posterior primary rami also can be used to inhibit pain within the spine (Grimsby 1994).

The articular cartilage of the apophyseal joint is important for function and is usually an area of degeneration that can lead to pathology. Poor articular health is usually attributable to some form of movement around nonphysiological planes. This causes poor load transfer throughout the cartilage and leads to articular degeneration. The optimal stimulation for regeneration of articular cartilage is compression/decompression and gliding. Gliding decreases viscosity of the synovial fluid and allows the synthesis of nutrition through the chondrosynovial membrane, whereas compression/decompression helps with protein synthesis and general articular health (Mow, Proctor, and Kelly 1989). Thus, movement is essential for normal articular cartilage health.

Paravertebral Muscles

The muscles of the spine fall into two functional groups: those that are slow twitch (tonics) and those that are fast twitch (phasics). Slow twitch fibers are oxygen dependent and usually are associated with postural stability, whereas the fast twitch fibers are glucose dependent, usually are used for gross movement (Janda and Jull 1987). Tonic fibers are fatigue resistant, whereas phasic fibers fatigue easily.

In many cases, the phasic muscles are recruited to perform postural duties. Because they are typically glucose dependent and fatigue easily, they spasm and create active trigger points within the muscle belly, thus becoming an origin of pathological pain. An example is the levator scapula which can offset anterior translation of the spinal segments resulting from gravity's effect in a typical forward-head posture. This causes excessive fatigue within the muscle and can lead to increased tone and pain. This is a general phenomenon throughout the spine but is most common within the cervical spine.

In general, the paravertebral muscles of the spine act as rotators and extensors and are antagonistic to the anterior musculature that flexes and counterrotates the spine. The balance between the opposing sets of muscles is the basis of the muscle imbalance theories of Janda (1987, 1988). For example, the multifidus extends the spine and counterrotates each segment within the spine. Its main antagonist is the abdominal musculature in the lower thoracic and lumbar segments. Proper balance in strength between these two muscle groups is essential for normal joint function and stability.

Functional Anatomy of the Cervical Spine

The cervical spine is the most mobile section of the spine. This mobility provides the ability to align sensory organs, such as the eyes and ears, quickly and efficiently.

Bony Characteristics

Although all spinal segments have similar bony anatomy, each region has characteristics specific to its function. The main differentiating factors of the cervical spinal segment are related to the orientation of the facet joints and the structure of the vertebral body. The body has a beaklike projection anterior and inferior that adds to stability and helps direct motions of flexion/extension and rotation (Kapandji and D'Aubigné 1974). The vertebral body also has two lateral projections on the superior surface that articulate with two indentions on the inferolateral aspect of the vertebra above. These two structures form the uncovertebral joints and help increase stability and direct motion.

The facet joints are oriented in the transverse plane, which promotes rotation between each segment. Just lateral to the facet joints and lodged in the transverse process is the transverse foramen, which houses the vertebral artery. This artery should be addressed when treatment is considered for the cervical spine.

Muscles of the Cervical Spine

The deep extensor muscles of the cervical spine are collectively known as the suboccipitals. They are arranged to move the occiput, atlas, and axis independently of the rest of the cervical spine (Porterfield and Derosa 1995). The deep extensor muscles are the rectus capitus posterior major, rectus capitus posterior minor, inferior oblique, superior oblique, and transversospinalis.

The suboccipital muscles symmetrically and bilaterally extend the cervical spine and accentuate the cervical curve (Kapandji and D'Aubigné 1974). Ipsilateral contraction of suboccipitals will cause ipsilateral side-bending and rotation of the cervical spine contralaterally.

The muscles in the cervical spine are a combination of both phasic and tonic muscle fibers, thus performing aerobic postural support and anaerobic prime movement of the upper cervical segments. Therefore, they must be trained for postural support as well as movement initiation.

The superficial muscles of the cervical spine consist of the trapezius, levator scapulae, and sternocleidomastoid. The trapezius acts on the cervical spine as well as the scapula. Symmetrical contraction of the left and right trapezius causes cervical extension or bilateral scapular elevation and upward rotation. A unilateral trapezius contraction extends the cervical spine with ipsilateral side-bending and contralateral rotation.

The levator scapulae muscle mimics the deep erector spinae muscles of the lumbar spine, in its ability to prevent anterior shear of the cervical vertebrae. The levator scapulae also functions as a lateral flexor of the cervical spine as well as a scapular elevator and downward rotator. As stated previously, a forward-head posture that creates anterior shear of the vertebrae causes the levator scapulae to fire continuously to offset this anterior position. This may be the reason palpation of this muscle is usually painful in patients with cervical pain.

The sternocleidomastoid actively causes upper cervical extension as well as lower cervical flexion with bilateral contraction. It also causes contralateral rotation and ipsilateral side bending. Its main passive function is to resist forceful extension of the cervical spine, typically seen with whiplash-type injuries (Porterfield and Derosa 1995). The scalene musculature acts as a lateral flexor of the cervical spine as well as a general cervical flexor. It also checks posterior shear of the cervical vertebrae. Along with the levator scapulae, the scalenes help to provide anteroposterior stability to the cervical spine. Weakness or tightness within the scalenes also can affect the neurovascular bundle of the thoracic outlet, which exits between the anterior and middle scalene (Kapandji and D'Aubigné 1974; Porterfield and Derosa 1995). The deep anterior muscles of the cervical spine function as flexors with some rotary components. The deep flexors also directly affect the function of the temporomandibular joint (TMJ).

Functionally, the cervical spine maintains the head in a position optimal for sight. Thus, the cervical spine can accommodate for any postural abnormality that would affect this relationship. Most of the motion of the cervical spine is a component of rotation. The orientation of the facet joints in the transverse plane promotes rotation. Flexion and extension occur but are not governed by the structure of the anatomy as much as are rotation and side-bending.

Elastic Resistance Exercises for the Cervical Spine

Elastic resistance exercises usually progress from isometric strengthening (figures 6.01-6.06) to more dynamic strengthening (figures 6.07-6.09). Finally, whole-body motions can add a "dynamic isometric" component to cervical spine exercises (figures 6.10-6.12). Conventional exercise machines for strengthening the cervical spine may not be specific to the upper or lower cervical region, therefore possibly overdosing and overstressing the muscles of the cervical region. With elastic resistance, patients can perform low-dose exercises in functional and comfortable positions that can be specific for each patient.

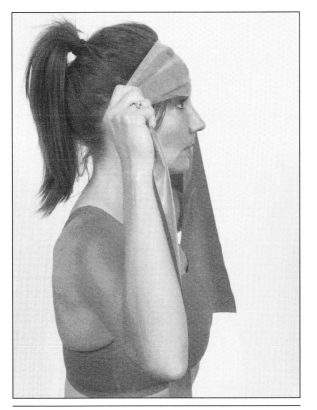

Figure 6.01 Isometric cervical flexion (start position).

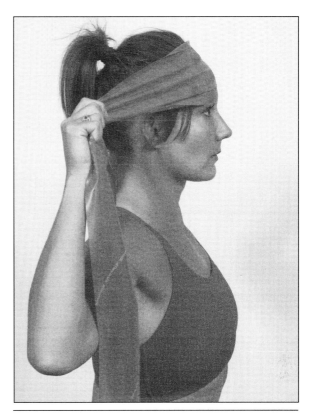

Figure 6.02 Isometric cervical flexion (end position).

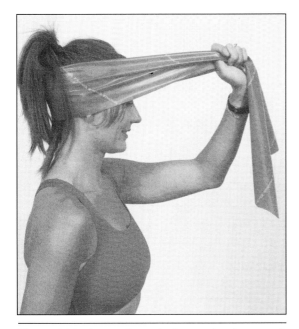

Figure 6.03 Isometric cervical extension (start position).

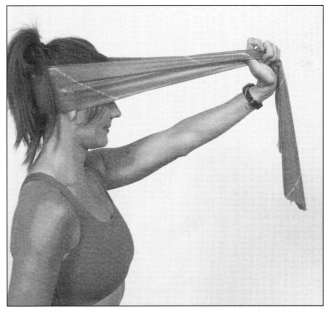

Figure 6.04 Isometric cervical extension (end position).

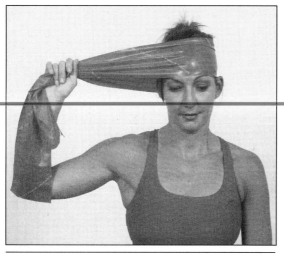

Figure 6.05 Isometric cervical lateral flexion (start position).

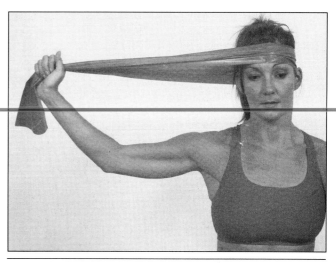

Figure 6.06 Isometric cervical lateral flexion (end position).

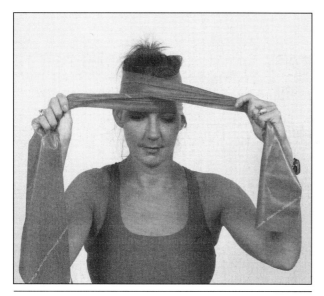

Figure 6.07 Cervical rotation in neutral.

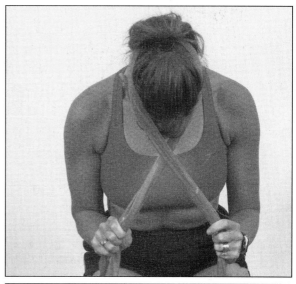

Figure 6.08 Cervical rotation in flexion.

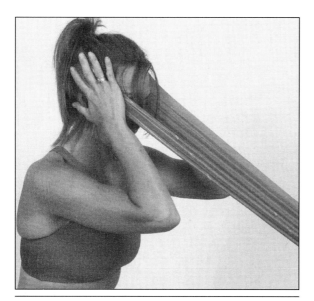

Figure 6.09 Cervical extension.

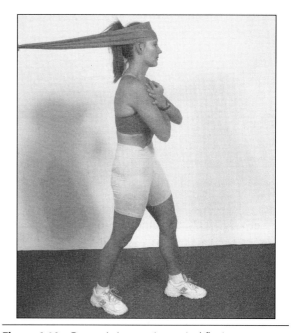

Figure 6.10 Dynamic isometric cervical flexion.

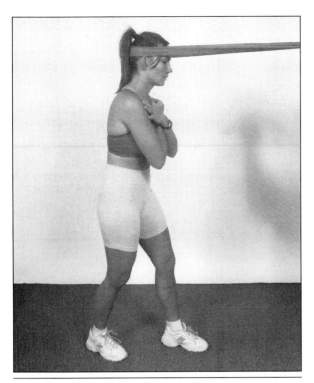

Figure 6.11   Dynamic isometric cervical exension.

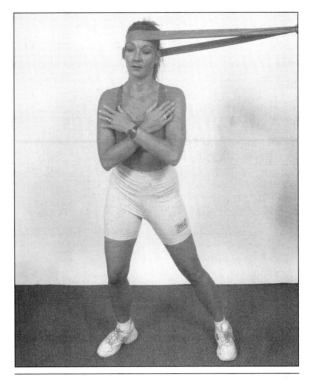

Figure 6.12   Dynamic isometric cervical side-bending. (Repeat on opposition slide.)

Functional Anatomy of the Thoracic Spine

The thoracic vertebrae are the least mobile segments of the spine. They are inherently more stable because of their costovertebral attachments to the ribs.

Bony Characteristics

The thoracic spine is a transitional zone of movement. Its upper segments have facet orientation similar to the lower cervical spine, whereas its lower segments allow for easy transition to the orientation of the lumbar spine (Soderberg 1997). The middle segments stabilize and anchor muscles for their actions on the very mobile cervical and lumbar vertebrae. In mobility studies on the spine, the middle thoracic spine has been shown to be the least mobile segment of the spine (Soderberg 1997). Segmental mobility progresses as one moves superior and inferior from the middle thoracic spine. The facet joints are oriented in the frontal plane and promote motions of side-bending and rotation, with flexion and extension as secondary motions. Rotation is a gliding function of the joints in the thoracic spine if one believes that the axis for rotation is in the

body of the vertebrae. This rotation would not cause approximation of the facet joints but in fact would promote gliding of the facets on each other (Kapandji and D'Aubigné 1974).

Muscles of the Thoracic Spine

The thoracic spine functions as a stabilizing entity. The deep muscles of the cervical and lumbar spine (longissimus, semispinalis, multifidus, and splenius) use their attachments in the thoracic spine as an anchor for actions on the head/neck and lumbar vertebrae, respectively. The rhomboids and trapezius muscles use the thoracic spine as an origin for action to the scapulae and shoulder as well. This rule holds true for the muscles of respiration such as the intercostal externi, interni, and intimi. They all use the stability of the thoracic vertebrae to increase their mechanical advantage on the ribs they are moving.

Another unique characteristic of the thoracic spine is its vital role in respiration. With exhalation and inhalation, the ribs elevate and rotate through their vertebral and sternal articulations. This movement of the ribs is initiated with the contraction of the diaphragm as well as the intercostal musculature. One must address rib mobility and sternocostal function when evaluating and treating the thoracic spine.

Elastic Resistance Exercises for the Thoracic Spine

Activation of the thoracic extensor muscles (figures 6.13-6.15) will improve stability and promote good facet joint gliding while promoting a posture that discourages the typical forward-head and rounded shoulder positions. Thoracic rotation with elastic resistance will train a normal functional position and movement that can be translated into general functional activities (figures 6.16 and 6.17).

The exercises in figures 6.18 through 6.21 all promote strengthening of the thoracic musculature in a position that will promote stability as well as mobility. These are easily used in a home program setting as well as in the clinic with minimal equipment.

Functional Anatomy of the Lumbar Spine

The lumbar region is the largest load-bearing area within the spine. The segments of the lumbar spine are larger and denser than those of the cervical and thoracic region. It is an area of the spine that must have a true balance of stability and mobility for proper function. This delicate balance between mobility and stability lends itself to dysfunction.

Bony Characteristics

The lumbar spine is made of five vertebrae that form a lordotic curve between the thoracic spine and the

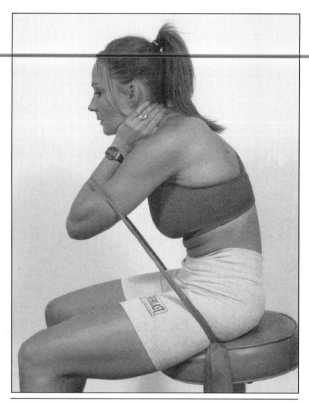

Figure 6.14   Seated thoracic extension (start position).

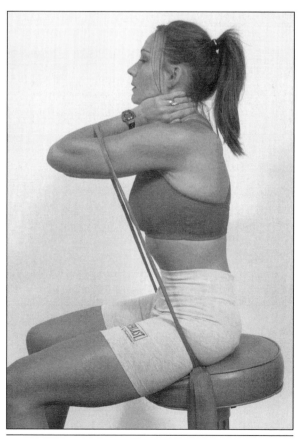

Figure 6.15   Seated thoracic extension (end position).

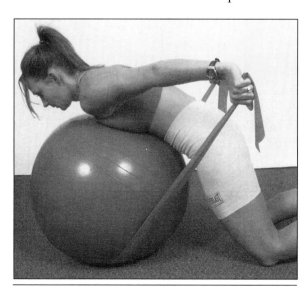

Figure 6.13   Prone thoracic extension.

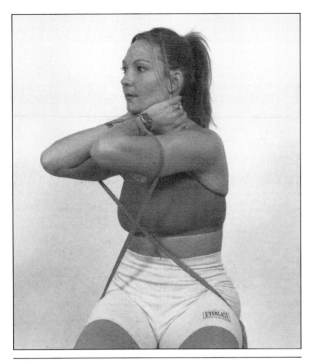

Figure 6.16 Seated thoracic rotation (start position).

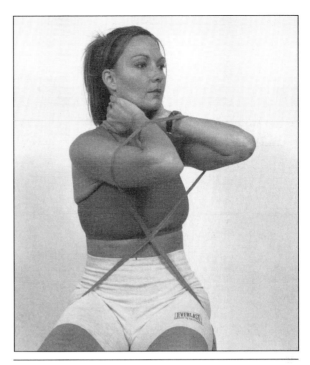

Figure 6.17 Seated thoracic rotation (end position).

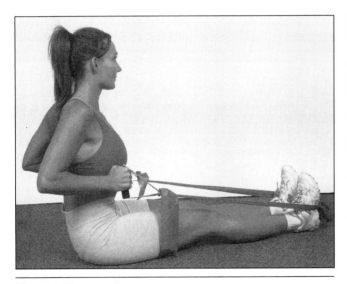

Figure 6.18 Seated row.

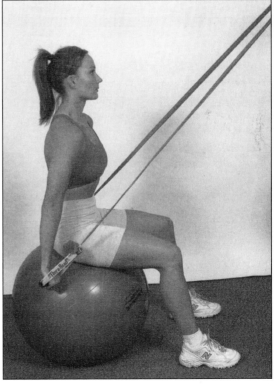

Figure 6.19 Seated bilateral shoulder extension.

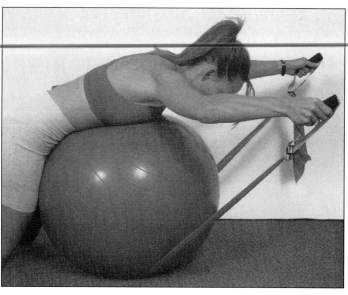

Figure 6.21 Prone flexion.

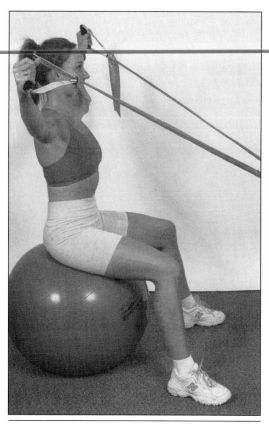

Figure 6.20 Seated reverse flies.

sacrum. The body of the typical lumbar vertebra is large and relatively square. It is a typical example of function governing structure. Because of the excessive loads to the lumbar spine, it must have a larger vertebral body and facet joint than the other aspects of the cervical or thoracic region. The facet joints in the lumbar spine are oriented in the sagittal plane. This promotes flexion and extension, and causes approximation of the facet joints with rotation.

Muscles of the Lumbar Spine

The abdominal muscles, along with the multifidus, provide an important method of dynamically stabilizing the lumbar spine (Janda and Jull 1987). The abdominal obliques insert into the lumbar fascia and have indirect effects on the lumbar spine and associated musculature. According to Janda and Jull (1987), the quadratus lumborum is a tonic muscle, but clinically it can demonstrate the same muscle irritation as a phasic would when used in a postural role.

The multifidus has both an antagonistic and a synergistic relationship to the abdominal muscles. As antagonists, the abdominals flex the spine and

the multifidus extends it, and synergistically they work together to control rotation. An imbalance between these muscles can cause functional pathology.

The lumbar spine is also greatly affected by the relationship of the lower extremities and their associated musculature. The gluteals, hamstrings, adductors, and abductors all have some primary or secondary affect on the spine. An imbalance of muscle function in the lower extremities can lead to hyper- or hypotonicity within the spinal musculature, which in turn can lead to either hypo- or hypermobilities within the kinetic chain. This can lead to subtle and chronic degenerative changes within the lumbar segments.

Elastic Resistance Exercises for the Lumbar Spine

There are more theories and methods of evaluation and treatment of lumbar pathology than for any other region of the spine. Exercise is the most universally accepted method of treatment of almost all lumbar pathologies.

Exercise should affect the joints as well as the muscles of the lumbar spine. One must also take into account the role of the abdominal muscles and lumbar fascia in lending stability to the spine. The exercises used in treating the spine also should stimulate the proprioceptive system to maintain proper muscle balance. Elastic resistance applies resistance to the lumbar musculature in many different planes of movement. Most exercise routines for the lumbar spine focus on single planar motions; however, the lumbar spine functions in three planes and must be trained to function in three planes. With the ability to change the attachment point and level of resistance, a clinician can train uniplanar and triplanar motions. Elastic resistance also provides concentric and eccentric resistance to movement. This is important, because many of the lumbar stabilizers work eccentrically to control movement. If they are not properly trained after injury, they can be reinjured.

Abdominal strength and endurance are vital for lumbar spine function. The abdominals are an important area for preventing lumbar pathologies and controlling lumbar dynamic stability. Patients should train the abdominals in different positions to target specific areas of the abdominal wall (figures 6.22 and 6.23). Patients then can progress to more functional strengthening positions to allow for control of the spine in all planes of movement (figures 6.24-6.26).

The paravertebrals are also important to train because of their function in maintaining dynamic stability and providing lumbar extension. Most patients demonstrate poor coordination of the paravertebrals during normal activities and tend to use larger, nonspecific muscles for function. Increasing the endurance and functional stability of the lumbar extensor musculature in multiple and dynamic planes is essential for functional progression (figures 6.27-6.30).

Another aspect of lumbar stabilization is the interaction of the core muscles during side-bending. The exercises in figures 6.31 and 6.32 apply resistance with side-bending to activate the quadratus lumborum and lateral abdominals.

A high percentage of patients have limited activity in their gluteals as well as poor firing sequence of the hamstrings (Janda and Jull 1987). Exercises must be performed that increase the activity of the gluteals and hamstrings during gait. Janda and Jull (1987) described muscle imbalances that can cause chronic low back pain. They associated tightness of one set of muscles with weakness of the antagonistic set of muscles. This imbalance will cause improper joint function and associated pain. An example of this theory is the relationship between tight hip flexors and weakness in the gluteus maximus. This is a common finding in patients with chronic lumbar pain. Restoring gluteal strength and decreasing hip flexor tightness substantially decrease pain and increase function. Bridging exercises are excellent for restoring hip extension strength and range of motion (figures 6.33 and 6.34).

The ability of joints to give proper feedback to the brain on their position and function in space is an essential component of lumbar spine function. The spine must be able to give mechanoreceptor feedback to coordinate functions of the lower extremities, pelvis, and spinal musculature. Proprioceptive

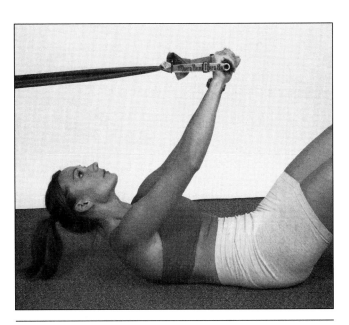

Figure 6.22   Abdominal crunch.

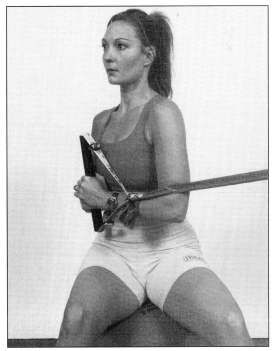

Figure 6.23   Seated rotation.

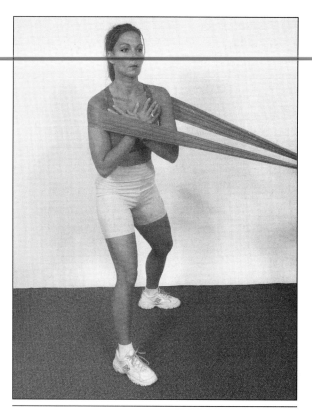

Figure 6.24 Standing rotation.

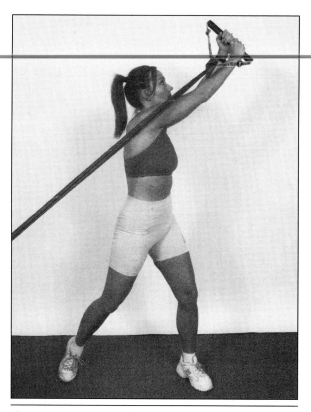

Figure 6.25 Diagonal lift.

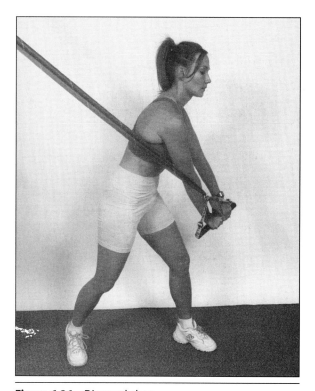

Figure 6.26 Diagonal chop.

training stimulates the joint mechanoreceptors and associated ligamentous structures and activates the paravertebrals in controlled and small-movement exercises. Figure 6.35 demonstrates the use of elastic resistance and the proprioceptive properties of the exercise ball to teach good postural awareness and stability while performing resisted pelvic tilts.

A general rule for exercising all regions of the spine should be to begin with uniplanar and uncomplicated exercises that may be muscle-specific and then to progress to functional exercises that are task-specific.

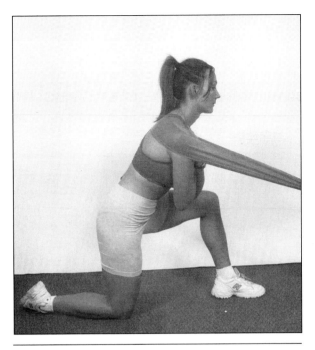

Figure 6.27 Kneeling extension (start position).

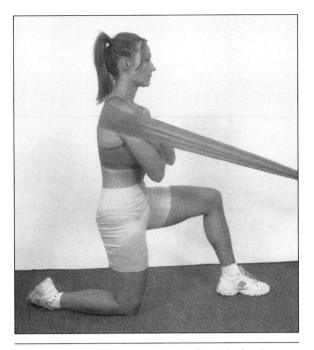

Figure 6.28 Kneeling extension (end position).

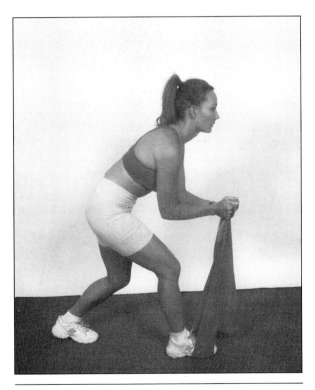

Figure 6.29 Standing extension (start position).

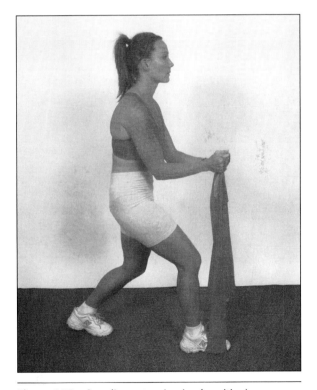

Figure 6.30 Standing extension (end position).

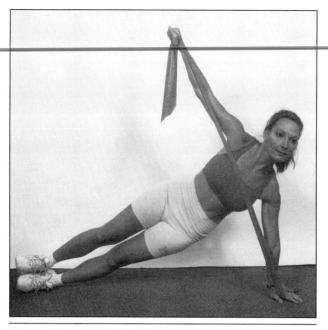

Figure 6.31 Sidelying bridge.

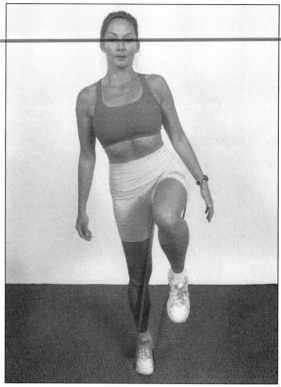

Figure 6.32 Standing quadratus hip hike.

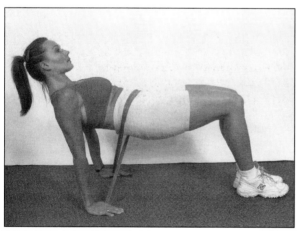

Figure 6.33 Bridge on hands.

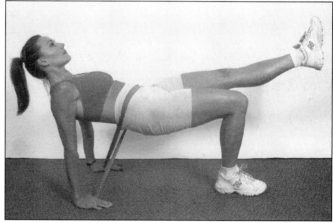

Figure 6.34 Bridge with leg extension.

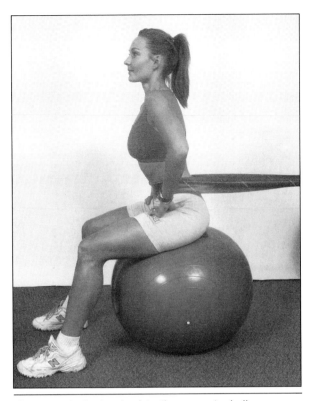

Figure 6.35 Resisted pelvic tilt on exercise ball.

Spine Pathology and Rehabilitation

Although the three regions of the spine are different functionally, the structures respond similarly within each region to both trauma and rehabilitation. Common pathologies in each region of the spine include postural impairment, degenerative joint disease, degenerative disk disease, and myofascial pain.

Postural Impairment

Poor posture itself is a pathology of the cervical, thoracic, and lumbar spine. It causes excessive wear on joints throughout the spine and activates phasic muscles to perform tonic duties. Pain is a common result of poor posture and is difficult to treat unless the posture is improved first.

The most common postural deficit in the cervical spine is the forward-head position (Porterfield and Derosa 1995). In this position, the lower cervical spine is flexed while the upper cervical spine is extended to maintain the forward-eye position. This shortens the suboccipitals, scalenes, and sternocleidomastoid and increases activity of the levator scapulae and lower cervical extensors. The levator scapulae and deep spinal extensors also have to offset the pull of gravity on the head when it is moved forward out of the balanced position. In this position, passive insufficiency and fatigue occur in the levator scapulae and upper fibers of the trapezius. There is also active insufficiency and fatigue of the suboccipitals as they work to maintain the head upright while in a relative shortened position. Elastic resistance can be used to dynamically retrain proper postural position and stability within that new position (figures 6.10-6.12)

At the spinal articulations, there is excessive loading of the cervical facet joints with little chance of unloading. This leads to degeneration of the articular cartilage as well as shortening of the posterior joint capsule. The forward-head position causes hypomobility of the occipitoatlantal joint and the C2 to C5 joints, with hypermobility of the posterior capsule of the lower cervical spine (C3-C7). This leads to abnormal motion about nonphysiological axes, thus causing abnormal load distribution and joint degeneration. Approximation of the posterior cervical bony structures may also occur, leading to bony spurring and pain.

Thoracic spine abnormalities are seen as either an increase or a decrease in thoracic kyphosis. Hyperkyphotic positions commonly are seen in the elderly and usually result in degeneration of the anterior vertebral bodies (Magee 1997). This forms a wedge abnormality in the anterior vertebral body that leads to increased kyphosis. Figures 6.13 through 6.21 demonstrate basic exercises that promote a better postural position throughout the hyperkyphotic thoracic spine. These exercises also can promote scapular stability and increase kinesthetic awareness and joint position sense.

In the lumbar spine, postural abnormalities present themselves in the degree of lumbar lordosis, as either hypo- or hyperlordotic positions. In hyperlordosis, shortening of the lumbar paravertebrals creates active insufficiency and places the pelvis in an anterior tilt, which lengthens the posterior hip musculature and shortens the anterior hip musculature. In hypolordosis, lumbar paravertebrals are lengthened and hamstring and gluteal muscles are shortened with lengthening of the hip flexors and shortening of the lower abdominals. Exercises in figures 6.22 and 6.23 help strengthen abdominal muscles that often are inhibited in muscle imbalances.

Degenerative Joint Disease

Degeneration of the apophyseal joints is usually secondary to microtraumas resulting from excessive loading of the joint. Postural abnormalities are the primary cause. Subchondral bone starts to invade the deepest layers of cartilage and reacts to the forces that the cartilage can no longer dissipate (Grimsby 1994). This leads to thinning of the cartilage and subsequent bony deformation. Pain associated with this pathology leads to muscle guarding and poor musculoskeletal function, thus increasing degeneration and increasing joint load.

Treatment of the joint must increase synovial fluid production to attenuate the load and increase joint nutrition. Increasing muscle activity and coordination will decrease load on the joint and further degeneration. The clinician should begin treatment by addressing postural abnormalities using different forms of exercise to stimulate normal postural positioning. Exercise should be dosed in a manner that will provide adequate repetitions to cause articular joint gliding for synovial fluid production without muscle fatigue. Exercise also can reinforce proper posture. Most people have demonstrated poor posture for many years, and it will take literally thousands of properly dosed repetitions to retrain the body for appropriate posture.

Because muscle imbalances often result in degenerative joint disease, the specific weaknesses of muscles prone to weakness should be addressed. These may include exercises in figures 6.01, 6.02, 6.10, 6.13, 6.18, 6.20, 6.21, 6.22, and 6.33.

Degenerative Disc Disease

Degeneration of the vertebral disc is a common spinal pathology that is usually associated with compromise of the posterolateral horn of the disk (Adams et al. 2000; Hadjipavlou et al. 1999; Modic 1999). The posterolateral horn is furthest away from the central load-bearing portion of the disc. Nuclear material also tends to migrate to this region under load. Excessive loading and immobilization caused by poor posture and mechanics can weaken the annular fibers of the disc. This annular deformation then will cause migration of the nuclear substance to the posterolateral horn with resultant bulging and herniation. Once herniation occurs, the imbibing properties of the nuclear material (its ability to absorb water) cause swelling in the space around the neural structures that are just posterior to the lateral horns (Adams et al. 2000; Hadjipavlou et al. 1999; Modic 1999). This causes neurological signs and symptoms as well as muscle guarding and pain.

Disc degeneration also is associated with a decrease in disc height secondary to decreased water content of Type 2 collagen within the nucleus. Decreased disc height can lead to degeneration of the vertebral end plates and spurring attributable to excessive loading of the associated bony structure (Adams et al. 2000; Hadjipavlou et al. 1999; Modic 1999) . The Type 2 collagen within the nucleus reacts well to compression and decompression, its main function when dispersing and absorbing compressive loads. This collagen degenerates when there is no unloading during activities of daily living, as typically seen in postural deficits or muscle imbalances. Nuclear collagen degeneration also can result from degeneration of the annular fibers that hold the nucleus in place. Treatment must be directed at unloading the neural tissue and increasing annular fiber strength. Because the annular fibers are made primarily of Type 1 collagen, they are strengthened by modified tension in the line of stress (Grimsby 1994). As stated previously, the annular fibers are oriented at 45 to 60° angles to the horizontal plane. With this fiber formation, rotation would be the best means of stimulation. Rotation applies mechanical stress to the Type 1 collagen, stimulates protein synthesis, and increases collagen strength. Rotational exercises (figures 6.07, 6.08, 6.16, 6.17, 6.23, and 6.24) also stimulate the surrounding musculature to support the segment. The alignment of the annular fibers also increases disc height with rotation and essentially unloads the nuclear fibers while increasing tension on the annular fibers.

Myofascial Pain

Myofascial pain within the spinal musculature usually is associated with an area of increased neuromuscular activity and local metabolism that manifests itself in the form of a trigger point (Travell and Simons 1983). This can be caused by some form of trauma or a chronic irritation. A true trigger point, according to Travell and Simons (1983), will refer pain along a specific pattern that is specific to a particular muscle. Myofascial pain also can be related to some of Janda's muscle imbalance theories (Janda and Jull 1987). A tight muscle usually is in a state of increased contractile activity. A sustained contraction (increased neuromuscular activity) can lead to trigger points as described by Travell and Simons (1983). Restoring normal muscle resting tone and length goes hand in hand with the muscle imbalance theories.

Treatment of myofascial pain involves manual techniques and modalities to decrease the activity of the involved musculature. Restoring normal muscle tone also can be associated with restoring normal length. Resistance training can be used to restore normal resting tone. Exercise increases the tolerance of the muscle to stretch and strain. Although resistance exercises may not eliminate the trigger point, they may increase the patient's tissue tolerance without activating the referred pain pattern. Myofascial pain is particularly prevalent throughout the spinal regions, particularly on the dorsal side. Therefore, exercises that target these muscles (figures 6.03, 6.04, 6.09, 6.11, 6.13-6.15, 6.18-6.21, and 6.27-6.30) may be effective in managing myofascial pain.

Conclusion

Clinicians should use these interventions to reduce impairments and ultimately progress patients to functional and task-oriented activities. The use of elastic resistance allows us to be as specific or as general with our exercises as needed. The use of elastic resistance also allows patients to begin exercises in the clinic and continue those same activities at home. Elastic resistance is a very effective, low-cost means to empower our patients to take charge of their own progress, succeed in therapy, and enhance their own wellness.

CASE STUDY

Ken is a 36-year-old male patient with chronic history of lumbar pain associated with lumbar flexion and rotation who was referred to physical therapy for evaluation and treatment.

History: Ken works as a ship loader on the docks of a grain shipping company and has to lift and throw bags of grain that are approximately 80 to 100 lb repetitively throughout the day. He has experienced a gradual increase in lumbar pain and symptoms over the past 5 years and is now to the point where it is affecting his job performance and normal activities of daily living. He reports no other significant medical history and states that he has had a 30-lb increase in body weight over the past 3 years. He reports symptoms of lumbar pain and intermittent right posterior leg pain.

Objective
Posture: Increased lumbar lordosis with area of increased extension at L3 to L4 level. He has abdominal protrusion and general decrease in abdominal resting tone. Right shoulder is slightly lower than the left and is internally rotated.

ROM: Flexion: decreased 40%
      Extension: decreased 30%
      Rotation: L, decreased 50%;
          R, decreased 30%
      Side-bending: L, decreased 60%;
          R, decreased 40%

Strength: Decreased activity of bilateral gluteal musculature and poor abdominal and lumbar paravertebral strength.

Neurological examination is within normal limits with no signs of paresthesia or associated myotome weakness.

Special tests: – Straight Leg Raise test
              – Slump test
              + Left quadrant test for joint
                approximation

Assessment and Plan: Ken presents with typical signs and symptoms of gradual degeneration of the lumbar spine with associated decreases in endurance and strength. He has no specific mechanism of injury and appears to have had a gradual degeneration of spinal strength and mobility. The plan was to initiate exercises to increase joint nutrition and mobility and gradually progress to functional activities with components of flexion and rotation.

Intervention: Initially soft tissue work and other manual techniques were used to restore muscle balance to decrease any associated hypertonicity. Ken was progressed to exercises on the first day of physical therapy. Trunk rotations were initiated on Day 1 (figure 6.23) to begin some joint nutrition and promote gliding of the facet joints. This exercise also increases tensile strength within the annular fibers that can prevent any further degeneration of the lumbar disk. He performed 4 sets of 30 repetitions 3 times a day with emphasis on pain-free and smooth motion. He was instructed to increase range as pain and mobility allowed.

(continued)

Case Study   *(continued)*

Gluteal strengthening also was initiated (figures 6.33 and 6.34) on the first day of physical therapy to begin promoting gluteal activity during daily activity, as well as lumbar pelvic tilt activities on the exercise ball to promote proprioception and postural awareness in the lumbar region (figure 6.35). Abdominal exercises (figure 6.22) also were initiated to promote functional stability in the lumbar region.

Ken was progressed to elastic resistance rotational activities while seated and standing (figures 6.23 and 6.24). As pain decreased, he then added diagonals and lifting simulation to the routine (figures 6.25 and 6.26). During this time, he performed regular aerobic activity such as walking, bicycle riding, and upper body ergometry.

Outcome: Ken was pain-free with no residual limitations and was able to return to normal activity. He was also able to continue with all of his therapeutic exercises at home.

In this case, Ken's body type had changed and adapted while he performed the same daily activity. Before treatment his spine was unable to recover from the daily activities, and injuries occurred that decreased gluteal and abdominal strength and balance while promoting adaptation within the body. With just a small activation of the lumbar and lower extremity musculature, his body could restore the coordination and control that had been lost.

References

Adams, M.A., B.J. Freeman, H.P. Morrison, I.W. Nelson, and P. Dolan. 2000. "Mechanical Initiation of Intervertebral Disc Degeneration." *Spine* 25: 1625-36.

Bogduk, N., and L. Twomey, eds. 1991. *Clinical Anatomy of the Lumbar Spine*. 2nd ed. Melbourne, Australia: Churchill Livingstone.

Cherkin, D., R. Deyo, M. Battie, J. Street, and W. Barlow. 1998. "A Comparison of Physical Therapy, Chiropractic Manipulation, and Provision of an Educational Booklet for the Treatment of Patients With Low Back Pain." *New England Journal of Medicine* 339: 1021-9.

Grimsby, O. 1994. "Scientific Therapeutic Exercise Progressions." *Journal of Manual and Manipulative Therapy* 2: 94-101.

Hadjipavlou, A.G., J.W. Simmons, M.H. Pope, J.T. Necessary, and V.K. Goel. 1999. "Pathomechanics and Clinical Relevance of Disc Degeneration and Annular Tear: A Point-of-View Review." *American Journal of Orthopaedics* 28: 561-71.

Jackson R. 2000. "Functional Causes of Low Back Pain." Presented at the American Physical Therapy Association Annual Meeting, June 14, 2000.

Janda, V. 1987. "Muscles and Motor Control in Low Back Pain Assessment and Management." Pp. 253-278 in *Physical Therapy of the Low Back*, ed. L. Twomey and J. Taylor. New York: Churchill Livingstone.

Janda, V. 1988. "Muscles and Cervicogenic Pain Syndromes." Pp. 153-166 in *Physical Therapy of the Cervical and Thoracic Spine*, ed. R. Grand. New York: Churchill Livingstone.

Janda, V., and G. Jull 1987. "Muscles and Motor Control in Low Back Pain." In *Therapy of the Low Back: Clinics in Physical Therapy*, ed. L. Twomey and J. Taylor. New York: Churchill Livingstone.

Kapandji, I., and R. D'Aubigné. 1974. *The Physiology of the Joints: Vol. 3, The Trunk and the Vertebral Column*. 2nd ed. London: Churchill Livingstone.

Magee, D.J. 1997. "Thoracic (Dorsal) Spine." Pp. 331-361 in *Orthopedic Physical Therapy*, 3rd ed. Philadelphia: Saunders.

Modic, M.T. 1999. "Degenerative Disc Disease and Back Pain." *Magnetic Resonance Imaging Clinics of North America* (7): 481-91.

Mow, V., C. Proctor, and M. Kelly. 1989. "Biomechanics of Articular Cartilage." Pp. 31-58 in *Basic Biomechanics of the Musculoskeletal System*, ed. M. Nordin and V. Frankel. 2nd ed. Philadelphia: Lea & Febiger.

Porterfield, J., and C. Derosa. 1995. *Mechanical Neck Pain: Perspectives in Functional Anatomy*. Philadelphia: Saunders.

Porterfield, J., and C. Derosa. 1998. *Mechanical Low Back Pain: Perspectives in Functional Anatomy*. 2nd ed. Philadelphia: Saunders.

Soderberg, G. 1997. *Kinesiology: Application to Pathological Motion*. 2nd ed. Baltimore: Williams & Wilkins.

Travell, J.G., and D.G. Simons. 1983. *Myofascial Pain and Dysfunction*. Baltimore: Williams & Wilkins.

Viru, A., and T. Smirnova. 1995. "Health Promotion and Exercise Training." *Sports Medicine* 19: 123-36.

PART III

SPECIFIC TRAINING APPLICATIONS

Traditionally, elastic resistance has been used only for strengthening muscle. Through its clinical use, several other applications have been developed to achieve several different training goals. The inherent properties of elastic resistance make it ideal for several types of training applications, as demonstrated in the following chapters. Plyometric training and speed training are effective with elastic resistance because of its resistive qualities at high exercise speeds. Elastic resistance also can be used for balance training, otherwise known as reactive neuromuscular training. Elastic resistance is popular for fitness programming. Stretching with elastic resistance can improve flexibility and muscle length. Finally, specialized applications of elastic resistance are presented, including use for assisted motion and use in microgravity environments.

CHAPTER 7

Plyometric Training With Elastic Resistance

• • • • •

Michael A. Clark, MS, PT, CSCS, PES
National Academy of Sports Medicine

Tyler W.A. Wallace, BS, CPT, PES
National Academy of Sports Medicine

The demands imposed during advanced phases of rehabilitation, reconditioning, and training must reflect those incurred during functional activity. This is referred to as the specificity of training concept (Allman 1974). Enhanced performance during functional activities requires the muscles to exert maximal force output in a minimal amount of time (rate of force production). Success in most functional activities depends on the speed at which muscular force is generated. Power and reactive neuromuscular control represent a component of function that is perhaps the most important component in activities requiring rapid force production.

The speed of muscular exertion is limited by neuromuscular coordination. This means that the body will only move within a range of speed set by the central nervous system (Voight and Draovitch 1991). Plyometrics improve neuromuscular efficiency and extend the body's range of speed. Optimum performance depends on the speed at which muscular forces can be generated. It is generally accepted that optimum performance in sports and other func-

tional activities requires both technical skill and power. Skill is the ability of the neuromuscular system to coordinate the kinetic chain to allow for quick and accurate movements in all directions. Power is the ability to exert maximal force in the shortest amount of time. Power is most efficiently increased by increasing the amount of force that the muscle can produce and decreasing the amount of time taken to produce that force (Voight and Brady 1992).

Integrated Performance Paradigm

All movements that occur during functional activities involve repetitive force reduction, stabilization, and force production. Specific functional exercises must be used to adequately prepare the athlete to return to the rigors of his or her specific activity (Blattner and Noble 1979; Cavagna and Kaneko 1977; Cavagna, Komarek, and Mazzoleni 1971). Traditional training, reconditioning, and rehabilitation, in which heavy loads are emphasized, induce greater hypertrophy and increase strength but do not improve maximal power output, functional strength, or neuromuscular efficiency (Åstrand and Rodahl 1970). The integrated performance paradigm, therefore, involves multijoint, multiplanar exercises performed in a proprioceptively enriched environment.

One of the most remarkable aspects of skeletal muscle is its adaptive potential. If a muscle is systematically and functionally stressed, it will allow continual adaptation and optimum performance. For example, a baseball pitcher uses the integrated performance paradigm to produce maximal explosive concentric contractions. To replicate these forces during training, reconditioning, and rehabilitation is beyond the scope of traditional training. For example, the Cybex 6000 isokinetic dynamometer reaches maximal angular velocities of 500 to 600°/s, which is nonspecific to the greater than 7,000 to 10,000°/s of shoulder angular velocity during baseball pitching (Pappas, Zawacke, and Sullivan 1985). Consequently, specific functional exercises should be an integral component of every training, reconditioning, and rehabilitation program to facilitate a complete functional return and allow optimum performance. The health and fitness professional should use plyometrics to replicate the explosive muscular contractions that occur during most functional movements.

Definition of Plyometrics

Plyometrics are defined as quick, powerful movements involving an eccentric contraction followed immediately by an explosive concentric contraction (Wilk and Voight 1993). This defines a stretch-shortening cycle or an eccentric-concentric coupling phase (integrated performance paradigm). Plyometric exercises stimulate the body's proprioceptive mechanism and elastic properties to generate maximal force output in the minimal amount of time (Wilk and Voight 1993).

Purpose of Plyometrics

All movement patterns that occur during functional activities involve a series of repetitive stretch-shortening cycles (integrated performance paradigm). The neuromuscular system must react quickly after an eccentric contraction to produce a concentric contraction and impart the necessary force (accel-

eration) in the appropriate direction. Muscles produce the necessary change in direction of the body's center of mass (Voight and Draovitch 1991). Specific functional exercises that emphasize a rapid change in direction must be used to prepare athletes for the functional demands of their specific activity. Plyometrics provide the ability to train specific movement patterns in a biomechanically correct manner, thereby strengthening the muscle, tendon, and ligaments more functionally. The ultimate goal of plyometrics is to decrease the amount of time (amortization phase) between yielding an eccentric contraction and initiating a concentric contraction (Voight and Brady 1992).

Phases of Plyometrics

By definition, a plyometric activity must incorporate a specific progression of muscular contractions. Three phases of plyometrics have been identified: the eccentric, amortization, and concentric phases.

Eccentric Phase (Force Reduction)

This phase increases muscle spindle activity by stretching the muscle before activation (Eldred 1967; Lundin 1985). Potential energy is stored in the elastic components of the muscle during the force reduction phase. Prolonged loading prevents optimum exploitation of the myotatic stretch reflex (Komi and Bosco 1978; Verhoshanski 1983).

Amortization Phase (Dynamic Stabilization)

This phase occurs between the eccentric contraction (force reduction) and the initiation of the concentric contraction (force production; Wilk and Voight 1993). The amortization phase is also referred to as the electromechanical delay between the eccentric and concentric contraction during which the muscle must switch from overcoming force to imparting the necessary force in the intended direction (Voight and Draovitch 1991). A prolonged amortization phase results in less than optimal neuromuscular efficiency secondary to a loss of elastic potential energy. The more rapidly an individual switches from an eccentric contraction to a concentric contraction, the more powerful the response (Wilk and Voight 1993).

Concentric Phase (Force Production)

This phase enhances muscular performance after the eccentric phase of muscle contraction. This is typically the functional phase of coordinated movement.

Physiological Principles of Plyometrics

Plyometrics use the elastic and proprioceptive properties of a muscle to generate maximum force production (Wilk and Voight 1993). Plyometrics stimulate the body's mechanoreceptors to increase muscle recruitment over a minimal amount of time (Wilk and Voight 1993). Mechanoreceptors are specialized sensory neurons located within the muscle that provide information to the central nervous system about the degree of muscular distortion. The central nervous system then uses this sensory information to influence muscle tone, motor execution, and kinesthetic awareness (Lundin 1985). Stimulation of these receptors can facilitate, inhibit, and modulate both agonist and antagonist muscle activity. This enhances neuromuscular efficiency and functional strength. Muscle spindles and Golgi tendon organs provide the proprioceptive basis for plyometrics (Åstrand and Rodahl 1970; Jacobson 1970; O'Connel and Gardner 1972; Schmidt 1982; Swash and Fox 1972).

Several authors (Assmussen and Bonde-Peterson 1974; Bosco and Komi 1979; Bosco, Tarka, and Komi 1982; Cavagna, Saibene, and Margaria 1971) have reported that an eccentric contraction immediately preceding a concentric contraction will significantly increase the force generated concentrically as a result of the storage of elastic potential energy. During muscle loading, the load is transferred to the elastic components (parallel elastic elements and series elastic elements) and stored as elastic potential energy. The elastic elements then can contribute to the overall force production by converting the stored elastic potential energy to kinetic energy, which is then used to enhance the contraction (Assmussen and Bonde-Peterson 1974; Bosco and Komi 1982; Bosko, Tarka, and Komi 1982). The muscle's ability to use the stored elastic potential energy is affected by several variables: time, magnitude of stretch, and velocity of stretch. Increased force generation during the concentric contraction is most effective when the preceding eccentric contraction is of short range and is performed quickly (Schmidt 1982).

Prestretching a muscle improves muscular performance through the combined effects of both the storage of elastic potential energy and the proprioceptive properties of the muscle (Assmussen and Bonde-Peterson 1974; Bosco and Komi, 1979; Cavagna, Disman, and Mararia 1968). The percentage that each component contributes is unknown (Bosco and Komi 1979). The degree of enhanced muscular performance depends on the time from the eccentric to the concentric contraction (Cavagna, Disman, and Mararia 1968). Integrated training enhances overall kinetic chain neuromuscular efficiency. Training that enhances neuromuscular efficiency decreases the time between the eccentric and concentric contraction, thereby improving performance.

Proposed Mechanisms to Enhance Performance

Several theories have been offered to describe the mechanism behind plyometrics. These include enhanced muscle spindle activity, desensitization of the Golgi tendon organ, and enhanced neuromuscular efficiency.

Enhanced Muscle Spindle Activity

The speed of a muscular contraction is limited by the neuromuscular system. The kinetic chain will only move within a set speed range regardless of the strength of a muscle (Wilk and Voight 1993). The faster a muscle is loaded eccentrically, the greater the concentric force production (Lundin 1985).

Desensitization of the Golgi Tendon Organ

Desensitization of the Golgi tendon organ would increase the stimulation threshold for muscular inhibition, ultimately allowing increased force production with a greater load applied to the musculoskeletal system (Wilk and Voight 1993).

Enhanced Neuromuscular Efficiency

Plyometrics may promote changes within the neuromuscular system to provide the individual better neuromuscular control of the contracting agonists and synergists, thus enabling the central nervous system to become more automatic (Voight and

Draovitch 1991; Wilk and Voight 1993). These neural adaptations enhance neuromuscular efficiency even in the absence of morphological adaptations. Exploiting the stretch reflex, inhibiting the Golgi tendon organ, and enhancing the ability of the nervous system to react with maximum speed to the lengthening muscle all optimize the force produced by the concentric contraction.

Elastic Resistance for Plyometrics

Because of its mechanical properties, elastic resistance is ideal for plyometric exercises. Elastic resistance inherently provides eccentric and concentric resistance regardless of its position in relation to gravity. The lack of inertia in elastic resistance makes it ideal for plyometric exercise. This allows for quick motions and rapid change of direction, thereby minimizing the amortization phase.

Program Requirements

Clinicians should consider several aspects of the plyometric exercise prescription. There are several requirements for an effective and safe plyometric program.

Specificity

The mechanical and physiological properties of the training activity and the functional activity should be similar for optimum carryover. When the patient performs plyometrics during integrated movement patterns, the exercise has specific physiological, biomechanical, metabolic, and neuromuscular carryover (Bielik et al. 1986; Chu 1984a, 1984b.).

Adequate Functional Strength

A greater functional strength base and greater neuromuscular efficiency will increase force production, resulting in optimum performance. Optimum levels of functional strength and neuromuscular efficiency allow optimum eccentric, isometric, and concentric contractions during integrated movement patterns (this is called the *muscle action spectrum*, whereby all muscles have the capacity to work isometrically, concentrically, or eccentrically in all three planes of motion to reduce force, stabilize, and produce force). Optimum eccentric neuromuscular control allows for more efficient use of stored elastic

potential energy and a greater concentric contraction. High levels of isometric stabilization strength and neuromuscular efficiency decrease the amortization phase. This decreases the amount of time between the eccentric contraction and the concentric contraction, thus decreasing tissue overload and that potential for injury.

Pretraining Assessment

Each individual must be thoroughly screened before beginning a training program. The individual must have an unremarkable medical history. The patient must receive a thorough kinetic chain assessment that includes evaluation of posture, muscle balance, core stability, neuromuscular status, and functional abilities.

Safety Requirements

Each individual should have supportive shoes, a resilient training surface, a proper program, and knowledgeable supervision before beginning a plyometric program (Chu 1992; Voight and Brady 1992).

Design and Implementation

A plyometric program is an essential component for all integrated training programs. The key to an effective, integrated plyometric program lies in the design and implementation. Each program should be progressive, systematic, multiplanar, and activity-specific.

Plyometric Program Variables

An integrated plyometric program can be varied like other types of training programs. Several training variables can be manipulated:

- Plane of motion: Integrated plyometric exercises should be performed in all three planes of motion—sagittal, frontal, and transverse planes.
- Range of motion: The exercise should be performed in the maximal range of motion that can be controlled. The range of motion should increase as the individual becomes competent within a certain range.
- External load: The external loads can vary in an effort to increase the resistance and difficulty of the exercise. The load progresses from body weight to external resistance. Examples of external resistance are elastic tubing, dumbbells, medicine balls, weighted balls, weight vest, and weight belt.

- Amplitude of movement: Movements should be simple in the early stages of plyometric training and progress to more complex movements.
- Contraction velocity: The patient should move from slow muscle contraction to fast muscle contraction. For example, a squat jump with a stabilized landing can progress to a quick repeat squat jump.
- Muscle action: The patient should progress from single muscle groups performing single-plane exercises to multiplanar exercises performed by multiple muscle groups.
- Intensity: The intensity of the exercise is controlled by the selection of the exercise. For example, a double-leg squat jump is less intense than a single-leg hop. Intensity also is controlled by the use of elastic resistance and by manipulating the duration, rest periods, and frequency of the exercise.
- Duration: Duration should be based on intensity, frequency, and external load, according to the plyometric stress continuum.
- Frequency: This is the number of training sessions per week. Each individual should have approximately 36 to 48 hr of rest between plyometric training sessions to facilitate maximum recovery and prevent overtraining.
- Training progression: The training program proceeds from simple to complex, stable to unstable, body weight to extra resistance, and low load to high load, all with proper use of the plyometric stress continuum.

It is important to assess an individual's power production and neuromuscular control before initiating an integrated training program to achieve a baseline. The vertical jump test and the "Shark Skill Test" can be used to assess power and reactive neuromuscular control, respectively (Clark 2000).

In any program, the clinician must evaluate for signs of overtraining. This is a pathological state that results from cumulative neuromuscular and metabolic fatigue. Signs of plyometric overtraining include prolonged foot contact, lack of neuromuscular control, decreased vertical height or horizontal displacement, and longer rest periods (Clark 2000).

Plyometrics for the Lower Extremity

Plyometrics are most commonly used in the lower extremity. A plyometric stress continuum for the lower extremity can be progressed in 3 levels.

Level 1

These exercises involve very little joint motion and are designed to establish optimum landing mechanics, postural alignment, and neuromuscular efficiency (figures 7.01-7.04).

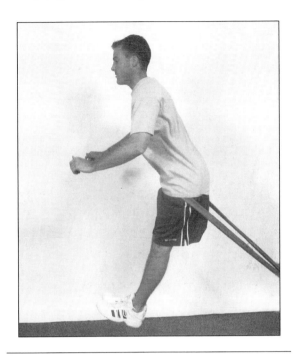

Figure 7.01 Ankle flips.

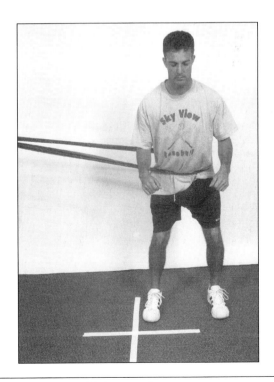

Figure 7.02 Double leg cross hops.

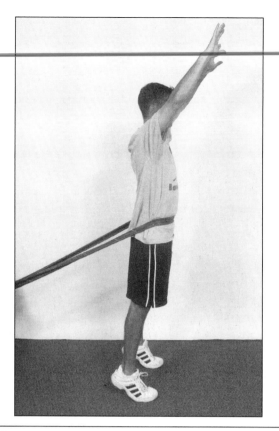

Figure 7.03   Vertical jump.

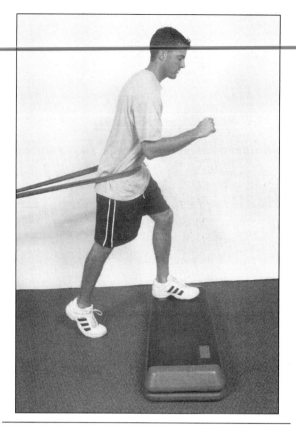

Figure 7.04   Run steps.

Physiological Rationale

Compression of the articular receptors facilitates reflex joint stabilization. In addition, optimum landing mechanics and postural alignment facilitate optimum neuromuscular efficiency.

Goals

These exercises create optimal joint stabilization reactions and teach optimum postural alignment, core stabilization strength, and optimum landing mechanics.

Level 2

Stabilization exercises are replaced with dynamic concentric and eccentric activities through a full functional range of motion (figures 7.05-7.08). The exercises are progressed to movements requiring dynamic control in multiple planes of movement.

Physiological Rationale

Linear movements stimulate articular receptors and create pressure changes. Activities in this phase are designed to stimulate postural responses, facilitate

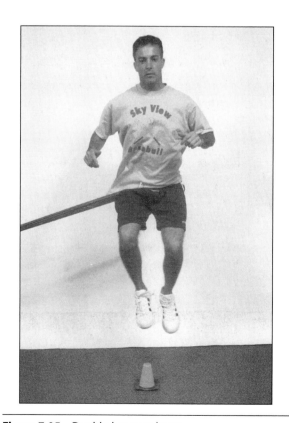

Figure 7.05   Double-leg cone hops.

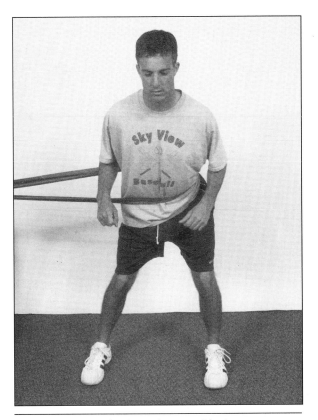

Figure 7.06 Ricochet jump (start position).

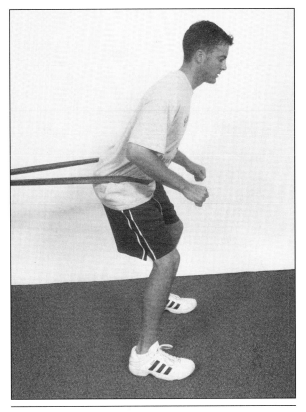

Figure 7.07 Ricochet jump (end position).

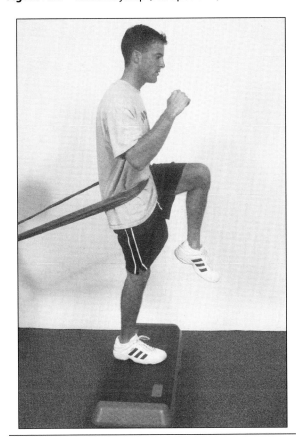

Figure 7.08 Power step-ups.

dynamic joint stabilization contractions, and enhance optimum force production.

Goals

These exercises establish optimum neuromuscular efficiency, joint stabilization, and power production in all planes of motion.

Level 3

This phase continues to follow the plyometric stress continuum. The specificity of the exercise increases as well as the neural demand (figures 7.09-7.11).

Physiological Rationale

Maximum neural adaptations occur with the dynamic plyometrics of Level 3.

Goals

These exercises enhance optimum force production and neuromuscular efficiency during functional movement patterns.

Level 4

At this level the individual performs specific functional activities at the same intensity that he or she will experience on return to sport (figures 7.12-7.14).

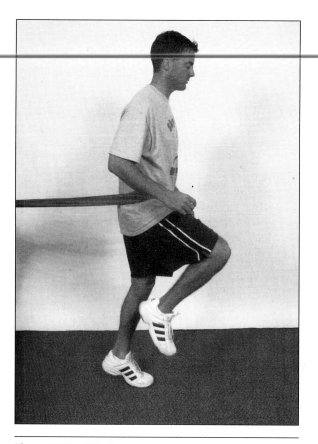

Figure 7.09 Skipping.

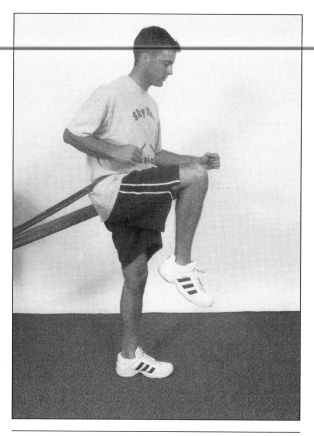

Figure 7.10 Alternate-leg bounding.

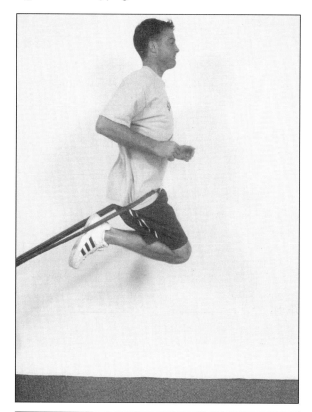

Figure 7.11 Buttkick.

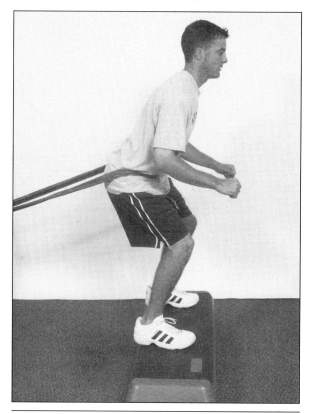

Figure 7.12 Repeat box jumps.

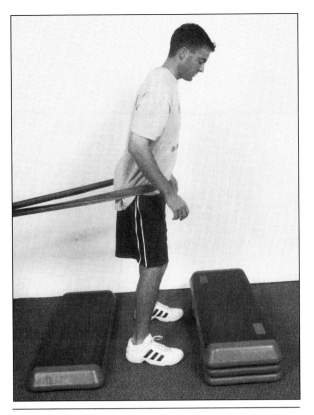

Figure 7.13   Multiple box jump.

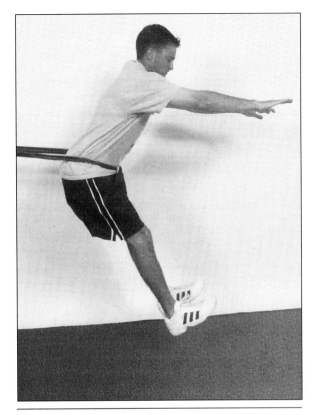

Figure 7.14   Repeat long jump.

Physiological Rationale

The neuromuscular system will adapt to the imposed demands placed on it during integrated training. The neuromuscular system needs to be trained appropriately and specifically to ensure optimal neuromuscular efficiency and injury prevention. Therefore, each client should follow the plyometric continuum to ensure consistent results and prevent injury.

Goals

These exercises establish optimum levels of reactive neuromuscular control, eccentric strength, reactive joint stabilization, dynamic neuromuscular efficiency, and force production.

Plyometrics for the Upper Extremity

Elastic resistance also can be used for plyometric training of the upper extremity. Because of the high velocities of functional activities that involve the upper extremity, elastic resistance can be used for velocity-specific training. Upper extremity plyometrics are particularly useful in training and rehabilitation of throwing athletes.

For example, baseball pitching at more than 7,000°/s requires rapid concentric and eccentric contractions of the posterior rotator cuff as the arm moves from the cocking to acceleration phase. Any sport that requires such a quick change of direction of motion should incorporate plyometric training. Figures 7.15 and 7.16 demonstrate examples of plyometric exercises for throwing athletes.

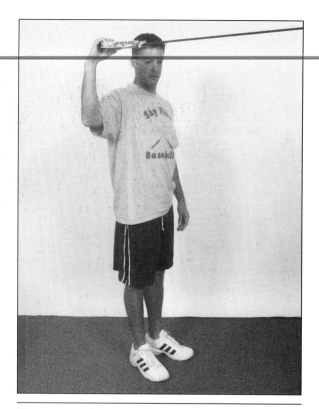

Figure 7.15 Plyometric shoulder external rotation at 90°.

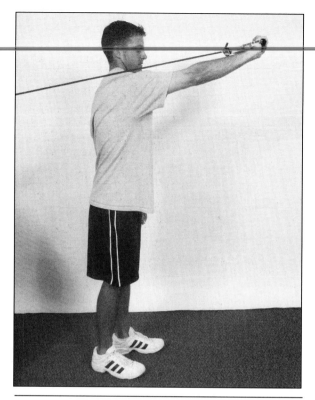

Figure 7.16 Plyometric shoulder press.

Conclusion

Plyometrics are an important component of all integrated training programs. All functional activities require efficient use of the integrated performance paradigm (eccentric deceleration → stabilization → concentric acceleration). Therefore, all programs should include plyometrics to enhance neuromuscular efficiency and prevent injury. The kinetic chain responds to the imposed demands of training. If the training program does not systematically and progressively challenge the neuromuscular system, results will be less than optimum.

References

Allman, F.L. 1974. *Sports Medicine*. New York: Academic Press.

Assmussen, E., and F. Bonde-Peterson. 1974. "Storage of Elastic Energy in Skeletal Muscle in Man." *Acta Physiologica Scandinavia* 91: 385-92.

Åstrand, P., and K. Rodahl. 1970. *Textbook of Work Physiology*. New York: McGraw-Hill.

Bielik, E., D. Chu, F. Costello, et al. 1986. "Roundtable. Practical Considerations for Utilizing Plyometrics. Part 1." *National Strength and Conditioning Association Journal* 8:14.

Blattner, S., and L. Noble. 1979. "Relative Effects of Isokinetic and Plyometric Training on Vertical Jumping Performance." *Research Quarterly* 50(4): 583-8.

Bosco, C., and P. Komi. 1979. "Potentiation of the Mechanical Behavior of the Human Skeletal Muscle Through Prestretching." *Acta Physiologica Scandinavia* 106: 467-72.

Bosco, C., and P. Komi. 1982. "Muscle Elasticity in Athletes." In *Exercise and Sports Biology*, ed. P.V. Komi. Champaign, IL: Human Kinetics.

Bosco, C., J. Tarka, and P.V. Komi. 1982. "Effects of Elastic Energy and Myoelectric Potentiation of Triceps Surca During Stretch-Shortening Cycle Exercise." *International Journal of Sports Medicine* 2: 137-40.

Cavagna, G., B. Disman, and R. Mararia. 1968. "Positive Work Done by Previously Stretched Muscle." *Journal of Applied Physiology* 24(1): 21-32.

Cavagna, G., and M. Kaneko. 1977. "Mechanical Work and Efficiency in Level Walking and Running." *Journal of Physiology* 268: 467-81.

Cavagna, G., L. Komarek, and S. Mazzoleni. 1971. "The Mechanics of Sprint Running." *Journal of Physiology* 217: 709-21.

Cavagna, G., F. Saibene, and R. Margaria. 1971. "Effect of Negative Work on the Amount of Positive Work Performed by an Isolated Muscle." *Journal of Applied Physiology* 217: 709-21.

Chu, D. 1984a. "The Language of Plyometrics." *National Strength and Conditioning Association Journal* 6(4): 30-1.

Chu, D. 1984b. "Plyometric Exercise." *National Strength and Conditioning Association Journal* 6(1): 56-62.

Chu, D. 1992. *Jumping Into Plyometrics*. Champaign, IL: Human Kinetics.

Clark, M.A. 2000. *Integrated Training for the New Millennium*. Thousand Oaks, CA: National Academy of Sports Medicine.

Eldred, E. 1967. "Functional Implications of Dynamic and Static Components of the Spindle Response to Stretch." *American Journal of Physical Medicine and Rehabilitation* 46: 129-40.

Jacobson, M. 1970. *Developmental Neurobiology*. New York: Holt, Rinehart and Winston.

Komi, P., and C. Bosco. 1978. "Utilization of Stored Elastic Energy in Leg Extensor Muscles by Men and Women." *Medicine and Science in Sports and Exercise* 10(4): 261-5.

Lundin, P.E. 1985. "A Review of Plyometric Training." *National Strength and Conditioning Association Journal* 7(3): 65-70.

O'Connel, A., and E. Gardner. 1972. *Understanding the Scientific Basis of Human Movement*. Baltimore: Williams & Wilkins.

Pappas, A.M., R.M. Zawacke, and T.J. Sullivan. 1985. "Biomechanics of Baseball Pitching: A Preliminary Report." *American Journal of Sports Medicine* 12(4): 216-21.

Schmidt, R. 1982. *Motor Control and Learning*. Champaign, IL: Human Kinetics.

Swash, M., and K. Fox. 1972. "Muscle Spindle Innervation in Man. " *Journal of Anatomy* (112): 61-80.

Verhoshanski, Y. 1983. "Depth Jumping in the Training of Jumpers." *Track Technique* 51: 1618-9.

Voight, M., and D. Brady. 1992. "Plyometrics. " Pp. 226-240 in *A Compendium of Isokinetics in Clinical Usage*, ed. G.J. Davies. Onalaska, WI: S&S.

Voight, M., and P. Draovitch. 1991. "Plyometrics. " Pp. 45-73 in *Eccentric Muscle Training in Sports and Orthopedics*, ed. M. Albert. New York: Churchill Livingstone.

Wilk, K.E., and M. Voight. 1993. "Plyometrics for the Overhead Athlete. " In *The Athletic Shoulder*, ed. J.R. Andrews and K.E. Wilk. New York: Churchill Livingstone.

CHAPTER 8

Speed and Agility Training With Elastic Resistance

• • • • •

James W. Matheson, MS, PT, CSCS
University of Montana Physical Therapy Clinic

George J. Davies, MEd, PT, SCS, ATC, CSCS
University of Wisconsin at La Crosse

Many athletes relate speed to sprinting performance. Others think of speed in terms of how fast a baseball can be thrown or a tennis ball served. In all cases, speed requires the rapid movement of the limbs, whether the legs of the sprinter or the arm of the pitcher. Nowhere is speed more visible than when we watch the 100-m sprint at an international track-and-field meet. However, most sports don't depend on sprinting speed alone. A football running back may have world-class sprinting speed but still lack the ability to explosively change direction. Because of this close association, speed often is confused with agility and quickness. Speed may be defined as either rapid arm or leg movement. In contrast, agility is the ability to decelerate, accelerate, or change direction quickly with good body control and without loss in speed or strength (Costello and Kreis 1993; Graham 2000; Twist and Benicky 1995). Agility depends on the components of quickness and reactive ability. Quickness is the ability of the central nervous system (CNS) to contract and relax or control muscle without any pre-

liminary stretch (Siff 2000). Siff operationally defined quickness as the time between the stimulus and the initiation of movement, whereas he described reaction time as the time from initiation of movement to the end of the movement (Siff 2000). Quickness is the ability of the athlete to hear the starter's pistol or the football snap and then initiate muscle firing. Quickness is determined largely by genetic factors and can be improved only minimally with training (Harbin, Durst, and Harbin 1989.). On the other hand, reactive ability or speed of movement depends on how the athlete can efficiently organize and coordinate her or his movements in response to the outside environment. Reactive ability has a far greater potential for improvement with specificity training than does quickness (Siff 2000). Specificity training and repetition can largely influence how well an athlete explodes out of the starting blocks or off the defensive line in a football game. Other chapters of this book provide details on how reactive ability may be improved with stretch-shortening or plyometric training.

In many sports, athletic ability depends on the combination of speed and agility. This chapter demonstrates the use of elastic resistance as a tool to help athletes increase both speed and agility. The drills and exercises described in this chapter are not meant to be an all-inclusive list; rather, we intend to provide the reader with examples of exercises to include in a variety of sport-specific speed training programs.

Elastic Resistive Devices and Sprint Speed Training

Speed training requires the use of devices that provide adequate resistance without significantly interfering with body mechanics or technique. The inert properties of elastic devices make them an asset to a speed coach's or clinician's inventory. However, optimum use of the elastic speed training devices currently on the market requires a sound knowledge of sprinting speed mechanics.

Components of Sprinting Speed

Sprinting has been described as a faultless, perfected series of finely tuned technical and motor coordinated skills. It involves the anaerobic energy system or 6 to 10 s of maximal sprinting effort (McFarlane 1994). Sprinting speed is determined by the product of stride rate and stride length (Allerheiligen 1994; Chu 1996; Chu and Korchemny 1989; Dintiman, Ward, and Tellez 1997; Faccioni 1994a, 1994b; Klinzing 1984; Lentz and Hardyk 2000). Stride length is the distance covered in one stride during running. Stride length is developed by increasing the speed-strength in the lower extremities (Chu 1996; Chu and Korchemny 1989; Dintiman, Ward, and Tellez 1997; Faccioni 1994a, 1994b). Speed-strength is the ability to exert maximal force during high-speed movement (Luhatenen and Komi 1978; Mann 1984). Stride rate is the number of steps taken in a given amount of time. All increases in sprint speed must come from an increase in stride rate or stride length. To improve stride rate, the athlete must decrease the time between strides. This has also been described as improving leg turnover (Luhatenen and Komi 1978; Mann 1984; McFarlane 1994; Mero and Komi 1986). Stride rate is more difficult for the athlete to increase than stride length. It is necessary to examine the two phases of sprinting stride to completely understand how leg turnover or stride rate can be in-

creased. The support phase represents the time from ground contact to takeoff. The flight, or nonsupport, phase represents the period when the feet do not touch the ground (Allerheiligen 1994; Chu and Korchemny 1989). If an athlete can decrease the amount of time in either of these phases, stride rate will increase. As an example, a hurdler is in the flight stage of sprinting as she goes over the hurdle. The goal is to get the lead foot back on the ground immediately after it is over the hurdle to decrease the flight stage and thus potentially increase sprint speed. Other means in which one may decrease overall sprint time include improving starting ability, acceleration time, and speed endurance. Coaches and athletes may use the dynamic resistance unique to elastic tubing or cords to train and maximize these components of sprint speed. Elastic devices can be used in an assisted speed exercise to help the athlete increase stride rate. They also can be used in resistance exercises to increase the required forces to sprint at a certain speed or accelerate from a starting position. Ideally, these elastic tubing–assisted methods or drills allow the athlete's neuromuscular system to adapt to the "assisted" high speed or "supramaximal" training. It is postulated that the motor skills learned in these assisted training periods may then be reproduced by the athlete, resulting in greater speed-strength during competition.

Supramaximal or Assisted Sprinting

Researchers (Mero and Komi 1986; Mero et al. 1987) have documented how stride length and stride rate do not increase in a linear relationship as sprinting speed increases from submaximal to supramaximal. In one study (Mero and Komi 1986) that used a towing system, investigators demonstrated that stride length plateaued as stride rate continued to increase during supramaximal sprinting. This implies that increasing leg turnover is necessary to attain faster speeds. Consequently, sprint-assisted training that involves sprinting at a supramaximal or increased linear speed may increase stride rate (Luhatenen and Komi 1978; Mann 1984; McFarlane 1994; Mero and Komi 1986; Mero et al. 1987). This type of training uses either a towing device, downhill sprinting, or high-speed treadmill sprinting to allow the athlete to reach a velocity greater than what could be accomplished under normal sprinting conditions. Reviews of the literature reveal that ground reaction forces, stride rate, muscle stiffness, stored elastic energy, and increased efficiency of muscle contraction are all present during supramaximal sprinting (Faccioni 1994a, 1994b; Mero and Komi 1986; Mero et al. 1987). Some researchers believe that increased muscle stiffness is an advantage during the eccentric stretch-shortening cycle (ground contact during sprinting) and may improve efficiency in sprint athletes (Faccioni 1994a, 1994b). Other scientists (Mero et al. 1987) used a rubber rope pulled by an electric motor at an angle of 10 to 17° from the horizontal. Subjects were pulled at 104.3 to 104.6% of their nonassisted maximal speeds. Results demonstrated increases in stride length and decreases in blood lactate and oxygen debt during supramaximal compared with maximal sprinting speeds. In addition, horizontal and vertical ground reaction forces were higher in the supramaximal group during impact. These results are interesting and demonstrate the need for further study of variables during supramaximal sprinting as well as the effect this type of training has on sprint speed.

To increase top speed and stride rate, partner-assisted speed sprinting may be performed (figure 8.01; Lentz and Hardyk 2000). Two athletes are connected by waist belts or harnesses attached to a 10- to 20-m length of elastic tubing. The athletes line up at a distance that stretches the tubing 20 to 30% of its original length. Sprints of 10 to 20 m are performed. The lead sprinter attempts to maintain the same lead distance to provide the rear athlete with a constant assisted or supramaximal sprinting speed.

A similar technique to increase stride rate involves using elastic resistance in partner-assisted to -unassisted speed sprints (Lentz and Hardyk 2000). First, two athletes are attached using 10 to 20 m of elastic tubing. They then line up at a predetermined distance to stretch the tubing 20 to 30% of its original length. Finally, the athletes begin sprinting forward simultaneously. For the first 10 to 20 m, the lead sprinter maintains a constant force on the tubing to provide assisted sprinting to the rear athlete (figure 8.01). In contrast to the assisted sprints described previously, at every subsequent 10- to 20-m interval, the lead athlete slows down to allow the rear athlete to sprint unassisted for 10 to 20 m. After this interval of unassisted sprinting, the lead athlete then speeds up in an effort to again provide assisted sprinting to the rear athlete. Sprinting unassisted allows carryover of the increased stride rate provided by the assisted sprinting.

To improve acceleration speed and quick leg recovery in the first few steps of a sprint, partner-assisted acceleration drills may be performed (figure 8.02; Lentz and Hardyk 2000). Two athletes are attached at the waist by a 10- to 20-m length of elastic tubing. In this drill, the second or "assisting" athlete is optional; the tubing may be attached to a stationary object such as a football goal post. The "assisted" athlete backs up to a distance that stretches the tubing 20 to 30% in length. After the stretching of the elastic cord, the athlete then gets into the sport-specific ready position. This may be a four-point sprint-start position or a three-point football stance position. The athlete explodes at the start signal and sprints 10 to 20 m with the assistance of the tubing.

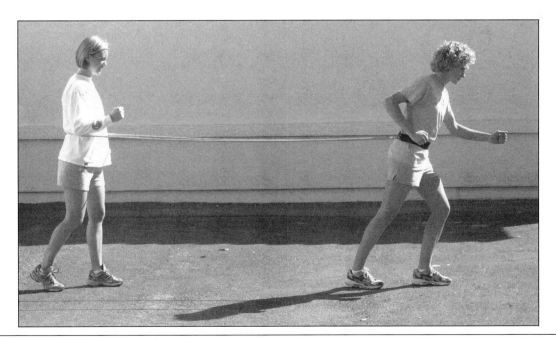

Figure 8.01 Partner tubing-assisted speed sprints.

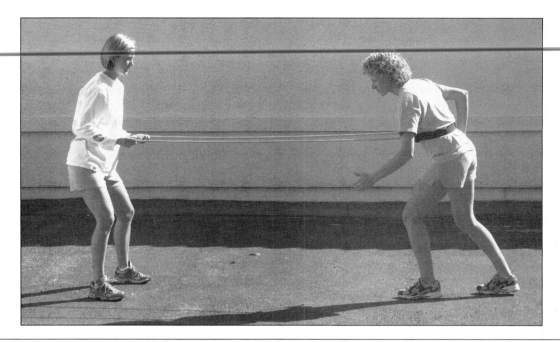

Figure 8.02   Partner tubing-assisted acceleration drill.

Resisted Acceleration or Sprinting

For longer assisted acceleration sprints, the athlete providing the assisting also can sprint at the start signal to provide continued assistance for a longer distance.

Athletes wishing to increase sprinting speed also must overcome the initial resistance (inertia) of the body through the acceleration phase of sprinting. The strong extensors of the lower extremity including the gluteals, hamstrings, quadriceps, and gastrocnemius muscles must help propel the athlete horizontally down the track (Chu and Korchemny 1989). These extensor groups also prevent the athlete's center of gravity from dropping too low during the support or ground contact phase of sprinting (Chu and Korchemny 1989; Faccioni 1994a, 1994b). Reducing the drop in the center of gravity allows for a greater eccentric prestretch in the extensor muscles. This large eccentric prestretch will increase the stretch reflex, which in turn will result in a larger concentric contraction during the push-off or driving phase of each stride (Faccioni 1994a, 1994b). This increase in the prestretch of the stretch-shortening cycle will allow the athlete to transfer greater explosive reactive strength to lower extremity concentric force production. This increased force production will increase stride length and therefore horizontal sprint speed. Resisted ac-

celeration training may be completed with uphill sprinting, resisted towing with sleds, or the use of weighted vests, elastic tubing, or parachutes (Dintiman, Ward, and Tellez 1997; Faccioni 1994a, 1994b; Lentz and Hardyk 2000; Siff 2000). Resisted towing with elastic tubing offers a distinct advantage over using weighted vests. Weighted vests, which provide resistance in a vertical direction, may alter the sprinting motion to such a degree that there is no carryover to the motor skill of sprinting (Siff 2000). In contrast, towing devices offer less resistance to sprinting form and therefore decrease the risk of skill interference. Elastic resistance also provides dynamic horizontal resistance that does not depend on the forces of gravity. Later we describe several different methods of resisted sprint training that use elastic cords or tubing.

Running form drills allow the athlete to focus on the isolated lower extremity movement involved in sprinting. These form drills may help the athlete improve stride frequency and strengthen lower extremity muscle groups in a sport-specific manner. Elastic tubing or cords can enhance this type of training by providing dynamic resistance in the direction of limb movement. Figures 8.03 and 8.04 demonstrate two running forms drills that use elastic resistance.

To enhance running strength and power in an effort to improve stride length, sprinters may use partner-assisted speed sprints (Lentz and Hardyk 2000) as a drill. Similar to partner-assisted speed

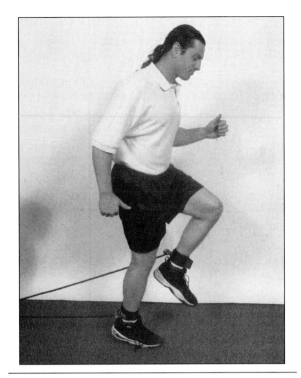

Figure 8.03 Resisted stationary skips (Level I).

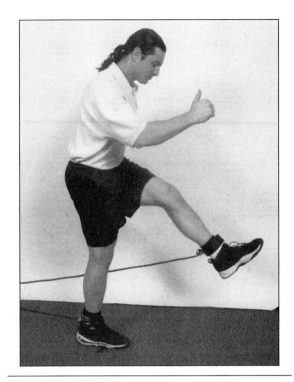

Figure 8.04 Resisted stationary skips (Level II).

sprints (figure 8.01), partner-resisted speed sprints use a 10- to 20-m section of elastic tubing connected to waist belts or harnesses. In this drill (figure 8.05), the lead sprinter rather than the rear sprinter is the focus of interest. In partner-resisted speed sprints, the rear athlete attempts to maintain the same distance behind the lead sprinter.

A quick-release belt can be used in conjunction with elastic tubing to provide "resisted-unassisted" or "contrast acceleration" sprint drills (figure 8.05). A quick-release belt contains a Velcro connecting strip. The quick-release belt allows the sprinter to accelerate against the stretched tubing until enough force is applied to break the Velcro strip holding the tubing to the athlete. This type of contrast training may teach quick transitions in speed and increase the stride rate of acceleration (Lentz and Hardyk 2000).

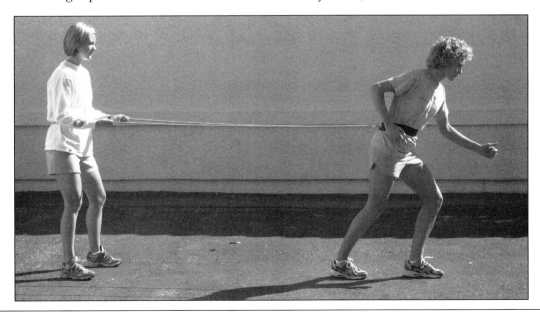

Figure 8.05 Quick-release belt training.

Precautions for Using Elastic Devices During Sprint Training

Trainers and athletes must follow several precautions when using elastic devices for assisted or resisted sprint training. These precautions are as follows:

- Ensure that the athlete has adequate strength and good sprinting form. Any defect in the athlete's sprinting form will be exaggerated during assisted or supramaximal sprinting.

- Ensure that the athlete wears proper footwear, and choose a proper training surface.

- Allow adequate recovery between supramaximal sessions. The recommended rest period is 2 to 3 days between speed sessions. Stop sessions immediately when the athlete begins to demonstrate fatigue or loss of form.

- Inspect the elastic tubing or cord before each use. Protect the tubing to avoid puncture and damage from spikes and other field equipment. Replace aged or damaged tubing when necessary.

- Avoid stretching the cord greater than the manufacturer's recommendations. If in doubt, don't stretch a cord by more than three times its resting length.

- When two athletes are working together, try to pair up athletes of the same body weight and ability.

- Begin each session of assisted or resisted training with a general warm-up that includes several low- to medium-intensity sprints.

- Ensure that the athlete maintains proper sprint mechanics. The pulled or towed sprinter should not brake, because this causes the athlete to land on the heels rather than the balls of his or her feet. It has been shown that supramaximal sprinting speeds greater than 5% of maximal sprinting speed are detrimental because the athlete usually begins to lose control of form (Dintiman, Ward, and Tellez 1997; Faccioni 1994a, 1994b; Lentz and Hardyk 2000).

- The athlete should try to maintain overspeed for 6 to 8 strides after the cord slackens or is released.

- End each session of assisted or resisted training with several unassisted maximal sprints to ensure carryover to the actual performance.

Elastic Resistance and Upper Extremity Speed Training

In addition to requiring lower extremity speed, many sports demand high levels of upper extremity speed and explosive power. Examples of sports in which upper extremity speed is key to performance are baseball, tennis, martial arts, boxing, and the throwing track-and-field events. As demonstrated for the lower extremity, elastic bands or tubes are useful tools to develop upper extremity speed and agility.

Upper Extremity Speed Training

All explosive, competitive, upper extremity throwing or punching actions involve a single or repeated series of stretch-shortening cycles. Other chapters in this book provide a more detailed explanation of these cycles or "reactive neuromuscular" events. The concept of upper extremity speed is illustrated perfectly in the violent upper extremity muscle actions of throwing a baseball. This sporting task demonstrates how elastic loading (prestretch) of the muscular connective tissues is used to produce a maximal explosive concentric muscle action and a subsequent rapid decelerative eccentric muscle action (Pezzullo, Karas, and Irrgang 1995; Wilk and Voight 1993; Wilk et al. 1993).

Upper Extremity Drills

To replicate the large forces and angular velocities of throwing a baseball, throwing a punch, or serving a volleyball, stretch-shortening (plyometric) training must be incorporated into the athlete's training program (Pezzullo, Karas, and Irrgang 1995; Wilk and Voight 1993; Wilk et al. 1993). Because of their inertial resistance, traditional weight machines or free weights are not recommended for stretch-shortening drills because this defeats the principle that the faster a muscle is forced to lengthen, the greater the tension it will exert. In contrast, elastic tubing or bands provide a dynamic resistance that is ideal for plyometric training of the upper extremity. Treiber et al. (1998) examined the use of slow-speed light dumbbell, and slow and fast elastic band training in elite tennis players. These exercises focused on training the shoulder internal and external rotators. When compared with a control group, the experimental group demonstrated a significant increase in peak and average serving speed after 4 weeks of training. An example of an upper extremity, stretch-shortening, elastic exercise similar to the one used in the study by Trieber et al. (1998) is shown in figures 8.06 and 8.07. The purpose of these types of stretch-shortening exercise is to provide the athlete with advanced strengthening exercises that are more aggressive and speed-specific compared with those provided by a light dumbbell program (Wilk and Voight 1993; Wilk et al. 1993)

Proprioceptive neuromuscular facilitation (PNF) patterns (Voight 1992; Voss, Knott, and Kabat 1953) have been used manually for years in the rehabilitation process and more recently into the conditioning phases. PNF involves many of the concepts of the stretch-shortening cycle, such as the quick prestretch to facilitate muscle recruitment. In conditioning for the overhead athlete, PNF patterns use the principles of stretch-shortening along with the functional specificity of replicating the various movement patterns incorporated in sports. Figures 8.08 and 8.09 demonstrate the use of elastic resistance in a diagonal 2 (D2) pattern incorporating the stretch-shortening concepts.

Another type of PNF training involves the concept of rhythmic stabilization (Voss, Knott, and Kabat 1953). Figure 8.10 demonstrates an example of rhythmic stabilization or perturbation training

that often is performed at different parts of the range of motion of the shoulder joint. The athlete maintains a position of resisted shoulder internal or external rotation while withstanding perturbations from a fellow athlete or coach. The perturbations may be progressed from a submaximal to maximum intensity and from a known to unknown pattern. The purpose of the perturbation training is to enhance the proprioceptive/kinesthetic abilities of the receptors around the joint. This in turn should translate into more effective neuromuscular reactive control (Wilk and Voight 1993; Wilk et al. 1993).

Resisted stretch-shortening drills that replicate an athlete's exact biomechanics are ideal and should be included in an upper extremity speed training program. Tom House, professional pitching coach, has created an elastic tubing drill that may increase a pitcher's speed and improve pitching mechanics. House has defined the "Flex-T" position as the position of the arms when the pitcher's front foot hits the mound. He believes the Flex-T is a position of optimal joint integrity for the pitcher's shoulders and elbows. In this position, the elbows are at shoulder height and are in line with the hips and balls of the feet (House 1996). The elastic tubing Flex-T pitching drill is shown in figures 8.11 and 8.12. The drill requires elastic tubing that reaches from elbow to elbow with both arms extended in 90° of shoulder ab-

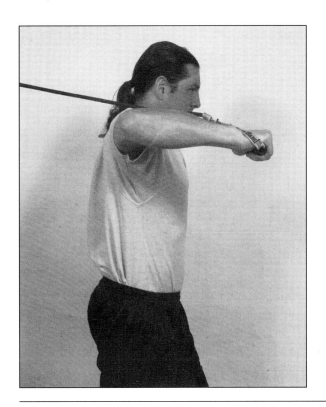
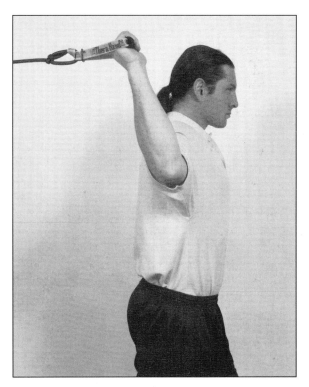

Figure 8.06-8.07 Stretch-shortening shoulder internal rotation exercise: start and end position (8.06); mid position (8.07).

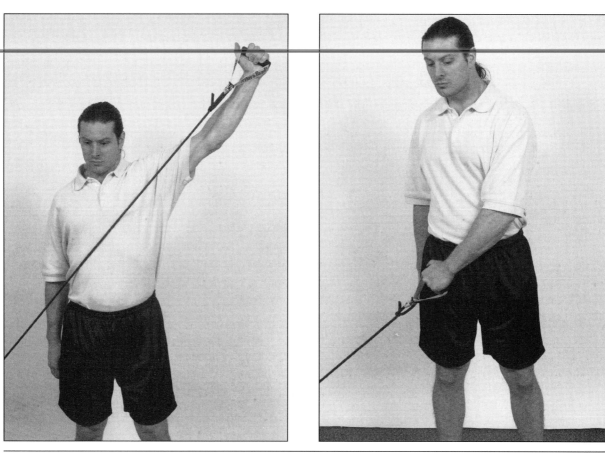

Figure 8.08-8.09 PNF D2 extension: start and end position (8.08); mid position (8.09).

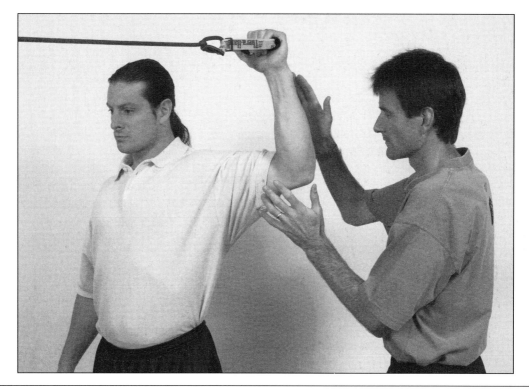

Figure 8.10 Rhythmic stabilization with resisted shoulder external rotation.

duction. The athlete attaches one end of the elastic tubing around the pitching wrist. The other end of the tubing is held or wrapped around the wrist of the athlete's glove hand. The athlete goes through the exact pitching motion, allowing the elastic tubing to provide increased arm and trunk speed. This type of assisted-speed drill is an excellent example of how elastic tubing can be used in a manner incorporating exact sport-specific mechanics.

Precautions for Using Elastic Devices During Upper Extremity Speed Training

Coaches, clinicians, and athletes should follow several precautions when integrating elastic tubing stretch-shortening drills for the upper extremity into training programs.

- The athlete's general strength should be adequate, and he or she must know the proper technique.
- The athlete should follow a proper warm-up with stretching exercises.

- The athlete should establish sport-specific goals.
- Drills should progress from low to high intensity.
- Drills should progress from low to high volume.
- When proper technique in the performance of the stretch-shortening activity can no longer be demonstrated, the exercise should be stopped.
- The greater the intensity of the workout with stretch-shortening drills, the greater the recovery time required.

Peak athletic performance in the overhead athlete depends on combining high speed and large muscular forces (i.e., power) into a sport-specific task. However, because power is a combination of strength and speed, a program to increase power must include exercises that both incorporate large muscular forces and decrease the time in which these forces are generated. Stretch-shortening drills for the upper extremity using elastic resistance offer the athlete a means to increase athletic power and improve sport-specific demands.

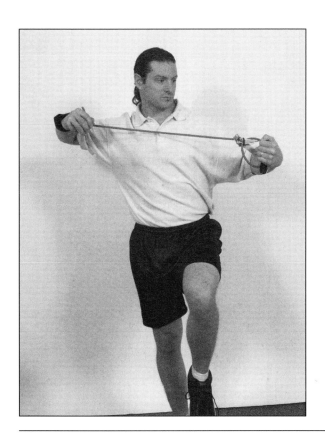 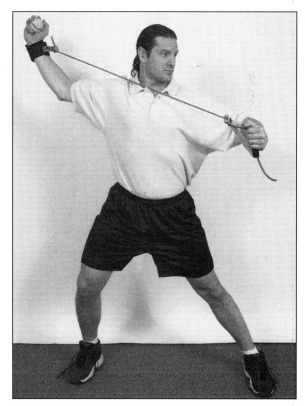

Figure 8.11-8.12 The "Flex-T" pitching drill: start position (8.11); release position (8.12).

Elastic Resistance and Agility Training

Earlier in this chapter, agility was defined as the ability to change direction without losing speed, strength, balance, and body control (Costello and Kreis 1993; Graham 2000; Twist and Benicky 1995). Costello and Kreis (1993) observed that there is a direct relationship between improved agility and athletic timing, rhythm, and movement. Other conditioning specialists (Graham 2000) have stated that agility is closely related to balance because it requires athletes to regulate dynamic changes in the body's center of gravity. Unlike sprinting, most sports demand quick, explosive burst of speeds with frequent changes in directions. A soccer player pulling to steal the opponent's ball and a basketball player cutting toward a pass exemplify two sport's requirements for athletic agility. Because most sports are games of multidirectional movement, agility training is essential to improve sport performance (Graham 2000). In addition, agility training can help prevent injury during sporting events. Studies have shown that female athletes are two to three times more likely than males to sustain noncontact anterior cruciate ligament (ACL) injuries (Hutchinson and Ireland 1995). High incidences of these noncontact ACL injuries occur in soccer and basketball programs. As one of the main stabilizing ligaments in the knee capsule, the ACL prevents anterior translation of the tibia on the femur. The ACL often is injured when the athlete twists the knee beyond its normal range of motion while pivoting, jumping, cutting, twisting, and jumping (Yap, Brown, and Woodman 2000). ACL injuries also tend to increase in college, because the level of sport competition becomes more demanding and athletes are forced to perform precise and automatic directional changes in an explosive manner. Agility drills may help the athlete develop and improve proprioception and kinesthetic sense. Improved kinesthetic sense allows the athlete to better understand the movements of his or her body. This heightened neuromuscular awareness may reduce the severity of an injury or even prevent an injury. Agility training drills incorporated during the season and off-season may help prevent these noncontact ligament injuries.

Agility Drills With Elastic Resistance

Programmable agility drills allow the athlete to know beforehand what movement combinations will be required. Examples of these types of agility drills include lateral shuffles, carioca, and figure-eight running. Elastic resistance can be used with these drills as a dynamic form of resistance to increase lower extremity strength and power. Balance is a very important part of agility training (Costello and Kreis 1993). Without adequate balance skills, athletes may not be able to maintain control of their bodies when quick directional changes are performed. The Fitter (figure 8.13), which uses four elastic cords for resistance, is an excellent device for sport-specific balance drills. Athletes using the Fitter should keep their knees bent and use an elastic tension that allows a controlled side-to-side motion to be performed. Ski poles can serve as balance aides when athletes are learning to use this agility training device.

Precautions for Using Elastic Devices During Agility Training

The precautions for resisted sprint training may be applied for agility training as well. It is key that ath-

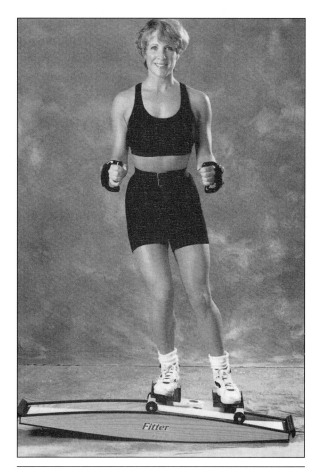

Figure 8.13   The Fitter®.

letes perform these drills without fatigue and with good form. Each drill should be performed at least once without elastic resistance after training to ensure carryover of the desired kinematics.

Periodization of Speed and Agility Training

Periodized training is a training plan that changes the workouts at regular intervals. Periodization is the gradual cycling of specificity, volume, intensity, duration, and frequency to achieve peak levels of sport-specific skills for the most important competitions (Davies et al. 1997; Fleck and Kraemer 1996; Wathen 1993). The traditional concept of periodization training usually manipulates the variables of volume, intensity, and skill training (Davies et al. 1997; Fleck and Kraemer 1996; Wathen 1993). The main reason for using periodized speed training is to prevent a plateau response during the athlete's competitive season. The theory behind periodization is that by manipulating the different strength, speed, and agility training variables throughout the year, a plateau response may be prevented. Year-round stimulation of the athlete is accomplished by establishing microcycles during the course of the training program. Cycles, as described in periodization programs, are accomplished by establishing long-term goals (macrocycles), intermediate goals, (mesocycles), and short-term goals (microcycles) for the athlete. Understanding the periodization model as the template of the athlete's progressively changing training program is an integral part of speed and agility training. The periodization speed training model also considers the sport the athlete is involved with, the speed-specific demands of the sport from a technical standpoint, and how to best integrate speed training to enhance athletic performance. Furthermore, the periodization model considers the time of the year such as preseason, in-season, and postseason and the need to peak for certain events. Manipulating the variables of volume, intensity, and skill training in a periodization model allows coaches to customize the speed and agility needs of each athlete at different times throughout their training cycles (Davies et al. 1997; Fleck and Kraemer 1996; Wathen 1993).

Conclusion

Speed and agility skills are paramount to successful athletic performance and the prevention of ath-

letic injury. For the best results, the speed and agility training program should be individualized as much as possible to the athlete and his or her sport. Assisted and resisted sprinting drills and stretch-shortening upper extremity drills always should be preceded by and coincide with other forms of resistance and flexibility training until an adequate foundation of strength and flexibility has been established. This needs to be done via the periodization model and by using common sense. Elastic resistance offers a dynamic method of enhancing speed and agility training. Several speed and agility drills for the athlete that incorporate elastic resistance have been shown in this chapter. The trainer and athlete should not feel limited to these drills alone. With its ability to provide resistance with sport-specific movements, elastic tubing may provide resistance for an unlimited amount of sport-specific speed and agility drills.

References

Allerheiligen, W.B., ed. 1994. "Speed Development and Plyometric Training." In *Essentials of Strength and Conditioning*, ed. T.R. Baechle. Champaign, IL: Human Kinetics.

Chu, D., ed. 1996. *Explosive Power & Strength*. Champaign, IL: Human Kinetics.

Chu, D., and R. Korchemny. 1989. "Sprinting Stride Actions." *National Strength and Conditioning Journal* 11(6): 6-8, 82-5.

Costello, F., and E.J. Kreis. 1993. *Sports Agility*. Nashville, TN: Taylor Sports.

Davies, G.J., M. Clark, D. Williams, K. Ward, V. Harding, R. Salinas, and M. Fortanasce. 1997. "Application of the Concepts of Periodization to Rehabilitation." Pp. 1-17 in *Sports Physical Therapy Section—APTA Home Study Course*, ed. W.D. Bandy. Alexandria, VA: American Physical Therapy Association.

Dintiman, G., B. Ward, and T. Tellez. 1997. *Sports Speed*. 2nd ed. Champaign, IL: Human Kinetics.

Faccioni, A. 1994a. "Assisted and Resisted Methods for Speed Development (Part I)." *Modern Athlete and Coach* 32(2): 3-6.

Faccioni, A. 1994b. "Assisted and Resisted Methods for Speed Development (Part II)." *Modern Athlete and Coach* 32(3): 8-11.

Fleck, S.J., and W.J. Kraemer. 1996. *Periodization Breakthrough*. Ronkonkoma, NY: Advanced Research Press.

Graham, J.F. 2000. "Agility Training." In *Training for Speed, Agility, and Quickness*, ed. L.E. Brown, V.A. Ferrigno, and J.C. Santana. Champaign, IL: Human Kinetics.

Harbin, G.L. Durst, and D. Harbin. 1989. "Evaluation of Oculomotor Response in Relationship to Sports Performance." *Medicine and Science in Sports and Exercise* 21(3): 258-62.

House, T. 1996. *Fit to Pitch*. Champaign, IL: Human Kinetics.

Hutchinson, M.R., and M.L. Ireland. 1995. "Knee Injuries in Female Athletes." *Sports Medicine* 1(4): 288-302.

Klinzing, J. 1984. "Improving Sprint Speed for All Athletes." *National Strength and Conditioning Association Journal* 6(4): 32-3.

Lentz, D., and A. Hardyk. 2000. "Speed training." In *Training for Speed, Agility, and Quickness,* ed. L.E. Brown, V.A. Ferrigno, and J.C. Santana. Champaign, IL: Human Kinetics.

Luhatenen, P., and P.V. Komi. 1978. "Mechanical Factors Influencing Running Speed." In *Biomechanics VI-B,* ed. E. Asmussen. Baltimore: University Park Press.

Mann, R. 1984. "Speed Development." *National Strength and Conditioning Association Journal* 5(6): 12-20, 72-3.

McFarlane, B. 1994. "Speed: A Basic and Advanced Technical Model." *Modern Athlete and Coach* 32(4): 11-4.

Mero, A., and P.V. Komi. 1986. "Force-, EMG-, and Elasticity-Velocity Relationships at Submaximal, Maximal and Supramaximal Running Speeds in Sprinters." *European Journal of Applied Physiology and Occupational Physiology* 55(5): 553-61.

Mero, A., P.V. Komi, H. Rusko, and J. Hirovenen. 1987. "Neuromuscular and Anaerobic Performance of Sprinters at Maximal and Supramaximal Speed." *International Journal of Sports Medicine* 8 (Suppl.): 55-60.

Pezzullo, D.J., S. Karas, and J.J. Irrgang. 1995. "Functional Plyometric Exercises for the Throwing Athlete." *Journal of Athletic Training* 30(1): 22-6.

Siff, M.C., ed. 2000. *Supertraining.* Denver: Supertraining Institute.

Treiber, F.A., J. Lott, J. Duncan, G. Slavens, and H. Davis. 1998. "Effects of Theraband® and Lightweight Dumbbell Training on Shoulder Rotation Torque and Serve Performance in College Tennis Players." *American Journal of Sports Medicine* 26(4): 510-5.

Twist, P.W., and D. Benicky. 1995. "Conditioning Lateral Movements for Multisport Athletes: Practical Strength and Quickness Drills." *Strength and Conditioning* 17(6): 43-51.

Voight, M.L. 1992. "Stretch-Strengthening: An Introduction to Plyometrics." *Orthopaedic Physical Therapy Clinics of North America* 1: 243-52.

Voss, D.E., M. Knott, and M. Kabat. 1953. "Application of Neuromuscular Facilitation in the Treatment of Shoulder Disabilities." *Physical Therapy Reviews* 33: 536-7.

Wathen, D. 1993. "Literature Review: Explosive/Plyometric Exercise." *National Strength and Conditioning Association Journal* 15: 17-8.

Wilk, K.E., and M.L. Voight. 1993. "Plyometrics for the Overhead Athlete." In *The Athletic Shoulder,* ed. J.R. Andrews and K.E. Wilk. New York: Churchill Livingstone.

Wilk, K.E., M. Voight, M. Keirns, V. Gambetta, J. Andrews, and C. Dillman. 1993. "Stretch-Shortening Drills for the Upper Extremities: Theory and Clinical Application." *Journal of Orthopaedic and Sports Physical Therapy* 17: 225-39.

Yap, C.W., L.E. Brown, and G. Woodman. 2000. "Development of Speed, Agility, and Quickness for the Female Soccer Athlete." *Strength and Conditioning* 22(1): 9-12.

CHAPTER 9

Reactive Neuromuscular Training With Elastic Resistance

Phillip Page, MS, PT, ATC, CSCS
Benchmark Physical Therapy, Baton Rouge, LA
The Hygenic Corporation

Balance and postural stability training have become popular interventions for injury prevention, fitness training, and rehabilitation. After injury or surgery, balance training helps restore function of the neuromuscular system for coordinated movement. Balance training is especially important in both athletes and older adults for performance and injury prevention. In particular, balance training is an important component of a fall prevention program in older adults (Tinetti et al. 1994).

Although elastic resistance is most commonly recognized as a resistance training device to improve strength, it can be used for balance training as well. Studies have demonstrated that elastic resistance strength training of the lower extremities improves balance (Docherty, Moore, and Arnold 1998; Duncan et al. 1998; Skelton and McLaughlin 1996; Topp et al. 1993). However, traditional strength training of muscles may not specifically target the neuromuscular system responsible for balance and coordinated movement. More recently, the specific use of elastic resistance for balance training was described as "reactive neuromuscular training" (RNT) (Cook, Barton, and Fields 1999). The purpose of this chapter is to provide a neurophysiological basis for balance training, the scientific basis for RNT, and a clinical progression of balance training with elastic resistance.

Neurophysiological Principles

Coordinated movement requires a constant interaction between the sensory and motor system. There are two basic pathways for neurological messages from the peripheral nervous system (PNS) to the central nervous system (CNS): the afferent system and the efferent system. These systems interact to provide certain levels of motor control from an unconscious, subconscious, or conscious level (table 9.01).

Afference

Afference is considered to be a sensory function. The afferent system consists of neuromuscular receptors in connective tissue, including receptors in musculotendinous structures (muscle spindles, Golgi tendon organs [GTO]) and receptors in capsuloligamentous tissue (joint mechanoreceptors). These receptors sense changes to the joint and muscle, and modify muscle tone through unconscious reflexes.

Table 9.01   Levels of Neuromuscular Control

Anatomic level	Sensory level	Functional level
Spinal reflex	Unconscious	Reflex joint stabilization
Lower brain	Subconscious	Postural control and righting reactions
Motor cortex	Conscious/unconscious	Coordinated movements

Efference

Efference is considered a motor function. There are two basic types of motor neurons: gamma and alpha motor neurons. Gamma motor neurons are responsible for unconscious control of the muscle. They work reflexively with the musculotendinous receptors and are responsible for resting tone and reflexive control of the muscles. Stimulation of mechanoreceptors in joint structures increases gamma motor activity, which may increase sensitivity of the muscle spindles in muscles surrounding the joint (Johansson, Sjolander, and Sojka 1991). Alpha motor neurons provide conscious control of muscle contraction. These motor neurons directly innervate groups of muscle fibers called motor units. Each motor unit is either facilitated (contracted) or inhibited (relaxed). The coordination of firing patterns of agonist and antagonistic muscles is essential for skilled and purposeful movement.

Proprioception

Proprioception is the cumulative afferent input from the PNS into the CNS, including information from the cutaneous, muscular, and joint receptors. There are two components of proprioception: kinesthesia and joint position sense (Lephart et al. 1997). The type of afferent receptor used characterizes each component.

Kinesthesia is an awareness of movement. Input from the musculotendinous receptors (muscle spindle and GTO) provides information on movement. In contrast, joint position sense is an awareness of position. Input from the joint mechanoreceptors provides information on joint position. Afferent information is then processed on one of three possible anatomic levels within the central nervous system (table 9.01): the spinal, lower brain, or motor cortex level (Biedert 2000). Once information is processed, an appropriate efferent response is mediated to the PNS.

Spinal Level Reflexes

When the muscle spindle is activated by a quick stretch, a reflexive facilitation in the muscle increases excitability via the gamma motor neurons. In contrast, a prolonged stretch activates the GTO to cause a reflexive inhibition or relaxation of the muscle. These activities occur only at the level of the spinal cord. The muscle spindles are also sensitive to joint mechanoreceptors, creating a reflex feedback loop. Stimulation of joint mechanoreceptors causes a reflexive spinal-mediated facilitation or inhibition in muscles surrounding the joint, thus directly influencing dynamic joint stabilization (Buchanan, Kim, and Lloyd 1996; Guanche et al. 1995; Kim et al. 1995).

Lower Brain

The lower brain encompasses the brain stem, cerebellum, and basal ganglia (Biedert 2000). Postural stability (the ability to maintain the center of gravity within the base of support) is maintained unconsciously at this level. Stability is maintained by automatic postural responses. Horak and Nashner (1986) described muscular synergies in response to postural sway on a flat surface. They found that the automatic postural response to forward sway consisted of concentric contraction of the paraspinals, hamstrings, and gastrocnemius. In contrast, a backward sway responded with automatic eccentric contraction of the abdominals, quadriceps, and tibialis anterior. Table 9.02 summarizes the characteristic reflexive and automatic postural responses to weight shifts.

Motor Cortex

The highest level of sensorimotor integration is within the cortex. At this level, kinesthesia and joint position sense are integrated to allow the body to perform coordinated movements. The cortex acts consciously to initiate movement or unconsciously to perform repetitive movements (Biedert 2000). Motor ingrams are stored within the motor cortex as preprogrammed

Table 9.02   Stabilizing Reflexive Reactions

Weight shift	Stabilizing reaction
Posterior weight shift	Trunk flexion Hip flexion Knee extension Ankle dorsiflexion
Anterior weight shift	Trunk extension Hip extension Knee flexion Ankle plantar flexion
Medial weight shift	Trunk side-bending Hip abduction Knee cocontraction Ankle eversion
Lateral weight shift	Trunk side-bending Hip adduction Knee cocontraction Ankle inversion

Data from F.B. Horak, and L.M. Nashner, 1986. "Central Programming of Postural Movements: Adaptation to Altered Support Surface Configurations." *Journal of Neurophysiology* 55: 1369-81.

subconscious repetitive movements. Therefore, the cortex acts in terms of movements rather than individual muscles.

Coordinated movement provides the ability to vary the type of muscular contraction and to coordinate and sequence movement with other body parts. This coordination is particularly important during changes in force production and reduction. When the athlete changes direction of motion, such as going from acceleration to deceleration, postural stability is required for efficient and coordinated movement. Optimal proprioceptive information and processing are crucial to restoring coordinated movement.

Balance Training

Neuromuscular coordination results from sensorimotor integration: an efferent response to peripheral afferent information resulting in purposeful movement. This coordination of information is important for joint stability, motor function, balance, postural stability, and coordinated movement.

Neuromuscular dysfunction occurs as a result of a disruption of the proprioceptive loops between afferent and efferent systems. These disruptions may be referred to as *deafferentation* or *de-efferentation* (Freeman, Dean, and Hanham 1965; Nitz, Dobner, and Kersey 1985). Commonly seen clinically as dynamic joint instability or movement impairments, these conditions may be caused by a number of

mechanisms. First, direct injury to the muscle or nerve may cause neuromuscular dysfunction. Joint effusion also may contribute to deafferentation (Spencer, Hayes, and Alexander 1984), thus inhibiting proper muscle function. More subtle disruptions in the proprioceptive loops are found in the cases of muscle imbalance and abnormal movement patterns.

Balance training is particularly important to prevent reinjury. Freeman, Dean, and Hanham (1965) used the term *functional instability* to describe joint instability resulting from injury to joint afferents that decreases balance and postural control. Individuals with functional instability may be more prone to reinjury. Balance training decreased the incidence of reinjury after acute ankle sprains (Holme et al. 1999), and decreased incidence of instability after ankle injury (Freeman, Dean, and Hanham 1965) and after anterior cruciate ligament tear (Fitzgerald, Axe, and Snyder-Mackler 2000).

Impairments in joint stability, motor function, balance, and postural stability require specialized interventions. The goal of balance training is to restore neuromuscular coordination by appropriately stimulating the maximal amount of afferent receptors to elicit a predictable physiological and functional response. This is done by progressively challenging the neuromuscular system to reestablish the reflex feedback loops, restore balance reactions and postural stability, and perform coordinated movement. Balance training should be initiated as soon as possible in the rehabilitation process.

Balance Training With Elastic Resistance

Tomaszewski (1991) first described the use of elastic resistance in balance training for ankle sprain rehabilitation. He used the term *T-Band kicks* to denote the use of Thera-Band elastic bands to resist hip motion of the uninvolved leg while the athlete balanced on the involved leg. Since then, several researchers have investigated the electromyographic responses during balance training with elastic resistance (Cordova, Jutte, and Hopkins 1999; Hopkins et al. 1999; Schulthies et al. 1998.). Cordova, Jutte, and Hopkins (1999) and Hopkins et al.(1999) found that elastic-resisted kicks induced greater muscle activity in the stance leg muscles compared with other types of balance training. Researchers (Hopkins et al. 1999; Schulthies et al. 1998) have noted reflexive actions in the stance leg during resisted kicking of the contralateral leg with elastic resistance (table 9.03). These reflexive muscular actions

## Table 9.03	Reflexive Muscle Activity to Elastic-Resisted Kicking

Kicking leg	Stance leg reflexive stabilization (electromyography)
Hip flexion	↑ Hamstrings
Hip extension	↑ Quadriceps
Hip abduction	↑ Lateral hamstrings
Hip adduction	↑ Medial hamstrings

Data from Hopkins, J.T., C.D. Ingersoll, M.A. Sandrey, and S.D. Bleggi, 1999. "An Electromyographic Comparison of 4 Closed Chain Exercises." *Journal of Athletic Training* 34(4): 353-7, and Schulthies, S.S., M.D. Ricard, K.J. Alexander, and J.W. Myrer, 1998. "An Electromyographic Investigation of 4 Elastic Tubing Closed Kinetic Chain Exercises After Anterior Cruciate Ligament Reconstruction." *Journal of Athletic Training* 33(4): 328-35.

are a result of automatic balance reactions to counteract changes in the center of gravity created by kicking against resistance.

Leiby and colleagues (1995) investigated the effect of T-Band kicks on hip strength of the stance leg. They reported that the stance leg gained significantly more strength than the exercise leg. Baker, Webright, and Perrin (1998) evaluated the effectiveness of T-Band kicks on healthy athletes and noted an improvement in postural stability, although not statistically significant from a control group. This may have been attributable to low training stimulus or a "ceiling effect" of balance training in athletic subjects.

Reactive Neuromuscular Training

T-Band kicks have progressed into the concept known as RNT, based on Newton's law of reaction: For every action, there is an equal and opposite reaction. Elastic resistance provides an extrinsic loading to stimulate appropriate stabilizing reactions and enhance proprioceptive pathways. The resistance imparts a weight shift to cause a predictable and reflexive reaction to maintain postural stability, therefore restoring the reflexive loops between receptors and muscles.

This approach restores the rapid and reflexive activation of the neuromuscular system that is important in protecting the joints, otherwise known as *dynamic stabilization*. By challenging the center of gravity, RNT is also used to teach better control and coordination during functional movements. Because of its newness, no clinical trials have evaluated the effectiveness of RNT. However, one case report (Cook, Burton, and Fields 1999) demonstrated the successful use of RNT in anterior cruciate ligament reconstruction.

RNT Progression

When prescribing a balance training intervention, the clinician should be concerned with control of movement rather than training volume (sets, reps, and resistance). Signs of fatigue or abnormal movement patterns, rather than repetitions or resistance, should indicate training volume. Proper posture and quality of movement are much more important than quantity of movement. Balance activities should be performed with bare feet to take advantage of the large number of receptors in the soles of the feet.

RNT has three stages: static, dynamic, and functional (table 9.04). Within each stage, the individual is progressed by changing the direction and magnitude of the weight shift as well as the base of support. The complexity and speed of the associated movement also can be progressed during exercise. Implements can be added to increase the difficulty of the exercise. In addition, the eyes can be progressed from open to closed to increase the challenge to the neuromuscular system.

Static

During the static phase, the individual remains stationary while the elastic resistance imparts a force to create a weight shift with minimal joint motion. Because of its relative safety, this activity can be performed very early in rehabilitation within weight-bearing limitations. This teaches the individual the relationship of gravity to his or her own center of gravity in preparation for postural stability and gait. Weight shifts created by the elastic resistance are progressed from the sagittal plane to the frontal plane. First, the sagittal plane is challenged with a posterior weight shift (PWS; figure 9.01) and an anterior weight shift (AWS; figure 9.02). It is important to note that the weight shift is defined by the direction of the force, not the reaction of the body. Characteristic reflexive stabilization during a PWS consists of trunk flexion, hip flexion, knee extension, and ankle dorsiflexion, whereas an AWS creates trunk extension, hip extension, knee flexion, and ankle plantar flexion (table 9.02).

Next, the frontal plane is challenged with a medial weight shift (MWS; figure 9.03) or lateral weight shift (LWS; figure 9.04). These are defined by the direction of the weight shift in relation to an injured extremity. Reflexive stabilization during a

Table 9.04   Reactive Neuromuscular Training Progression

Stage	Challenge	Base of support	Activity
Static	Stance	Bilateral → unilateral → foam	Weight shifts
Dynamic	Upper extremity motion	Bilateral → unilateral → foam	Upper extremity exercises: Planar → diagonal No resistance → elastic resistance
	Lower extremity motion	Unilateral → foam	Leg kicks: sagittal plane → frontal plane → diagonal No resistance → elastic resistance
	Oscillation	Bilateral → unilateral → foam	Oscillation device + weight shifts
	Perturbation	Bilateral → unilateral → foam	Wobble board + weight shifts Weighted ball toss + weight shifts
Functional	Squat	Bilateral → unilateral → foam	Weight shifts
	Lunge	Unilateral → foam	Weight shifts
	Jog		Weight shifts
	Laterals		Weight shifts
	Plyometrics	Bilateral → unilateral	Weight shifts

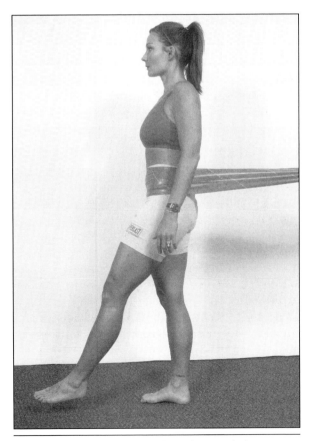

Figure 9.01   Static phase: unilateral, sagittal plane posterior weight shift.

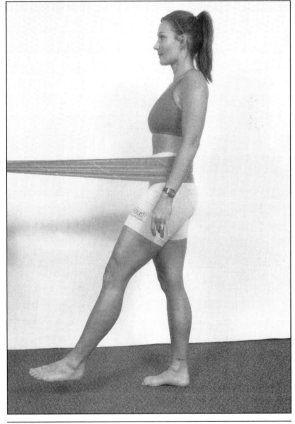

Figure 9.02   Static phase: unilateral, sagittal plane anterior weight shift.

147

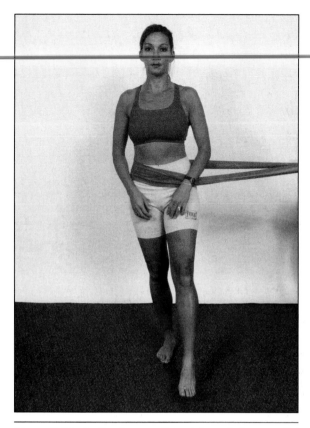

Figure 9.03 Static phase: unilateral, frontal plane medial weight shift.

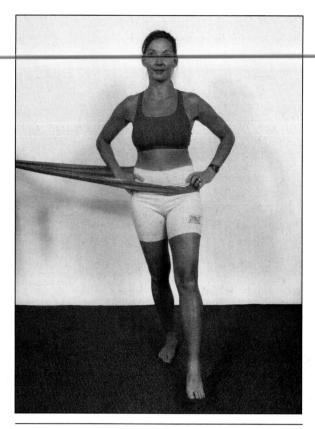

Figure 9.04 Static phase: unilateral, frontal plane lateral weight shift.

balance reaction for an MWS consists of trunk side-bending, hip abduction, knee cocontraction, and ankle eversion. The reaction for a LWS is trunk side-bending, hip adduction, knee cocontraction, and ankle inversion.

The individual also may increase the degree of weight shift by increasing the stretch on the elastic band or tubing. As the athlete's control of the center of gravity improves, resistance of the band or tubing can be increased. Once the individual is able to maintain postural stability with these weight shifts, the base of support is challenged: Exercises are progressed from bilateral stance to unilateral stance and then to stance on a compliant surface such as foam. Exercises also can be performed with the eyes open or closed for more challenge to postural stability.

Dynamic

The next progression of RNT is the dynamic phase. Static weight shifts in the sagittal and frontal planes are combined with extremity movement or dynamic challenges. The amount of extremity movement can progress from limited to full range of motion with resistance. The base of support also is progressed

from bilateral to unilateral stance to standing on foam. The speed of the activities can be progressed toward more functional velocities. During the dynamic phase, five general classifications of balance exercise are performed.

Upper Extremity.

Upper extremity motions begin without resistance in cardinal planes and are progressed to diagonal motions. These motions then are progressed by adding elastic resistance in the sagittal, frontal (figure 9.05), and diagonal (figure 9.06) planes. Upper extremity activities can be performed bilaterally or unilaterally. In addition, the base of support is progressed from bilateral to unilateral to standing on foam, and eyes are progressed from open to closed.

Lower Extremity.

Lower extremity motion also is progressed from planar kicking motions to diagonal kicking motions. Each kicking motion creates a reflexive reaction caused by the weight shift (table 9.03). Elastic resistance is added for progression (figures 9.07 and 9.08). The base of support for the stance leg also can be challenged with foam. The eyes can be closed for more challenge.

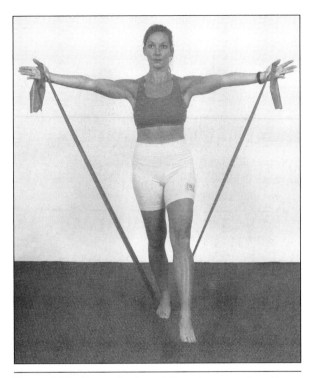

Figure 9.05 Dynamic phase: bilateral upper extremity exercise in frontal plane in unilateral stance.

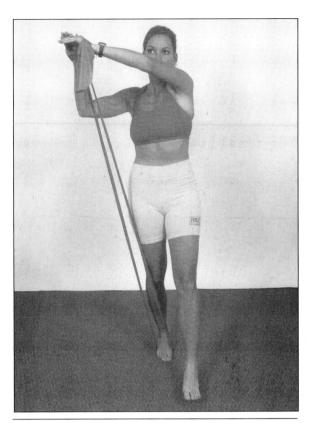

Figure 9.06 Dynamic phase: bilateral upper extremity exercise in diagonal plane in unilateral stance.

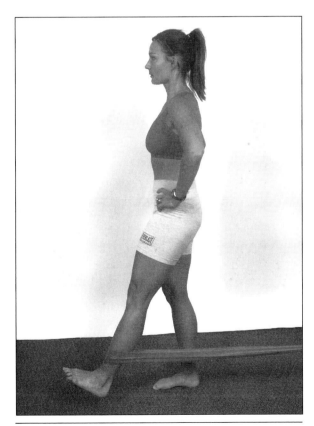

Figure 9.07 Dynamic phase: lower extremity posterior weight shift.

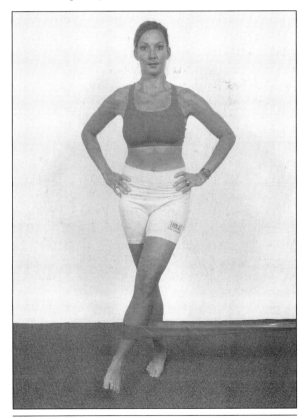

Figure 9.08 Dynamic phase: lower extremity lateral weight shift.

Weighted Balls.

Implements such as weighted balls are used to impart dynamic weight shifts in addition to the static weight shifts of the elastic resistance. For example, throwing a weighted ball forward creates a reactive posterior weight shift that must be stabilized reflexively to maintain balance (figure 9.09). This is because the individual must overcome the inertia of the implement to impart acceleration. If the weighted balls are also caught by the individual (such as tossing at a mini-trampoline), a posterior weight shift must also be stabilized reflexively to maintain balance. The weight of the ball can be progressively increased for challenge. The base of support also can be progressed with the weighted ball toss from bilateral stance to unilateral stance and to standing on foam.

Oscillation.

Recently, oscillatory equipment (FlexBar, Boing) has been used in conjunction with balance training. With this technique, weight shifts are created with elastic resistance in different directions while the individual holds onto an oscillatory device (figure 9.10). Oscillatory equipment also works on the basis of inertia. By quickly accelerating and decelerating the hand-held device within a small range of motion, the individual must maintain balance as the direction of inertia changes. Oscillation training occurs at a certain frequency or rate based on the excursion of the device. This rate can be increased for more challenge to control the center of gravity.

Perturbation.

Another progressive challenge to balance training involving weight shifts is perturbation training. In conjunction with elastic-resisted weight shifts, an unstable surface such as a wobble board can be used to quickly displace the base of support (figure 9.11). During RNT, the elastic resistance also can be used to quickly perturb the center of gravity by repetitively and quickly stretching the band or tubing attached to the individual. External perturbations by the clinician can also be implemented.

Functional

The final stage of balance training incorporates functional movements. These functional movements are performed with progressive weight shifts and progressive challenges to the base of support. Again, the eyes can also be progressed from open to closed to increase the challenge.

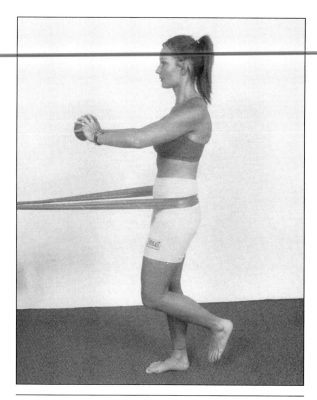

Figure 9.09 Dynamic phase: weighted ball toss with unilateral anterior weight shift.

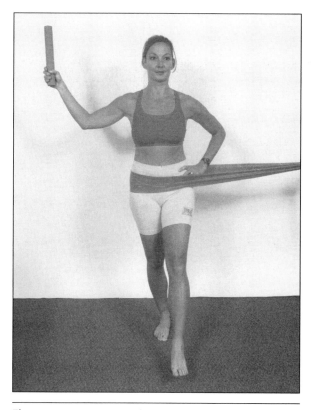

Figure 9.10 Dynamic phase: oscillation with FlexBar in frontal plane and unilateral medial weight shift.

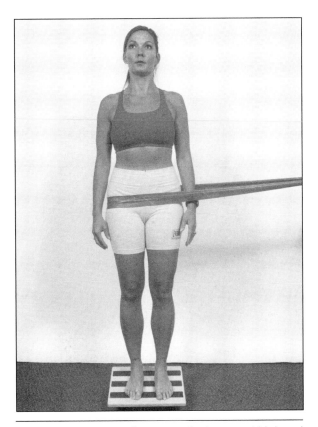

Figure 9.11 Dynamic phase: perturbation on wobble board and bilateral stance with medial weight shift.

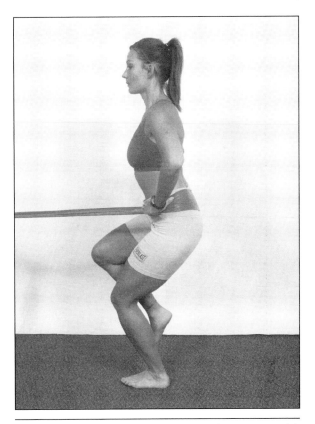

Figure 9.12 Functional phase: unilateral mini-squat with anterior weight shift.

Squat.

A mini-squat is performed first with sagittal plane weight shifts (AWS, PWS). Frontal plane weight shifts (MWS, LWS) are then performed. The base of support is progressed from bilateral stance to unilateral stance (figure 9.12) and finally to standing on foam. The depth of the squat also can be increased as the individual progresses.

Lunge.

A lunge performed with an AWS (figure 9.13) is considered to be a "resisted" lunge, whereas a PWS lunge (figure 9.14) is considered an "assisted" lunge. Frontal plane weight shifts (MWS, LWS) are then performed with a lunge. Lunging onto foam can be used as a progression.

Run/Jog.

For athletic rehabilitation and performance enhancement, balance during running and agility is important. Weight shifts are first imparted with a stationary running motion. Stationary running with a PWS simulates acceleration (figure 9.15), whereas an AWS simulates deceleration (figure 9.16). Medial and lateral weight shifts then can be implemented

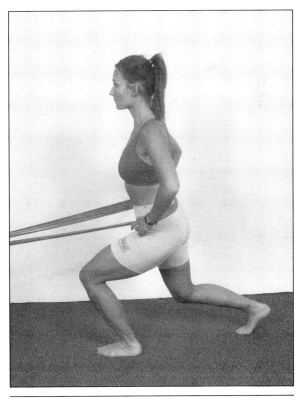

Figure 9.13 Functional phase: resisted lunge with anterior weight shift.

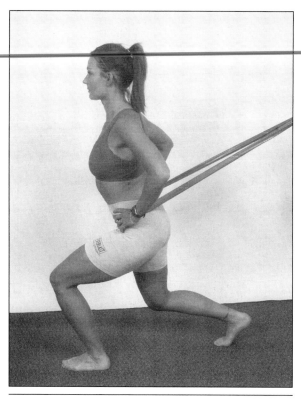

Figure 9.14 Functional phase: assisted lunge with posterior weight shift.

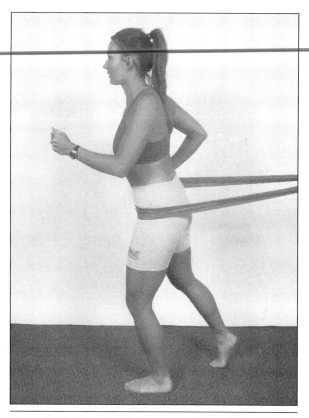

Figure 9.15 Functional phase: posterior weight shift with jogging.

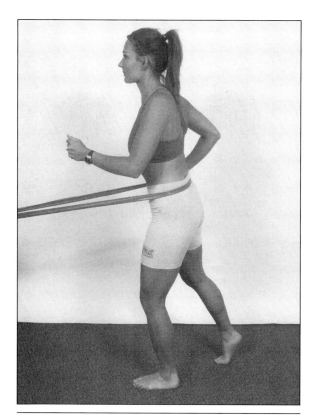

Figure 9.16 Functional phase: anterior weight shift with jogging.

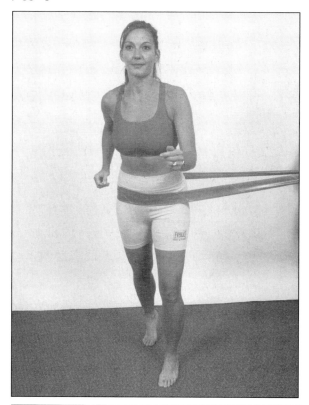

Figure 9.17 Functional phase: medial weight shift with jogging (relative to right leg).

with stationary running to simulate agility. Jogging in place with an MWS, for example, simulates cutting away from the injured extremity (figure 9.17); an LWS simulates cutting toward the injured extremity (figure 9.18). Stationary running motion can be progressed to assisted or resisted running against elastic resistance.

Laterals.

Elastic resistance can be used to impart weight shifts to resist or assist a lateral shuffle exercise. The resisted lateral shuffle emphasizes concentric control (figure 9.19), whereas the assisted lateral shuffle emphasizes eccentric control. The direction of the weight shift (MWS or LWS) is defined by the involved extremity. An AWS or a PWS also can be used with lateral movements (figure 9.20).

Plyometrics.

The final progression for RNT is plyometric training. This is particularly important for athletes returning to jumping activities. Vertical hops and jumps are performed with weight shifts created by elastic resistance (figure 9.21). These are progressed from bilateral to unilateral.

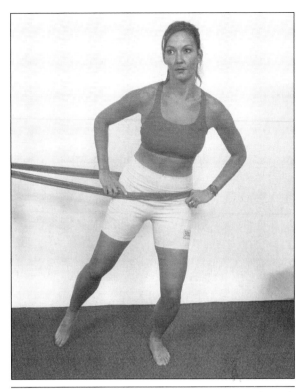

Figure 9.19 Functional phase: resisted lateral shuffle with medial weight shift (relative to left leg).

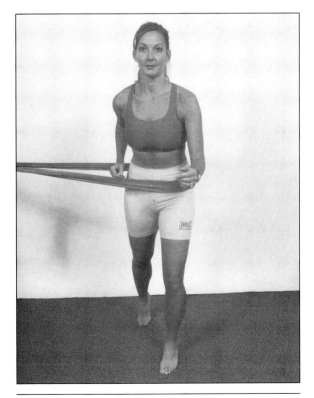

Figure 9.18 Functional phase: lateral weight shift with jogging (relative to right leg).

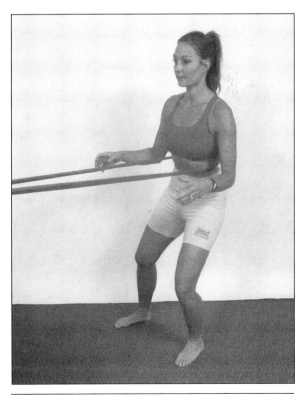

Figure 9.20 Functional phase: lateral shuffle with anterior weight shift.

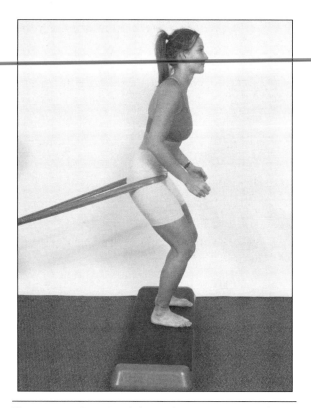

Figure 9.21 Functional phase: plyometric jumps with posterior weight shift.

Conclusion

Elastic resistance can be a valuable tool in balance training. When specific weight shifts are imparted, reflexive dynamic stabilizing reactions can be created. Other equipment can be used to increase challenges to the neuromuscular system, including foam pads, wobble boards, weighted balls, and oscillation devices. These balance reactions are necessary for proper function, optimal performance, and prevention of injury. Although there is some evidence to support these interventions, we should continue to study their use in improving balance impairments and functional ability.

References

Baker, A.G., W.G. Webright, and D.H. Perrin. 1998. "Effect of a 'T-Band' Kick Training Protocol on Postural Sway." *Journal of Sport Rehabilitation* 7: 122-7.

Biedert, R.M. 2000. "Contribution of the Three Levels of Nervous System Motor Control: Spinal Cord, Lower Brain, Cerebral Cortex." Pp. 23-30 in *Proprioception and Neuromuscular Control in Joint Stability*, ed. S.M. Lephart and F.H. Fu. Champaign, IL: Human Kinetics.

Buchanan, T.S., A.W. Kim, and D.G. Lloyd. 1996. "Selective Muscle Activation Following Rapid Varus/Valgus Perturbations at the Knee." *Medicine and Science in Sports and Exercise* 28(7): 870-6.

Cook, G., L. Burton, and K. Fields. 1999. "Reactive Neuromuscular Training for the Anterior Cruciate Ligament-Deficient Knee. A Case Report." *Journal of Athletic Training* 4(2): 194-201.

Cordova, M.L., L.S. Jutte, and J.T. Hopkins. 1999. "EMG Comparison of Selected Ankle Rehabilitation Exercises." *Journal of Sport Rehabilitation* 8: 209-18.

Docherty, C.L., J.H. Moore, and B.L. Arnold. 1998. "Effects of Strength Training on Strength Development and Joint Position Sense in Functionally Unstable Ankles." *Journal of Athletic Training* 33(4): 310-4.

Duncan, P., L. Richards, D. Wallace, J. Stoker-Yates, P. Pohl, C. Luchies, A. Ogle, and S. Studenski. 1998. "A Randomized, Controlled Pilot Study of a Home-Based Exercise Program for Individuals With Mild and Moderate Stroke." *Stroke* 29: 2055-60.

Fitzgerald, G.K., M.J. Axe, and L. Snyder-Mackler. 2000. "The Efficacy of Perturbation Training in Nonoperative Anterior Cruciate Ligament Rehabilitation Programs for Physically Active Individuals." *Physical Therapy* 80(2): 128-40.

Freeman, M.A.R., M.R.E. Dean, and I.W.F. Hanham. 1965. "The Etiology and Prevention of Functional Instability of the Foot." *Journal of Bone and Joint Surgery* 47B: 678-85.

Guanche, C.A., T. Knatt, M. Solomonow, R.V. Baratta, and Y. Lu. 1995. "The Synergistic Action of the Capsule and the Shoulder Muscles." *American Journal of Sports Medicine* 23: 301-6.

Holme, E., S.P. Magnusson, K. Becher, T. Bieler, P. Aagaard, and M. Kjaer. 1999. "The Effect of Supervised Rehabilitation on Strength, Postural Sway, Position Sense and Re-Injury Risk After Acute Ankle Ligament Sprain." *Scandinavian Journal of Medicine and Science in Sports* 9: 104-9.

Hopkins, J.T., C.D. Ingersoll, M.A. Sandrey, and S.D. Bleggi. 1999. "An Electromyographic Comparison of 4 Closed Chain Exercises." *Journal of Athletic Training* 34(4): 353-7.

Horak, F.B., and L.M. Nashner. 1986. "Central Programming of Postural Movements: Adaptation to Altered Support Surface Configurations." *Journal of Neurophysiology* 55: 1369-81.

Johansson, H., P. Sjolander, and P. Sojka. 1991. "A Sensory Role for the Cruciate Ligaments." *Clinical Orthopaedics* 268: 161-78.

Kim, A.W., A.M. Rosen, V.A. Brander, and T.S. Buchanan. 1995. "Selective Muscle Activation Following Electrical Stimulation of the Collateral Ligaments of the Human Knee." *Archives of Physical Medicine and Rehabilitation* 76: 750-7.

Leiby, K.W., P.J. Neece, S.H. Phipps, and C.J. Hughes. 1995. "A Comparison of Two Methods of Resistance Training on Ipsilateral/Contralateral Hip Abduction Strength" (Abstract). *Journal of Orthopaedic and Sports Physical Therapy* 21(1): 52.

Lephart, S.M., D.M. Pincivero, J.L. Giraldo, and F.H. Fu. 1997. "The Role of Proprioception in the Management and Rehabilitation of Athletic Injuries." *American Journal of Sports Medicine* 25(1): 130-7.

Nitz, A.J., J.J. Dobner, and D. Kersey. 1985. "Nerve Injury and Grades II and III Ankle Sprains." *American Journal of Sports Medicine* 13: 177-82.

Schulthies, S.S., M.D. Ricard, K.J. Alexander, and J.W. Myrer. 1998. "An Electromyographic Investigation of 4 Elastic Tubing Closed Kinetic Chain Exercises After Anterior Cruciate Ligament Reconstruction." *Journal of Athletic Training* 33(4): 328-35.

Skelton, D.A., and A.W. McLaughlin. 1996. "Training Functional Ability in Old Age." *Physiotherapy* 82(3): 159-67.

Spencer, J.K., K.C. Hayes, and I.J. Alexander. 1984. "Knee Joint Effusion and Quadriceps Reflex Inhibition in Man." *Archives of Physical Medicine and Rehabilitation* 65: 171-7.

Tinetti, M.E., D.I. Baker, G. McAvay, E.B. Claus, P. Garrett, M. Gottschalk, M.L. Koch, K. Trainor, and R.I. Horwitz. 1994. "A Multifactorial Intervention to Reduce the Risk of Falling Among Elderly People Living in the Community." *New England Journal of Medicine* 331(13): 821-7.

Tomaszewski, D. 1991. "'T-Band Kicks' Ankle Proprioception Program." *Athletic Training* 26(3): 216-9.

Topp, R.A., A. Mikesky, J. Wigglesworth, W. Holt, and J.E. Edwards. 1993. "The Effect of a 12-Week Dynamic Resistance Strength Training Program on Gait Velocity and Balance of Older Adults." *Gerontologist* 33(4): 501-6.

CHAPTER 10

Fitness Programs With Elastic Resistance

• • • • •

Terri Mitchell, PTA

Austin, Texas

Strength training is an important fitness component that can significantly improve a person's functional health, appearance, resistance to injury, and sport performance. Everyday activities that require muscular strength include climbing stairs, lifting a bag of groceries, or simply moving one's body or limb against a force (such as gravity). A listing of fitness classes offered at most health clubs, however, indicates an emphasis on aerobic conditioning. Although the cardiorespiratory endurance component of fitness is important for decreasing heart disease risk, lowering blood pressure, reducing bad cholesterol, and providing other healthful benefits, adding effective strength training exercises is recommended for quality exercise programs (ACSM 2000).

Muscle Balance

The muscles in the body are arranged in opposing pairs to create movement. When one muscle in the pair is stronger than the other, muscle imbalance occurs, which leads to improper body alignment or possible injury. Muscle imbalance distorts alignment and sets the stage for undue stress and strain on joints, ligaments, and muscles (Kendall et al. 1993). For example, we use our arms in front of our body to lift, carry, eat, drive, and work on the computer. This causes the development of stronger and shorter anterior deltoids and pectorals (front of shoulder) compared with the posterior deltoids and rotator cuff (back of shoulder). Hours of sitting at a desk with slumped posture can further aggravate this muscle imbalance by weakening and stretching the posterior deltoids, middle trapezius, and rhomboids. This in turn produces rounded shoulders with tight pectoralis major, latissimus dorsi, and anterior deltoid (Clippinger-Robertson 1989). Correction involves strengthening the upper back and stretching the chest. To promote flexibility, joint stability, and muscle balance, the fitness professional must include exercises that strengthen and stretch the muscle pairs appropriately.

Benefits of Strength Training

According to the American College of Sports Medicine (ACSM 2000), the functional benefits of strength training include the following:

- Improved muscular strength and power—muscles play a key role in determining the ability to perform activities of daily living at home, work, and play.

- Improved posture—keeping muscles strong can help prevent back pain.
- Improved specificity for sport performance—strength training enhances an individual's ability to perform a variety of athletics-related skills.
- Increased metabolic rate to help decrease body fat—the amount of lean muscle mass helps determine basal metabolic rate, which in turn affects the number of calories burned with exercise (Heyward 1997).
- Increased bone mass—strength training strengthens bones as well as muscles.
- Improved balance and coordination—strength training can improve coordination and increase the effective strength of the muscles by making the resultant movements more efficient (Bird 1992).

To be fully effective, the strength program should use equipment. This promotes the characteristics desired while providing variation of training stimulus (Heyward 1997). In other words, provide exercises of appropriate intensity so that muscular strength and muscular endurance improve while injuries are avoided (Clippinger-Robertson 1989).

Types of Resistance Exercise

In traditional strength training, athletes achieve adequate overload by adding external resistance such as free weights, wall pulleys, or weight machines. In fitness or aerobics classes, the increased overload is achieved with light weights, elastic bands, or tubes, in conjunction with slower reps, increased range of motion (ROM), or isometric contractions (Love 1995).

Using hand-held weights for strength training requires storage for the equipment, an inventory of different weights to accommodate different fitness levels, constant cueing, and perhaps supervision of participants to ensure proper form. Weight machines can be intimidating to participants and require space with an adequate supply of machines for class participants. Because elastic bands are portable, are inexpensive, and can be used in the seated, standing, supine, or prone position, professional fitness instructors, personal trainers, or therapists can incorporate many beneficial strengthening exercises into classes by using elas-

tic resistance equipment. Exercises that use elastic resistance bands or tubes also can complement a variety of aerobic programs including step, hi-lo, kickboxing, circuit training, abdominal classes, and water fitness classes.

Elastic resistance usually is provided in a color-coded progression from light to heavy resistance. For example, the color sequence for Thera-Band exercise bands is tan, yellow, red, green, blue, black, silver, and gold. Thera-Band exercise tubing follows the same sequence, with a range in colors from yellow to silver. Therefore, elastic resistance bands or tubes can accommodate exercisers of varying ages and abilities.

Goals of Resistance Exercise

Strength training must be specific, which means that exercises should relate to the demands of performance. In other words, athletes should perform a particular exercise for a specific reason. The goals of resistance exercise are as follows:

- Increase muscle size and strength. This refers to the maximum amount of force a muscle or group of muscles can generate in a single maximum contraction.
- Increase muscular endurance. This refers to the individual's capacity to repeat or sustain muscular contractions over time.
- Improve flexibility, or the ability of the limbs to move at the joints through a normal range of motion. Strength training encourages performing each exercise through the entire ROM.
- Improve body composition, which is the body's relative percentage of fat compared with lean tissue. Dynamic resistance training is effective for decreasing percentage body fat and increasing fat-free mass of men and women (Heyward 1997).

Guidelines for Resistance Exercise

The ACSM (2000) has determined standard guidelines for resistance training for apparently healthy individuals:

- Perform a minimum of 8 to 10 separate exercises that train the major muscle groups.
- Perform 1 set of 8 to 12 repetitions of each of these exercises to the point of fatigue.

- Perform these exercises at least 2 days per week.
- Adhere as closely as possible to the specific techniques for performing a given exercise.
- Perform every exercise through a full ROM.
- Perform both the lifting (concentric phase) and lowering (eccentric phase) portion of the resistance exercises in a controlled manner.
- Maintain a normal breathing pattern, because breath holding can increase blood pressure excessively.
- If possible, exercise with a training partner who can provide feedback, assistance, and motivation (instructor, personal trainer, therapist, friend).

In addition to the ACSM guidelines, the following should be considered by the fitness professional:

- Understand the body's anatomy and work all the major muscles to prevent muscle imbalance.
- Promote proper form with each movement.
- Emphasize working from a neutral pelvis position to stabilize the trunk and create good posture during each movement.
- Begin each class with a 5- to 7-min warm-up of rhythmic exercises.
- Promote control and quality of movement, rather than quantity.
- Use the principle of progressive overload.

The ACSM's guidelines (2000) are simple and basic. Following these guidelines does not require a lot of time. Including strength training in an aerobics/fitness class may take 10 to 20 min, based on the goals of the class, the participants' ability level, and the length of the class.

Elastic Resistance Recommendations for Fitness

Following are some recommendations for using elastic resistance for muscular strength training or muscular endurance exercises in aerobics/fitness classes:

- The fitness professional or instructor must provide appropriate resistance, cues for proper technique, and options of resistance training to meet the needs of the participants.

- Use low resistance and high reps in beginner classes, emphasizing muscular endurance. Gradually increase resistance and decrease or maintain reps as students adapt to the workload. This uses the principle of progressive overload.
- Maintain exercise at a higher resistance in intermediate or advanced classes.
- Combine higher and lower resistances by varying the colored bands or tubes, and alternate muscular strengthening with muscular endurance exercises within the same workout.
- Emphasize a specific fitness component based on the participant's ability and skill level as well as the fitness professional's aptitude.
- The participant should mimic movements done with free weights and machines when using the bands and should maintain similar form with bands as with weights.
- The participant should avoid using momentum but focus on "squeezing" the working muscles with every repetition.
- Adjust the band or tubing so there is resistance through the full range of motion, preventing any slack in the band or tubing.

Exercises With Elastic Resistance

All major muscle groups can be exercised with elastic resistance as effectively as with machines or free weights. Foot placement, length of elastic resistance, and tautness of elastic resistance will determine the intensity of the exercise. When the feet are close together, or if only one foot is used, the intensity is less (Mantia 1995). Moving the feet apart, shortening the length of the band or tube, and increasing the tautness will increase intensity. Basic exercises with elastic resistance are listed next:

- Biceps (figure 10.01)
- Triceps (figure 10.02)
- Anterior shoulder/pectoralis (figure 10.03)
- Posterior shoulder/ upper back (figure 10.04)
- Quadriceps and gluteus (figure 10.05)
- Gluteals (figure 10.06)
- Latissimus (figures 10.07 and 10.08)
- Anterior tibialis (figure 10.09)
- Gastrocnemius (figure 10.10)
- Trunk extensors (figures 10.11 and 10.12)

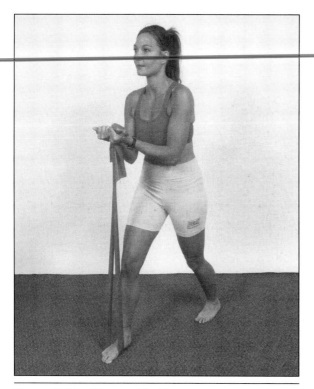

Figure 10.01 Elbow curl for biceps.

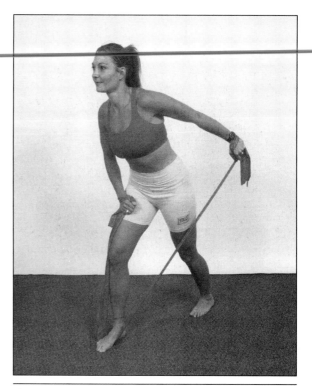

Figure 10.02 Elbow press for triceps.

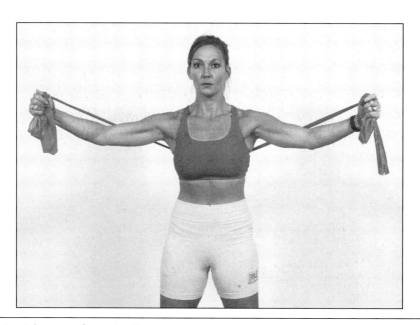

Figure 10.03 Horizontal squeeze for pectoralis.

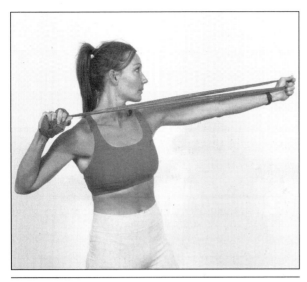

Figure 10.04 Archery pull for posterior shoulder.

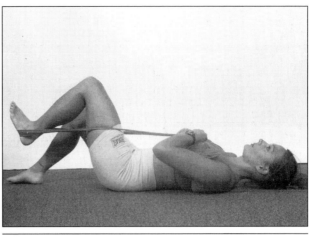

Figure 10.05 Leg press for glutes and quads.

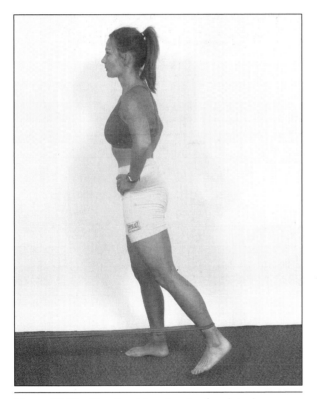

Figure 10.06 Standing hip extension for gluteals.

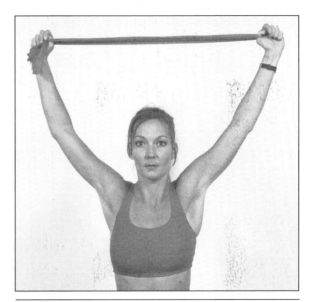

Figure 10.07 Lat pull-down for latissimus (start position).

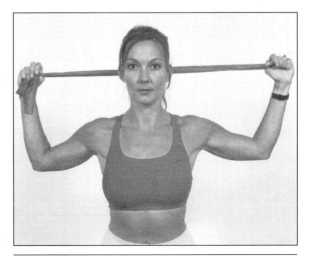

Figure 10.08 Lat pull-down for latissimus (end position).

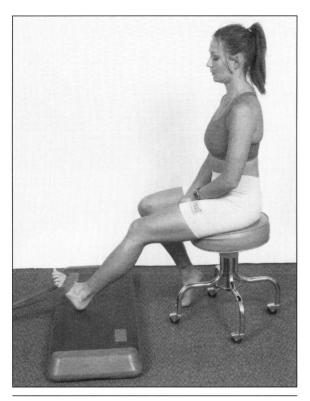

Figure 10.09 Ankle dorsiflexion for anterior tibilias.

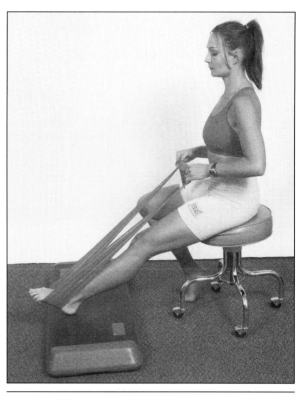

Figure 10.10 Ankle plantar flexion for gastrocnemius.

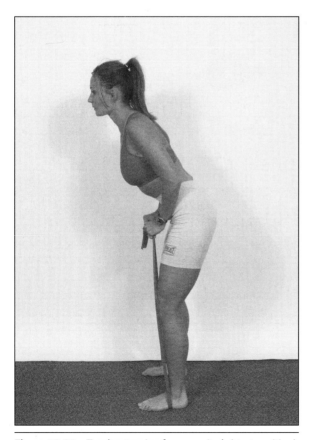

Figure 10.11 Trunk extension for paraspinals (start position).

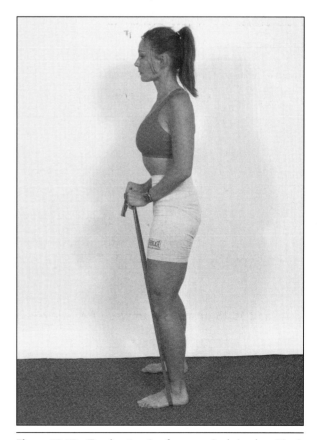

Figure 10.12 Trunk extension for paraspinals (end position).

Specific Fitness Programs That Use Elastic Resistance

Applying elastic resistance training to fitness programs such as a step class, a circuit format, or a hi-lo aerobics class with a partner can provide effective strength training exercises and add variety to current programs. For participants who prefer the water, elastic resistance bands or tubes can be taken into the pool.

The number of exercises is endless. The exercise professional must understand muscle balance, use imagination, be safe, have fun, and follow ACSM guidelines. The following are some ideas to try in certain fitness settings.

Integration With the Step

Use the step as a tool to assist and provide variety for lower and upper body exercises. For example, a step-up with resistance (figure 10.13) can be used for lower body training, whereas a bench press with resistance (figure 10.14) can be used for upper body training.

Integration With Circuit Training Format

Circuit classes could include as few as 5 or as many as 15 stations depending on time, space, and structure of the class. The goal is to complete as many repetitions (15-20) as possible within a specified duration at each station to fatigue the specific muscle or muscle group being worked (Filer 1995). The next station should work a different muscle or muscle group, alternating between aerobic and strengthening stations. Two examples of strength stations are provided in Figures 10.15 and 10.16.

Integration With a Partner

Elastic resistance training with a partner can add fun and motivation to the exercise session. Figures 10.17 and 10.18 provide examples of elastic resistance training with partners.

Therarobics

Fitness and therapy experts from Switzerland and Germany developed a workout that combines the popularity of aerobics with the versatility of elastic bands, called Therarobics (Cumming 1998). This

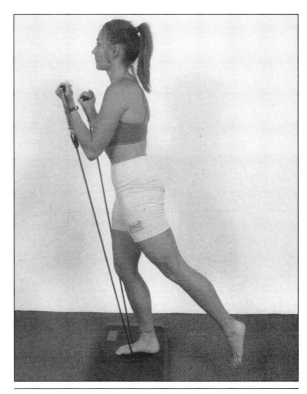

Figure 10.13   Step-up with biceps curl.

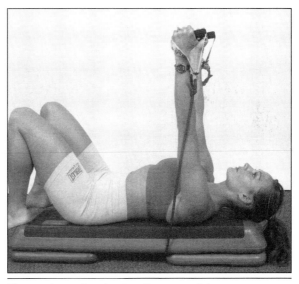

Figure 10.14   Bench press (for pectoralis).

program incorporates multiple joint and externally rotated movements to improve body posture, muscle balance, and movement. Secured to specially developed attachments for arms and feet (figure 10.19), the elastic resistance offers full freedom of movement as well as resistance for muscular workouts. Sample exercises are provided in figures 10.20 through 10.22. The arm movements can be performed alone or with added dynamic movements

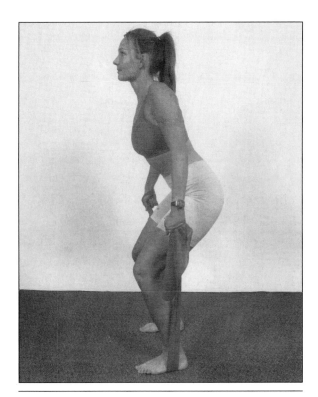

Figure 10.15   Squats for glutes, quads, gastrocs.

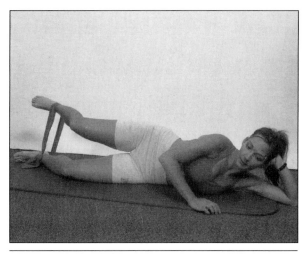

Figure 10.16   Hip abduction for gluteus medius.

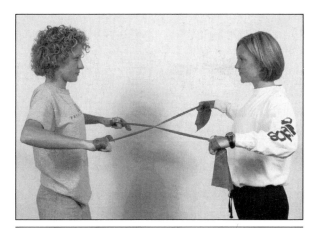

Figure 10.18   Partner pull.

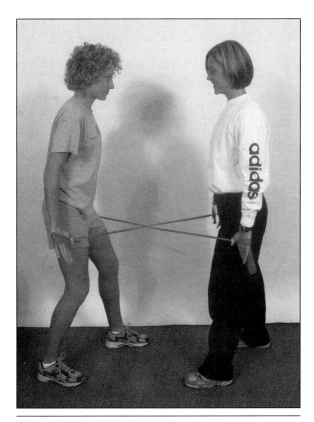

Figure 10.17   Partner extension.

of the legs to increase cardiorespiratory endurance as well as resistance in the lower extremities. Adding a directional component (forward, backward, sideways) to the leg movements further increases intensity.

Power in the Pool Program

The Power in the Pool (PIP) program was designed to use elastic bands in the pool. Although using bands or tubes in the water does not necessarily use the physical properties of buoyancy, hydrostatic pressure, or turbulence, the density of the water itself creates additional resistance to submerged elastic resistive bands or tubes (Lindle 1998). Elastic resistance can add variety and strength training to an aquatic fitness program. The emphasis is on trunk stabilization and strengthening. The PIP

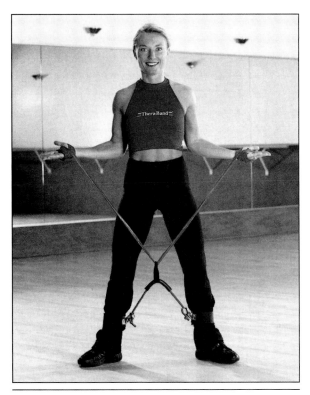

Figure 10.19 Therarobics assembly.
Reprinted by permission from The Hygenic Corporation.

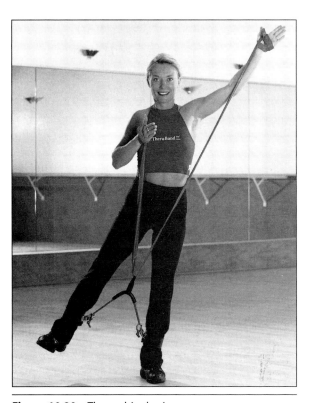

Figure 10.20 Therarobics basic move.
Reprinted by permission from The Hygenic Corporation.

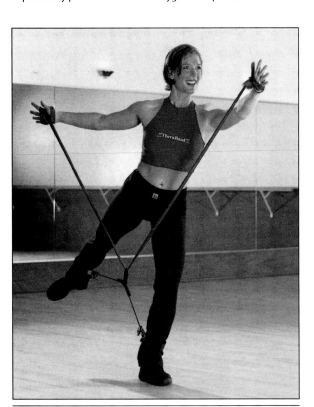

Figure 10.21 Therarobics diagonal move.
Reprinted by permission from The Hygenic Corporation.

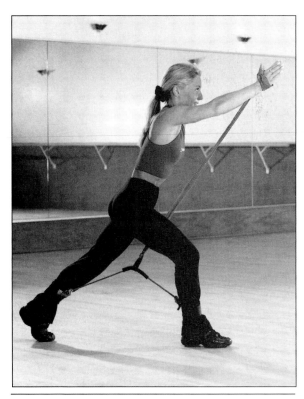

Figure 10.22 Therarobics lunge.
Reprinted by permission from The Hygenic Corporation.

program can be done as an aerobic format, as a strengthening segment, or as circuit training. Before beginning the PIP program, the participant should perform a proper warm-up without the bands, making sure to prestretch all major muscles in the upper and lower body. Finally, a poststretch after the PIP program will ensure long-term flexibility. Figure 10.23 demonstrates assembly of the equipment at the feet and hands.

The PIP exercise examples work both upper and lower body. The upper body movements can vary to change the muscles worked during the exercise. Following are some examples:

- Diagonal jumping jacks with horizontal shoulder abduction/adduction (figure 10.24)
- Jogging with alternating punches (figure 10.25)
- Cross-country skiing with shoulder flexion and extension (alternating or symmetrical; figure 10.26)

Finally, when elastic devices are used in an aquatic fitness program, the participant should rinse the band or tubing in fresh water after use and store in a bucket of fresh water. This will keep the bands from drying out and will prolong their life.

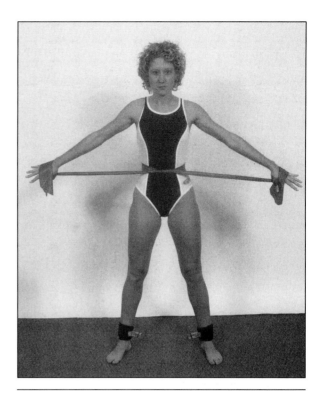

Figure 10.24   Power-in-the-pool diagonal jumping jacks.

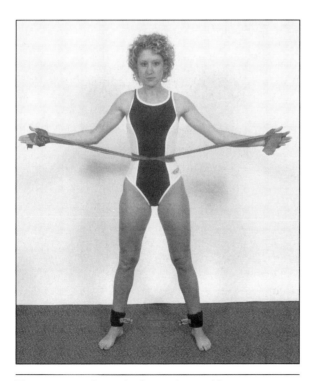

Figure 10.23   Power-in-the-pool assembly.

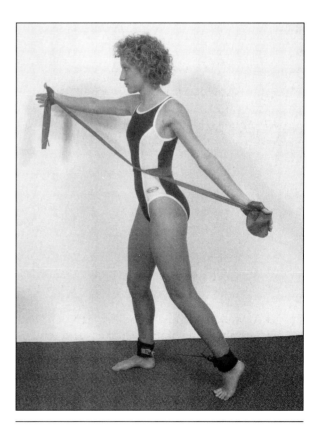

Figure 10.25   Power-in-the-pool jogging with alternating punches.

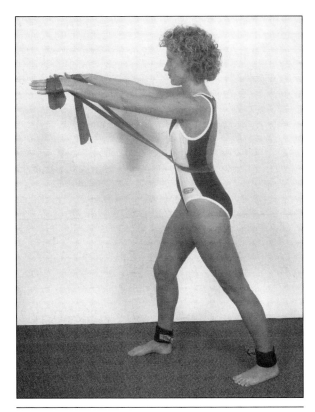

Figure 10.26 Power-in-the-pool cross-country skiing (alternating or symmetrical).

Precautions for Strengthening Programs

As with any exercise program, precautions are advised when elastic resistance is used for strength training.

Valsalva

Participants should avoid the Valsalva maneuver, which involves holding the breath during strenuous activity such as strength training. Performing the Valsalva maneuver causes the glottis to close and the abdominals to contract. This increases thoracic pressure, which interrupts venous return to the heart, blood flow to the coronary arteries, and oxygen supply to the brain. Dizziness and temporary loss of consciousness may occur (Mantia 1995). Therefore, participants must remember to breathe.

"No Pain, No Gain" Is Nonsense

Muscle soreness is common when an individual begins an elastic resistance strength training pro-

gram because isolated muscle groups are being overloaded beyond normal use (Heyward 1997). Pain, however, could signal a common injury such as tendinitis or ligament injury. Rest, ice, compression, and elevation (RICE) are recommended as a remedy. If pain persists for more than 3 days despite RICE, a medical professional should be consulted. Also, seek medical attention when there is a loss of joint motion, any joint swelling, or a feeling of "giving way" or if the pain is sharp and the participant is unable to use the joint because of pain (Ban-Pillarella 1995).

Stabilization

The participant should apply stabilization techniques to avoid substitution of movements. These include maintaining proper alignment by keeping the spine in neutral; stabilizing the spine with tight abdominals and low back muscles held in a slight contraction; and keeping the chest open and the shoulders down and back.

Special Populations

Use caution with persons who are pregnant or who have arthritis. External resistance may be too strenuous these people's joints.

Stretching

Stretch the muscles that have been strengthened by moving the joint to the end of its ROM. ACSM recommends holding the stretched position as long as it feels comfortable (usually 10-30 s; ACSM 2000). Participants should keep breathing slowly and rhythmically while holding the stretch.

Conclusion

Participating in an exercise program that combines aerobic exercise with resistance training is an effective way to improve or maintain functional fitness. Strength training allows common activities of daily living (such as carrying groceries, shoveling snow, lifting small children) to be performed with less effort. Strengthening postural muscles and enhancing postural stability can prevent low back problems. Elastic resistance bands are versatile, mobile, and adaptable and can be an enjoyable way to strength train.

References

American College of Sports Medicine. 2000. *ACSM's Guidelines for Exercise Testing and Prescription.* 6th ed. Hagerstown, MD: Lippincott, Williams & Wilkins.

Ban-Pillarella, D. 1995. "Training for Plyometrics and Power." Pp. 115-121 in *Fitness: Theory and Practice, The Comprehensive Resource for Fitness Instruction*, ed. P. Jordan. 2nd ed. Sherman Oaks, CA: Aerobics and Fitness Association of America. Stoughton: Reebok University Press.

Bird, S. 1992. *Exercise Physiology for Health Professionals.* London: Chapman & Hall.

Clippinger-Robertson, K. 1989. "Components of an Aerobic Dance-Exercise Class." Pp. 127-168 in *Aerobic Dance-Exercise Manual*, ed. N. Van Gelder. San Diego: IDEA International Dance-Exercise Association.

Cumming, C. 1998. *Therarobics™ Body Evolution Concept—The World's Latest Fitness Concept.* Hadamar, Germany: Therarobics™ Information International.

Filer, T. 1995. "Circuit Training." Pp. 421-424 in *Fitness Theory and Practice, The Comprehensive Resource for Fitness Instruction*, ed. P. Jordan. 2nd ed. Sherman Oaks: Aerobics and Fitness Association of America. Stoughton: Reebok University Press.

Heyward, V. 1997. *Advanced Fitness Assessment and Exercise Prescription.* 3rd ed. Champaign, IL: Human Kinetics.

Kendall, F., E. McCreary, and P. Provance. 1993. *Muscles Testing and Function.* 4th ed. Baltimore: Williams & Wilkins.

Lindle, J., ed. 1998. *A Guide to Aquatic Rubberized Resistance Exercises.* Mundelein, IL: SPRI Products.

Love, C. 1995. "Resistance Tubing." Pp. 404-408 in *Fitness Theory and Practice, The Comprehensive Resource for Fitness Instruction*, ed. P. Jordan. 2nd ed. Sherman Oaks: Aerobics and Fitness Association of America. Stoughton: Reebok University Press.

Mantia, P. 1995. "The Cardiopulmonary System." Pp. 95-106 in *Fitness Theory and Practice, The Comprehensive Resource for Fitness Instruction*, ed. P. Jordan. 2nd ed. Sherman Oaks: Aerobics and Fitness Association of American. Stoughton: Reebok University Press.

CHAPTER 11

Therapeutic Stretching With Elastic Resistance

• • • • •

Phillip Page, MS, PT, ATC, CSCS
Benchmark Physical Therapy, Baton Rouge, LA
The Hygenic Corporation

Vladimir Janda, MD, DSc
Charles University Hospital, Prague, Czech Republic

Stretching has become a popular activity among the active and well population; stretching is also necessary to prevent and treat various pain syndromes of the locomotor system and to treat various injuries. In some diseases such as progressive muscular dystrophy, the maintenance of appropriate muscle lengths is essential in maintaining functional ability. Stretching for fitness is used to enhance performance or prevent soft tissue injury and is commonly performed as part of the warm-up or cool-down (Ekstrand and Gillquist 1983). Therapeutic stretching can be defined as a specific intervention with the specific anticipated outcome to elongate or relax muscles or soft tissue, such as connective tissue within the muscle, muscle fibers, fascia, tendons, or ligaments. Although it is generally accepted that stretching is an important part of any exercise routine, many questions remain concerning its optimal dose-response (ACSM 2000). There are also many contradictory findings as to the most effective stretching techniques and their mechanisms. In addition, very little literature exists evaluating therapeutic stretching interventions on dysfunctional or injured tissue. The purpose of this chapter is to review the research on therapeutic stretching and to provide a scientific basis for the use of elastic resistance in stretching.

Mechanical Properties of Soft Tissue

Stretching techniques generally are used to elongate different types of soft tissue within the body. The mechanical properties of soft tissue determine its specific response to stretching; therefore, the stretching technique must be specific to the tissue type. These tissue types include both contractile (muscle) and noncontractile (tendon, ligament, fascia) structures.

Noncontractile Components

Each type of human tissue demonstrates a particular load-deformation curve, where tissue deformity

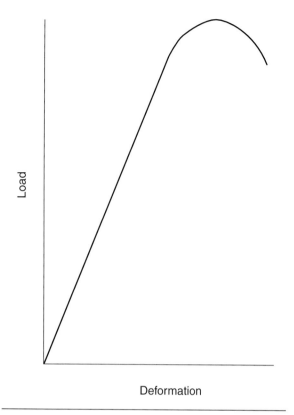

Figure 11.01 Load-deformation curve.

increases as load increases (figure 11.01). The load-deformation curve is the basis for passive stretch techniques: As load increases, tissue elongates.

Viscoelasticity is a property of connective tissue (including muscle, tendon, ligament, and fascia) where the tissue deforms at a certain rate, regardless of its load. This characteristic is known as rate-dependent behavior (Carlstedt and Nordin 1989). Two mechanical properties that demonstrate this viscoelastic behavior are load-relaxation and creep. In both load-relaxation and creep, a low load is applied to the tissue over time. In the load-relaxation response, the length remains constant and the stress in the tissue decreases over time. In the creep response, the load remains constant while the tissue deforms.

Disuse and immobilization promote atrophy and scar tissue formation after 7 weeks (Cummings and Tillman 1992). Connective tissue dysfunctions, including abnormal collagen crosslinks and shortened interfiber distances, are associated with the lack of motion (Amiel et al. 1982; Kottke, Pauley, and Ptak 1966). To prevent joint contracture after injury, collagen must be remodeled parallel to the lines of tension.

Viscoelastic properties are mostly responsible for length increases associated with stretching (Taylor,

Brooks, and Ryan 1997; Taylor et al. 1990). These viscoelastic characteristics of soft tissue are a result of its composition. The proper balance of collagen, elastin, and ground substance helps maintain normal tissue mobility. Factors such as fatigue, aging, immobilization, and medication can decrease tissue elasticity and cause tightness in soft tissue (Carlstedt and Nordin 1989). When noncontractile elements become tight in the body, this is referred to as *structural shortening*.

Contractile Components

In regard to tension, contractile tissue (muscle) has both a passive and an active component (figure 11.02).

This means that muscle can demonstrate increased tension by either structural shortening or by contractile shortening. Muscle is susceptible to the same means of structural shortening as described previously because of changes in the connective tissue surrounding the contractile components.

Muscle also can demonstrate contractile shortening as a result of increased tone within the muscle. Changes in tone are mediated unconsciously by the gamma motor neuron via the intrafusal muscle fibers. Hypertonicity can develop as a result of an altered function of some part of the nervous system, which can be recognized clinically as muscle spasm, myofascial trigger points, or taut bands within the muscle. These changes also can result from a structural lesion of the upper motor neuron that is then recognized as spasticity or rigidity (Janda and Jull 1987). Increased muscle tone attributable to an altered function is considered an important factor in the genesis of pain of the locomotor system. Pain from the viscera almost always is associated with muscle spasm in a specific area.

Neurophysiological Properties

Optimal function of the musculoskeletal system requires an intricate balance between antagonistic muscle groups. This interaction involves simultaneous and reflexive coordination of opposing muscle facilitation and inhibition. The quality of function of the muscle spindles and of the Golgi tendon organs (GTO), among others, is directly responsible for this coordination. The muscle spindle reflex facilitates muscle (increases tone), whereas the GTO reflex inhibits muscle (decreases tone).

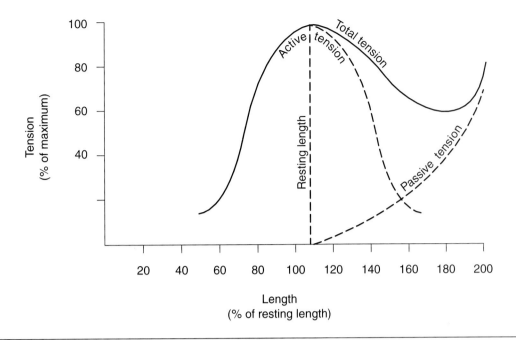

Figure 11.02 Active/passive tension components.

Reciprocal inhibition was first described by Sherrington (1906) as the relaxation of the antagonist during agonist motion, allowing movement within the agonistic pattern. *Autogenic inhibition* has been described as agonist relaxation following contraction resulting from the GTO reflex (Kabat 1950; Tanigawa 1972). This brief postfacilitation inhibitory period (which lasts 1-10 s) occurs immediately after maximal isometric contraction (Carter et al. 2000; Moore and Kukulka 1991).

Muscle Imbalances

Muscle imbalances represent an altered relationship between specific muscle groups; one group is prone to tightness, and the other is prone to inhibition. Muscle imbalance develops for many reasons but mainly results from a sedentary lifestyle. Muscle imbalances directly affect the joint biomechanics and quality of movement and consequently alter distribution of pressures, particularly in non-weight-bearing joints.

Any imbalance in muscle length or strength provokes a response in opposing muscle groups that predisposes the muscle to functional pathology. This muscle imbalance alters the quality of motor performances, resulting in faulty movement patterns that may lead to chronic pain. All parts of the motor system, either central or peripheral, function as one entity, and, thus, any "local" dysfunction within the system is reflected immediately by an adaptive response in all parts of the motor system; therefore, impairments are never strictly localized.

Although there is no histological correlation, clinicians find that certain muscle groups are predisposed to inhibition or weakness, whereas others are prone to facilitation or tightness (Janda 1988; Janda and Jull 1987; table 11.01).

Muscles prone to weakness are predominantly phasic in function; they atrophy readily, they are primarily single-joint muscles, and they are associated with extensor reflexes. Muscles prone to tightness have a predominant postural function, resist atrophy, are primarily double-joint muscles, and are associated with flexor reflexes.

Because tight muscles are more easily remedied, treatment of tight muscles with stretching should precede strengthening of inhibited or weakened muscles (Janda 1986; Janda and Jull 1987). Muscle tightness inhibits antagonistic muscles and further activates tight muscles during any movement. Therefore, in the presence of tight muscles, it is impossible to strengthen specific weakened muscles. Failure to stretch tight muscles is one reason why an exercise program fails. Once normal muscle length is reestablished, opposing muscles that initially were assessed as inhibited and weak often spontaneously improve (Janda and Jull 1987). Finally, normal movement patterns should be restored

Table 11.01   Muscular Predisposition to Imbalances

Muscles prone to inhibition or weakness	Muscles prone to facilitation or tightness
Peroneus longus	Gastrocnemius and
Peroneus brevis	Soleus
Tibialis anterior	Tibialis posterior
Vasti (mainly medialis)	Short hip adductors
Gluteus maximus, medius, minimus	Hamstrings
Rectus abdominis	Rectus femoris
Serratus anterior	Iliopsoas
Rhomboids	Erector spinae
Middle and lower trapezius	Tensor fascia lata
Short/deep cervical flexors	Quadratus lumborum
Extensors of upper limb	Upper trapezius
	Pectoralis major
	Levator scapulae
	Suboccipitals
	Sternocleidomastoid
	Scalenes
	Flexors of upper limb

through proprioceptive training before inhibited muscles are strengthened.

Stretching Techniques

Because mechanical properties govern the specific tissue response to stretching, it is important to identify the underlying cause of the tissue shortening to prescribe the appropriate stretching technique. The clinician must begin by thoroughly evaluating muscle lengths and differentiating which muscle component is responsible for the shortening. In particular, muscles prone to tightness, listed in table 11.01, should be evaluated. Joint range of motion (ROM) also can be measured and compared with so-called norms of the particular joint to note any decrease in ROM.

Once a tight structure has been identified, the clinician should identify the appropriate intervention by first determining if the contractile or noncontractile components are limiting motion. A quick test involves having the patient perform a manual contract-relax technique of the shortened muscle. If the ROM of the joint or muscle length improves,

then the clinician can assume that the contractile components are mainly responsible for the tissue tightness caused by increased tone (contractile shortening). If there is almost no change after this screening, then the passive noncontractile structures are responsible (structural shortening). The contract-relax technique almost always decreases tone of contractile muscle so that a certain degree of muscle lengthening will occur; therefore, the muscle must be thoroughly palpated and the duration of the tone decrease noted. This test is important to perform when any limitation is found because contractile muscle spasm often mimics the clinical presentation of noncontractile capsular restriction (Simons, Travell, and Simons 1999), and vice-versa.

The stretching intervention can be either passive (no muscular contraction) or active (involves muscular contraction). There are many different approaches to stretching, including combinations of each. The two most popular, advocated, and researched stretching interventions are passive static stretching and active proprioceptive neuromuscular facilitation (PNF) stretching (contract-relax or hold-relax techniques; Voss, Ionta, and Myers 1985). Each intervention has a particular indication and prescription. These techniques are summarized in Table 11.02.

Static Stretching

In structural shortening, the viscoelastic properties are responsible for the tightness; therefore, these structures should respond best to passive static stretching. The viscoelastic property of stress-relaxation is used when applying typical passive, static stretching techniques (Taylor et al. 1990); the load and length remain constant. In the case of severe hypomobility (such as joint contracture), more aggressive stretching techniques may be necessary to take advantage of the creep response. Low-load, long-duration stretching is the most effective means of restoring normal tissue length through collagen deformation (Kabat 1950; Sapega et al. 1981; Warren, Lehmann, and Koblanski 1971, 1976). This technique often is preceded with passive heating (Sapega et al. 1981) to denature the collagen and allow for proper remodeling.

Sapega et al. (1981) described a program designed to lengthen functional connective tissue structures in an atraumatic fashion. They advocated a moderate but tolerable force with the joint at end range to stretch contractures for 20 to 60 min, depending on tolerance. This method, which had been used for many years previously, is called *positioning* and is

Table 11.02 Therapeutic Stretching Interventions

Stretching intervention	Target tissue	Indications	Benefit	Technique
Passive	Non-contractile	Hypomobility Contracture Joint restriction	↑ Tissue length ↑ ROM ↓ Cross-links	Static stretch
Active	Contractile	Hypertonicity Spasm Atrophy	↓ Spasm ↓ Pain ↑ ROM	PNF, PFS, PIR (Contract-relax/hold-relax)

ROM = range of motion; PNF = proprioceptive neuromuscular facilitation; PFS = post-facilitation stretch; PIR = post-isometric relaxation.

still widely practiced in progressive muscular dystrophy. Several 30-s breaks can be incorporated into the method. A 3° increase of joint motion per week is an acceptable standard (Cummings and Tillman 1992).

Muscle fibers in primary muscle diseases have a different adaptability to stretch and thus respond differently to stretching. In spasticity, on the other hand, the muscle spindle stretch reflex cannot be suppressed sufficiently, and stretching may increase tone.

PNF Stretching

In contractile shortening, muscle spasm is mainly responsible for the shortening. Therefore, an inhibitory active stretching technique (contract-relax or hold-relax) should be used. Tension produced during a maximal isometric contraction results in less resistance to length changes in the muscle (Moore and Hutton 1980; Osternig et al. 1990; Prentice 1983). This reflex relaxation allows active shortening of a weakened antagonistic muscle; therefore, PNF stretching is particularly important in treating muscle imbalances.

In muscle imbalances, spasm or trigger points must be addressed first through PNF stretching. Any attempt to passively stretch a hypertonic structure or spasm may activate the muscle spindle reflex, causing further tightness and pain. In the presence of spasm or myofascial trigger points, care must be taken to avoid aggravating these trigger points with maximal contract-relax or hold-relax stretching (Simons, Travell, and Simons 1999).

Lewit and Simons (1984) described an active stretching technique similar to the hold-relax technique, termed *post-isometric relaxation (PIR)*. Rather than using the PNF technique of maximal contraction, Lewit and Simons used a minimal contraction (10-25% of maximal) to inactivate trigger points with an osteopathic technique. The researchers

noted that 94% of 244 myofascial patients treated experienced immediate pain relief with this technique. Through the use of minimal resistance, the specific muscle fibers are activated and then specifically inhibited; thus, the degree of manual resistance depends on the number of fibers involved in the trigger point or spasm. The resistance will fluctuate, therefore, for a specific response. Lewit and Simons' technique was based on the muscle energy technique, described by Mitchell, Moran, and Pruzzo (1979).

Unfortunately, controversy exists regarding the use of PNF stretching techniques. Although most studies comparing the two types of stretching have shown that PNF stretching results in greater increases than static stretching (Cornelius 1983; Holt, Travis, and Okita 1970; Moore and Hutton 1980; Osternig et al. 1987, 1990; Prentice 1983; Sady, Wortman and Blanke 1982; Tanigawa 1972; Wallin et al. 1985), the exact mechanism behind PNF is unclear. There are several possibilities for this.

First, most studies examining the mechanism behind PNF have been performed on laboratory animals or healthy (non–neurologically impaired) individuals. Few published studies (Lewit and Simons 1984) have evaluated specific therapeutic stretching interventions with injured or dysfunctional individuals.

Second, the neurophysiological basis of PNF has come under question. Electromyographic research (Condon and Hutton 1987; Cornelius 1983; Moore and Hutton 1980; Osternig et al. 1987, 1990) has cast doubt on the concept of "autogenic inhibition" as the mechanism behind PNF stretching. However, these studies only looked at passive electromyographic responses; more recent studies on PNF stretching noted a decrease in reflexive muscle spindle activity (Carter et al. 2000) and depressed Hoffman reflexes (indicating less muscle excitability; Moore and Kukulka 1991) immediately after contract-relax stretching.

These findings indicate that factors other than muscle relaxation are important for increasing ROM (Moore and Hutton 1980; Osternig et al. 1990) when PNF is used. PNF stretching is likely effective because of both reflexive and viscoelastic properties (Osternig et al. 1990; Taylor, Brooks, and Ryan 1997; Taylor et al. 1990). It is also possible that the warming effect of the muscular contraction during PNF stretching may help increase tissue length. Safran et al. (1988) noted that an isometric contraction of muscle increased tissue temperature by $1°$ C and improved the muscle's ability to tolerate greater force and length increases compared with unconditioned muscles when pulled to failure.

Clinical Application

The clinical use of elastic resistance for stretching techniques is fairly new. There is very little literature on the role of elastic resistance in stretching. Several authors have described the use of elastic resistance in providing low-load stretching for the shoulder and elbow (Donatelli and McMahon 1997; Greenfield 1994; Stralka and Brawsel 1994; Tonino 1998), but none have researched its effectiveness. Only one study has evaluated the use of elastic resistance in PNF stretching (Page, Wake, and Rice 2000), noting a nonsignificant increase in contract-relax stretching of the gastrocnemius compared with static stretching.

Traditionally, elastic resistance has been used for strengthening muscle. However, its properties make elastic resistance ideal for providing load during stretching techniques. First, the appropriate amount of load can be prescribed by adapting the resistance of the band or tubing (usually expressed by different colors) to the individual's strength or tolerance. For example, in static stretching, a low load can be applied to a contracture for a long period of time and can be adjusted easily as tolerance and ROM increase. Second, the patient can perform stretching at home without the assistance of another individual. This also helps ensure that appropriate loads are provided consistently, rather than varying loads being provided by another individual. Lewit and Simons (1984) noted that patients performing stretching as part of a home exercise program experienced more lasting pain relief.

Static Stretching

Elastic resistance can be used to assist individuals in general passive stretching techniques. The litera-

ture has shown that in healthy individuals, the most effective method of static stretching includes 15- to 30-s holds (Bandy and Irion 1994; Bohannon 1984; Taylor et al. 1990) repeated 3 to 5 times (Taylor et al. 1990). For a general fitness program, the ACSM (2000) recommends stretching major muscle groups a minimum of 2 to 3 days per week for 10 to 30 s, repeated 3 to 4 times for each stretch.

In the case of joint contractures, Sapega et al. (1981) suggested a moderate but tolerable load with the joint at end range for 20 to 60 min, depending on tolerance. The elastic resistance can be adjusted easily by shortening or lengthening the band or tubing to accommodate different tolerances within one session or between multiple sessions. Stretching of joint contractures may be uncomfortable but should not be painful. It is particularly important to remind individuals to breathe while they stretch. Clinically, several common joint contractures can be addressed through low-load static stretching with elastic resistance, including frozen shoulder (figure 11.03), elbow flexion contractures (figure 11.04), and knee flexion contractures (figure 11.05).

PNF Stretching

The general prescription for PNF stretching involves an initial passive stretch followed by an isometric (hold-relax) or agonist contraction (contract-relax) for 5 to 10 s, which is followed by a final stretch at end range. We advocate an initial isometric contraction performed at midrange for 7 s, followed immediately by a final stretch for 10 s at end range. This is termed a "post-facilitation stretch" (PFS). This should be repeated for 5 repetitions, once a day. By performing the contraction at midrange rather than end range, the patient uses the muscle to its best mechanical advantage and the greatest numbers of motor units are activated; therefore, the greatest possible inhibition is achieved. Therefore, less resistance to stretch is provided by the contractile units, and more stretch can be isolated to the non-contractile elements. These recommendations are based on clinical experience; no experimental studies have investigated the optimal dosing parameters and prescription of PFS stretching in a therapeutic setting.

Once the patient has mastered partner PNF stretching, elastic resistance can be prescribed to continue a home exercise program or maintenance program. Figures 11.06 through 11.23 demonstrate contract-relax stretching techniques with elastic resistance for muscle groups prone to tightness and facilitation.

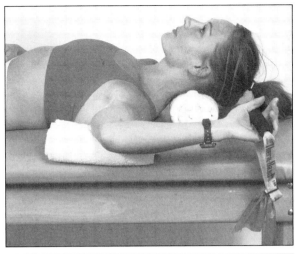

Figure 11.03 Shoulder anterior contracture stretch.

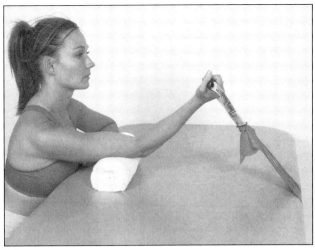

Figure 11.04 Elbow flexion contracture stretch.

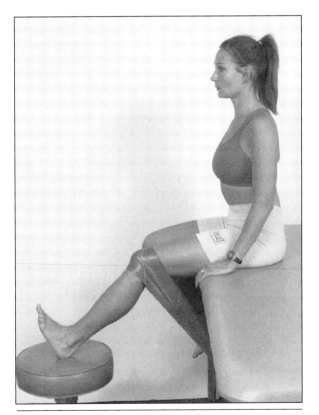

Figure 11.05 Knee flexion contracture stretch.

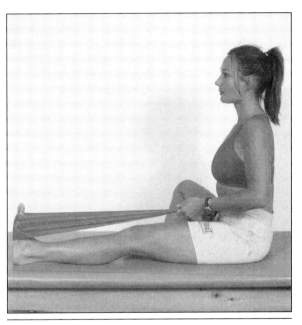

Figure 11.06 Gastroc/soleus contract-relax.

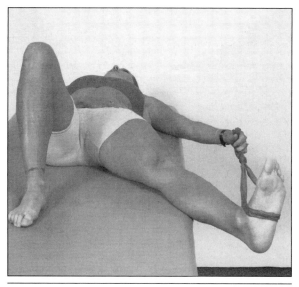

Figure 11.07   Hip adductor contract relax.

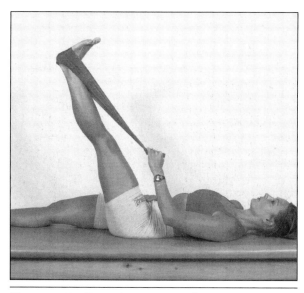

Figure 11.08   Hamstring contract-relax.

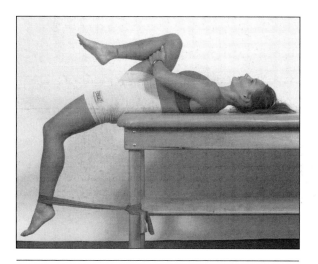

Figure 11.09   Rectus femoris contract-relax.

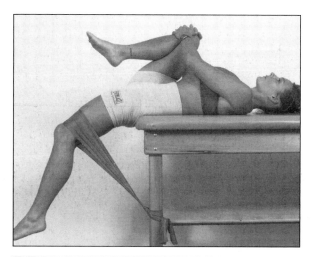

Figure 11.10   Iliopsoas contract-relax.

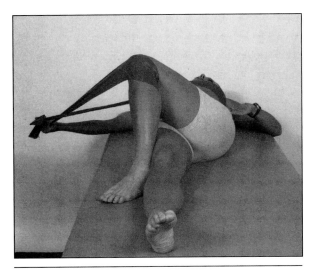

Figure 11.11 Piriformis contract-relax.

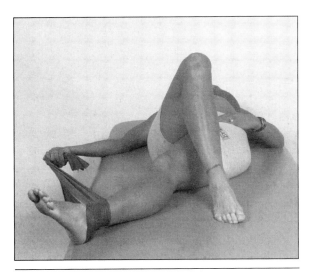

Figure 11.12 Tensor fascia lata contract relax.

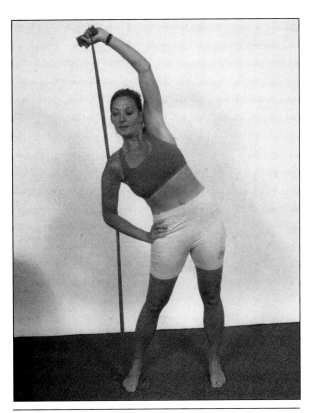

Figure 11.13 Quadratus lumborum contract-relax: stretch.

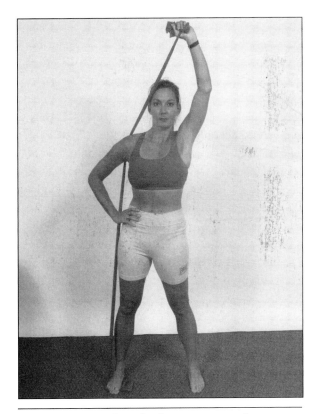

Figure 11.14 Quadratus lumborum contract-relax: contract.

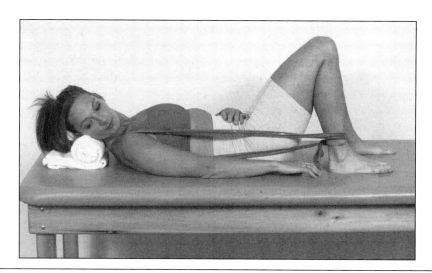

Figure 11.15 Upper trapezius contract-relax: stretch.

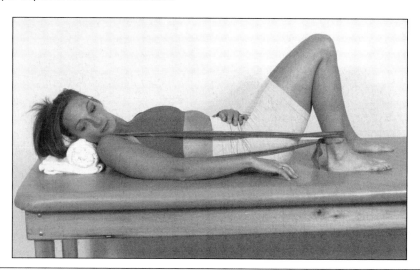

Figure 11.16 Upper trapezius contract-relax: contract.

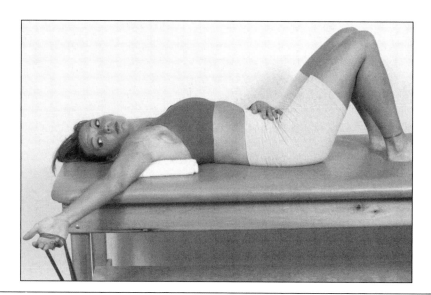

Figure 11.17 Pectoralis major contract-relax.

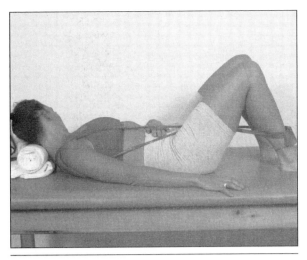

Figure 11.18 Levator scapulae contract-relax (stretch).

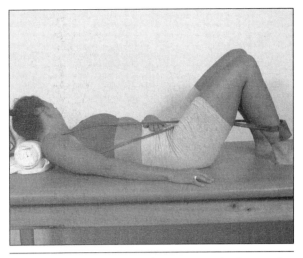

Figure 11.19 Levator scapulae contract-relax (contract).

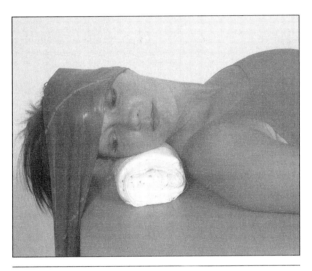

Figure 11.20 Sternocleidomastoid contract-relax: stretch.

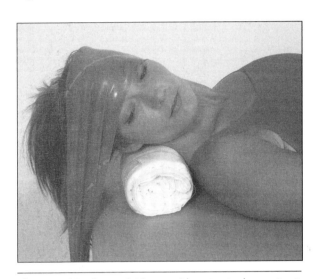

Figure 11.21 Sternocleidomastoid contract-relax: contract.

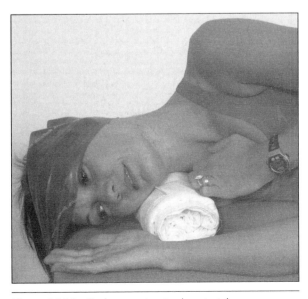

Figure 11.22 Scalene contract-relax: stretch.

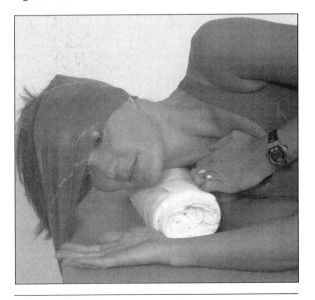

Figure 11.23 Scalene contract-relax: contract.

Conclusion

Therapeutic stretching should address the tissues that are used during functional activity. A thorough evaluation to differentiate tight structures should be performed before any stretching intervention is established. Static stretching is indicated for general fitness or hypomobility (joint contracture). PNF stretching is indicated for hypertonicity associated with muscle imbalances. Although the literature has shown that PNF stretching produces greater gains than static stretching, the mechanism responsible remains unclear; it seems evident that each technique influences different structures of the muscle, ligaments, and joint capsule. Elastic resistance can be used safely and effectively in stretching programs for both static and PNF routines, if the patient has been instructed properly and understands the procedure.

References

American College of Sports Medicine. 2000. *Guidelines for Exercise Testing and Prescription.* 6th ed. Philadelphia: Lippincott, Williams & Wilkins.

Amiel, D., S.L. Woo, F.L. Harwood, and W.H. Akeson. 1982. "The Effect of Immobilization on Collagen Turnover in Connective Tissue: A Biochemical-Biomechanical Correlation." *Acta Orthopaedica Scandinavica* 53(3): 325-32.

Bandy, W.D., and J.M. Irion. 1994. "The Effect of Time on Static Stretch on the Flexibility of the Hamstring Muscles." *Physical Therapy* 74(9): 845-50.

Bohannon, R.W. 1984. "Effect of Repeated Eight-Minute Muscle Loading on the Angle of Straight-Leg Raising." *Physical Therapy* 64(4): 491-7.

Carlstedt, C.A., and M. Nordin. 1989. "Biomechanics of Tendons and Ligaments." In *Basic Biomechanics of the Musculoskeletal System*, ed. M. Nordin and V.H. Frankel. 2nd ed. Philadelphia: Lea & Febiger.

Carter, A.M., S.J. Kinzey, L.F. Chitwood, and J.L. Cole. 2000. "Proprioceptive Neuromuscular Facilitation Decreases Muscle Activity During the Stretch Reflex in Selected Posterior Thigh Muscles." *Journal of Sport Rehabilitation* 9: 269-78.

Condon, S.M., and R.S. Hutton. 1987. "Soleus Muscle Electromyographic Activity and Ankle Dorsiflexion Range of Motion During Four Stretching Procedures." *Physical Therapy* 67(1): 24-30.

Cornelius, W.L. 1983. "Stretch Evoked EMG Activity by Isometric Contraction and Submaximal Concentric Contraction." *Athletic Training* 18(2): 106-9.

Cummings, G.S., and L.J. Tillman. 1992. "Remodeling of Dense Connective Tissue in Normal Adult Tissue." In *Dynamics of Human Biologic Tissues*, ed. D.P. Currier and R.M. Nelson. Philadelphia: Davis.

Donatelli, R.A., and T.J. McMahon. 1997. "Manual Therapy Techniques." In *Physical Therapy of the Shoulder*, ed. R. Donatelli. 3rd ed. New York: Churchill Livingstone.

Ekstrand, J., and J. Gillquist. 1983. "The Avoidability of Soccer Injuries." *International Journal of Sports Medicine* 4: 124-8.

Greenfield, B. 1994. "Special Considerations in Shoulder Exercises: Plane of the Scapula." In *The Athlete's Shoulder*, ed. J. Andrews and K.E. Wilk. New York: Churchill Livingstone.

Holt, L.E., T.M. Travis, and T. Okita. 1970. "Comparative Study of Three Stretching Techniques." *Perceptual and Motor Skills* 31(2): 611-6.

Janda, V. 1986. "Muscle Weakness and Inhibition (Pseudoparesis) in Back Pain Syndromes." In *Modern Manual Therapy of the Vertebral Column*, ed. G. Grieve. New York: Churchill Livingstone.

Janda, V. 1988. "Muscles and Cervicogenic Pain Syndromes." In *Physical Therapy of the Cervical and Thoracic Spine*, ed. R. Grand. New York: Churchill Livingstone.

Janda, V., and G. Jull. 1987. "Muscles and Motor Control in Low Back Pain." In *Therapy of the Low Back: Clinics in Physical Therapy*, ed. L. Twomey and J.R. Taylor. New York: Churchill Livingstone.

Kabat, H. 1950. "Studies on Neuromuscular Dysfunction XIII. New Concepts and Techniques of Neuromuscular Re-Education for Paralysis." *Permanente Foundation Medical Bulletin* 8: 121-143.

Kottke, F.J., D.L. Pauley, and R.A. Ptak. 1966. "The Rationale for Prolonged Stretching for Correction of Shortening of Connective Tissue." *Archives of Physical Medicine and Rehabilitation* 47(6): 345-52.

Lewit, K., and D.G. Simons. 1984. "Myofascial Pain: Relief by Post-Isometric Relaxation." *Archives of Physical Medicine and Rehabilitation* 65(8): 452-6.

Mitchell F.L, P. Moran, and N. Pruzzo. 1979. *An Evaluation of Osteopathic Muscle Energy Procedures.* Valley Park, MO: Pruzzo.

Moore, M.A., and R.S. Hutton. 1980. "Electromyographic Investigation of Muscle Stretching Techniques." *Medicine and Science in Sports and Exercise* 12(5): 322-9.

Moore, M.A., and C.G. Kukulka. 1991. "Depression of Hoffmann Reflexes Following Voluntary Contraction and Implications for Proprioceptive Neuromuscular Facilitation Therapy." *Physical Therapy* 71(4): 321-9.

Osternig, L.R., R. Robertson, R. Troxel, and P. Hansen. 1987. "Muscle Activation During Proprioceptive Neuromuscular Facilitation (PNF) Stretching Techniques." *American Journal of Physical Medicine* 66(5): 298-307.

Osternig, L.R., R.N. Robertson, R.K. Troxel, and P. Hansen. 1990. "Differential Responses to Proprioceptive Neuromuscular Facilitation (PNF) Stretch Techniques." *Medicine and Science in Sports and Exercise* 22(1): 106-11.

Page, P., V. Wake, and J. Rice. 2000. "Thera-Band Contract-Relax Versus Static Stretching on Ankle Dorsiflexion" (Abstract). *Journal of Orthopaedic and Sports Physical Therapy* 30(1): A47.

Prentice, W.E. 1983. "A Comparison of Static Stretching and PNF Stretching for Improving Hip Joint Flexibility." *Athletic Training* 18: 56-9.

Sady, S.P., M. Wortman, and D. Blanke. 1982. "Flexibility Training: Ballistic, Static or Proprioceptive Neuromuscular Facilitation?" *Archives of Physical Medicine and Rehabilitation* 63(6): 261-3.

Safran, M.R., W.E. Garrett, Jr., A.V. Seaber, R.R. Glisson, and B.M. Ribbeck. 1988. "The Role of Warmup in Muscular Injury Prevention." *American Journal of Sports Medicine* 16(2): 123-9.

Sapega, A.A., T.C. Quedenfeld, R.A. Moyer, and R.A. Butler. 1981. "Biophysical Factors in Range of Motion Exercise." *The Physician and Sportsmedicine* 9(12): 57-65.

Sherrington, C. 1906. *The Integrative Action of the Nervous System.* New Haven, CT: Yale University Press.

Simons, D.G., L.G. Travell, and L.S. Simons. 1999. *Myofascial Pain and Dysfunction: The Trigger Point Manual.* 2nd ed. Philadelphia: Lippincott, Williams & Wilkins.

Stralka, S.W., and J.G. Brawsel. 1994. "Elbow." In *Clinical Orthopaedic Physical Therapy,* ed. J. Richardson and Z. Iglarsh. Philadelphia: Saunders.

Tanigawa, M.C. 1972. "Comparison of the Hold-Relax Procedure and Passive Mobilization on Increasing Muscle Length." *Physical Therapy* 52(7): 725-35.

Taylor, D.C., D.E. Brooks, and J.B. Ryan. 1997. "Viscoelastic Characteristics of Muscle: Passive Stretching Versus Muscular Contractions." *Medicine and Science in Sports and Exercise* 29(12): 1619-24.

Taylor, D.C., J.D. Dalton, Jr., A.V. Seaber, and W.E. Garrett, Jr. 1990. "Viscoelastic Properties of Muscle-Tendon Units. The Biomechanical Effects of Stretching." *American Journal of Sports Medicine* 18(3): 300-9.

Tonino, P.M. 1998. "Athletic Injuries of the Elbow." In *Rehabilitation in Sports Medicine,* ed. E. Canavan. Stamford, CT: Appleton & Lange.

Voss, D.E., M.K. Ionta, and B.J. Myers. 1985. *Proprioceptive Neuromuscular Facilitation.* 3rd ed. Philadelphia: Harper & Row.

Wallin, D., B. Ekblom, R. Grahn, and T. Nordenborg. 1985. "Improvement of Muscle Flexibility. A Comparison Between Two Techniques." *American Journal of Sports Medicine* 13(4): 263-8.

Warren, C.G., J.F. Lehmann, and J.N. Koblanski. 1971. "Elongation of Rat Tail Tendon: Effect of Load and Temperature." *Archives in Physical Medicine and Rehabilitation* 52(10): 465-74.

Warren, C.G., J.F. Lehmann, and J.N. Koblanski. 1976. "Heat and Stretch Procedures: An Evaluation Using Rat Tail Tendon." *Archives of Physical Medicine and Rehabilitation* 57(3): 122-6.

CHAPTER 12

Integrated Uses
of Elastic Resistance

● ● ● ● ●

Phillip Page, MS, PT, ATC, CSCS
Benchmark Physical Therapy, Baton Rouge, LA
The Hygenic Corporation

E lastic resistance traditionally has been used for strength training in therapy and fitness. The most common strengthening applications are for the upper and lower extremities; however, there are several other applications of elastic resistance. This book has discussed several applications of elastic resistance, including balance training, plyometrics, speed and agility training, and stretching. The purpose of this chapter is to describe other clinical applications of elastic resistance as well as its integration with other exercise equipment or in other environments.

Other Clinical Applications of Elastic Resistance

In addition to traditional clinical applications such as strengthening and balance training, elastic resistance can be used in a variety of other ways. These include assisted range of motion (ROM), unloading tissue, providing multiple forces, and for functional strength assessments.

Assisted ROM

Because of its inherent property to return to a resting state when elongated, elastic resistance can be used in a "reverse" action, whereby, instead of using a resisted application, the participant uses an assisted action of the band or tubing. In this application, the elastic resistance is used to support the limb to complete the ROM. This is particularly useful in patients with adequate ROM but inadequate strength to complete the ROM, such as those with a strength grade of less than 3/5 (completing the ROM against gravity) or in shoulder patients demonstrating a "painful arc." Elastic resistance can help the patient complete the ROM to promote normal arthrokinematics in the presence of severe muscle weakness or pain.

For example, shoulder patients with rotator cuff weakness often substitute with the upper trapezius to complete shoulder abduction, causing a compensatory shoulder shrug to complete the motion. By using elastic resistance to support the weight of the arm, the patient can correctly perform shoulder abduction without upper trapezius substitution. If the patient and the elastic resistance are positioned correctly, the force of the band or tubing can be used to assist the motion rather than resist it, thus facilitating proper arthrokinematics (figures 12.01 and 12.02). This technique is useful for persons with weaknesses, particularly near the end range. The band or tubing also can be positioned so that resistance is provided during part of the motion and assistance is provided during the remaining motion (figures 12.03 and 12.04). This position is particularly useful for patients with a painful arc to assist them through the painful ROM.

Jayaprakash and Geiser (1993) used elastic bands to assist patients with frozen shoulder in performing shoulder flexion. The researchers placed the elastic bands over the top of the shoulder to assist normal scapular mechanics in these patients (figure 12.05). The band was attached to the patient's heel, pulled up over the scapula, and held in the front of the body with the opposite arm. The band assisted with inhibiting the upper trapezius and posteriorly rotating the scapula to promote normal scapulohumeral rhythm. The authors noted a significant increase in shoulder flexion and abduction in these patients, including improvements in shoulder pain and function (Jayaprakash and Geiser 1993).

Another application of assisted motion is for gait training in the lower extremity. The elastic band is wrapped around the foot, knee, and hip to promote a functional synergistic movement during gait (figure 12.06). During each step, the band assists with ankle dorsiflexion, knee flexion, and hip flexion. These are the main components of the swing phase during the gait cycle. Anecdotally, this application has been used successfully in neurologic patients with gait impairments.

Unloading

Often, pain is associated with excessive stress on the joints and musculotendinous structures during daily activities. This is particularly true of overuse syndromes, where repetitive, low loads are encountered by the tissue. For example, lateral epicondylitis of the elbow and chronic Achilles tendinitis are caused by repetitive low loads such as grasping and walking, respectively. Because physiologic loads are necessary to perform activities of daily living, overuse injuries can be difficult to treat because the tissue is continuously exposed to these forces.

To treat these overuse injuries effectively, the tissue first must be unloaded. Although braces and splints are effective for totally unloading tissue, immobilization can harm healing tissue in some instances. An alternative to immobilization is to unload the tissue with elastic resistance. This allows a protected ROM and unloads the tissue by removing excessive stresses from daily activity. An elastic band is secured above and below the joint to be unloaded with athletic tape. The elastic band then helps the muscles move the joint, taking some load off the injured or healing tissue.

Clinically, this method has been used particularly well for Achilles tendinitis (figure 12.07). By assisting with plantar flexion during the push-off phase of the gait cycle, the elastic band functionally assists the Achilles, thus placing less stress on the triceps

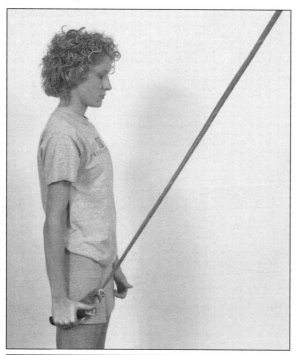

Figure 12.01 Assisted shoulder flexion: beginning range (start position).

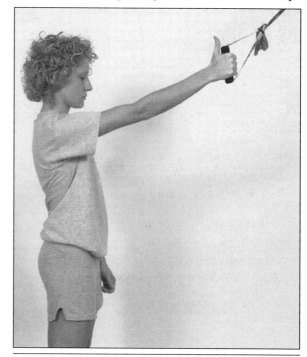

Figure 12.02 Assisted shoulder flexion: beginning range (end position).

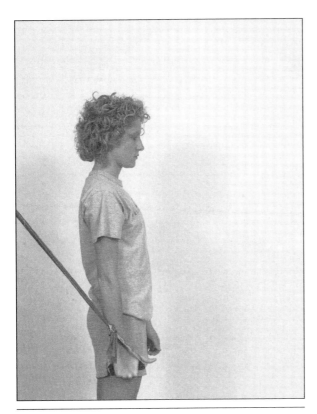

Figure 12.03 Assisted shoulder flexion: mid to end range (start position).

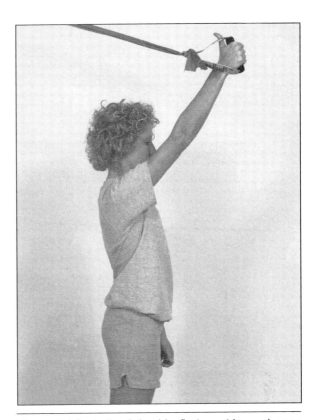

Figure 12.04 Assisted shoulder flexion: mid to end range (end position).

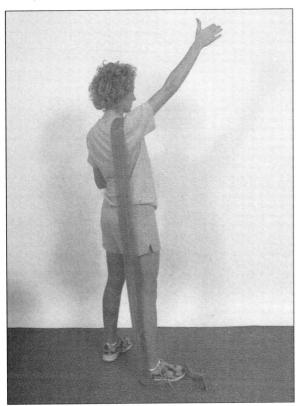

Figure 12.05 Assisted shoulder flexion for frozen shoulder. Elastic band assists shoulder depression and scapular rotation.

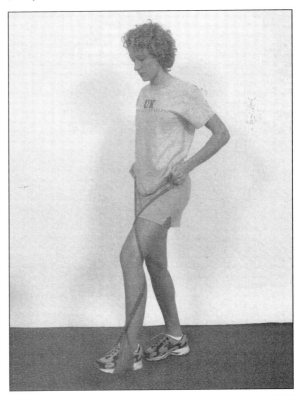

Figure 12.06 Assisted swing phase of gait. Elastic band assists with ankle dorsiflexion, knee flexion, and hip flexion during the swing phase.

surae to complete the push-off. Thera-Band taping also can be used for unloading of the wrist extensors in patients with tennis elbow (figure 12.08).

Multiple Force Application

Functional movement occurs in multiple joints, planes, and directions, requiring multiple muscles to work together synergistically. Traditional resistance training uses gravity-based resistance, which only provides resistance in one direction and one plane. Elastic resistance can be used to impart multidirectional resistance in multiple planes during a

single exercise. For example, when an athlete performs shoulder internal rotation at 90° of abduction, resistance can be applied against internal rotation and abduction (figure 12.09). This exercises the subscapularis as well as the deltoid. Multiple forces also can be applied to increase the challenge of an exercise at different lengths on the lever arm (figure 12.10). Applying the resistance at multiple locations of the moving limb challenges more muscles throughout the kinetic chain.

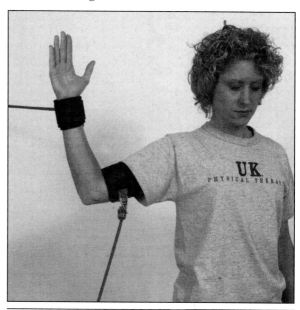

Figure 12.09 Multiple force application for shoulder internal rotation. Resistance is applied to strengthen both the shoulder abductors and the internal rotators.

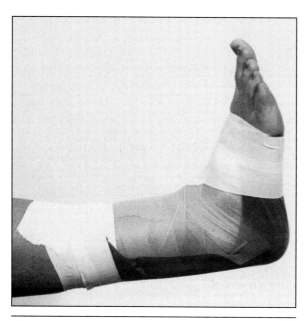

Figure 12.07 Thera-Band taping unloading for the Achilles. Adhesive tape secures the ends of the elastic band to assist the plantar flexion of the Achilles tendon.

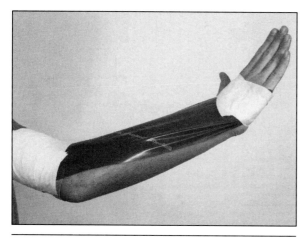

Figure 12.08 Thera-Band taping unloading for tennis elbow. Adhesive tape secures the ends of the elastic band to assist the wrist extension function of the wrist extensors.

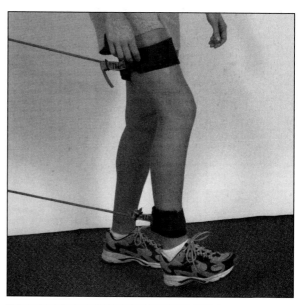

Figure 12.10 Multiple force application for leg kicks. This placement challenges both the hip flexors and knee extensors during a kicking motion.

Functional Strength Assessment

Elastic resistance can be used to quantify strength and functional ability. Topp, Mikesky, and Thompson (1998) described the "strength index" to quantify strength in older adults. Subjects completed certain exercises using Thera-Band resistive bands. The researchers then multiplied the number of repetitions completed by the resistance of the bands at full elongation. Mikesky and colleagues (1996) reported that techniques to assess muscular strength with elastic resistance yielded correlations from .48 to .93. Topp, Mikesky, and Thompson (1998) also noted that the seated row, squats, and hip flexion strength indexes correlated with functional tasks in older individuals.

Elastic resistance has been described to assess functional performance in patients with anterior cruciate ligament injuries. Lephart et al. (1991) used elastic resistance during a lateral movement in patients with anterior cruciate ligament insufficiency. The "co-contraction test" required subjects to complete five 180° semicircles with elastic tubing attached at the waist (figure 12.11) and attached 60 in. from the floor. This test was designed to reproduce the rotational forces at the knee (Lephart et al. 1991).

Applications With Other Equipment or Environments

Elastic resistance becomes even more useful and adaptable when used with other equipment or in different settings. For example, elastic resistance can be used with sports implements and other equipment, or it can be used in aquatic or microgravity environments.

Sports Implements

Elastic resistance often is used in conjunction with sports implements (Behm 1988). This provides more functional and sport-specific training for the athlete in a variety of sports. For example, elastic resistive bands or tubing can be attached to a tennis racket, baseball bat, or golf club (figure 12.12). Elastic resistance also allows for higher speed resistance training at sport-specific velocities.

Integration With Other Equipment

Elastic resistance is also a valuable adjunct to other types of exercise equipment such as oscillation

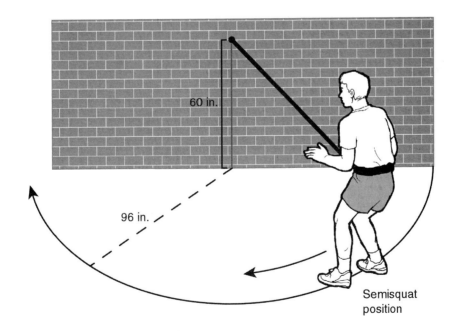

60 in.

96 in.

Semisquat position

Figure 12.11 Co-contraction test. Tubing (96") is attached to the waist and at 60" above floor. Athlete performs lateral shuffle in semi-circle.

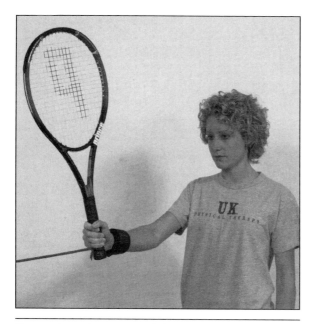

Figure 12.12 Integration of elastic resistance with the tennis racquet while swinging. Resistance is applied to the handle, rather than the end of the racquet to avoid excessive lever arm.

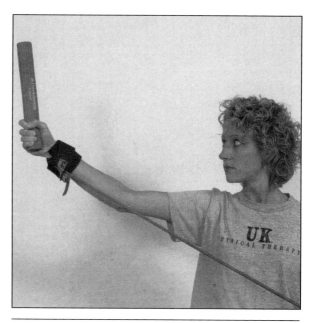

Figure 12.13 Integration with FlexBar for oscillation training. The "Statue of Liberty" exercise targets the posterior rotator cuff by oscillating in full D2 flexion.

devices, balance foam, and exercise balls. When the athlete uses elastic resistance with other exercise devices, the challenge to the neuromuscular system increases. This theoretically results in greater increases in proprioception and balance. For example, using elastic resistance with an oscillatory device (FlexBar) may increase proprioceptive input to joint mechanoreceptors. In performing the "Statue of Liberty" exercise (figure 12.13), the athlete uses the FlexBar with elastic resistance to overload the posterior rotator cuff and scapular muscles with oscillation. Adding elastic resistance exercise to balance training on foam (figure 12.14) may improve balance and coordination. Finally, athletes can use exercise devices to add challenge to elastic resistance training, such as performing shoulder exercises while on an exercise ball (figure 12.15).

Aquatic Resistance Training

During aquatic exercise, elastic bands or tubing can be used to add resistance to training in the pool. Thein and Brody (1998, 2000) described the use of elastic resistance in aquatic exercise. In particular, they recommend that the athlete use elastic resistance to challenge trunk stability in shallow water while performing a throwing or swinging motion against elastic resistance. Elastic resistance also can be used as a tether to resist swimming or jogging in water.

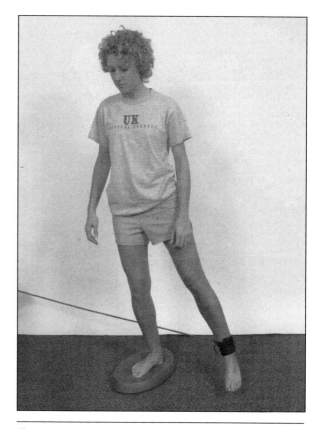

Figure 12.14 Integration with stability trainer for balance training. Balance while performing kicks against elastic resistance.

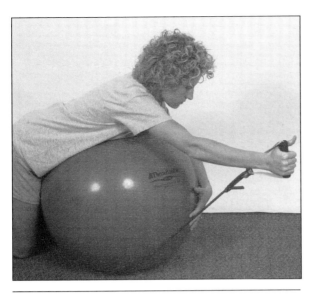

Figure 12.15   Integration with exercise ball for strengthening lower trapezius. Prone shoulder flexion.

Microgravity Applications

In the absence of gravity, muscle atrophies and weakens (Thorton and Rummel 1977). Traditional strength training equipment that relies on isotonic weights is ineffective in microgravity environments. Other types of resistance, such as pneumatic or hydraulic resistance equipment, only offer resistance in the concentric direction. Elastic resistance is an alternative strengthening method for astronauts because it provides both concentric and eccentric resistance and provides a lighter alternative to bulky resistance training equipment.

Astronauts also have used elastic resistance as a tethering device in space (Convertino 1990). Astronauts are attached to the treadmill by elastic straps to keep the individual in place and to increase the mechanical load on the legs (figure 12.16).

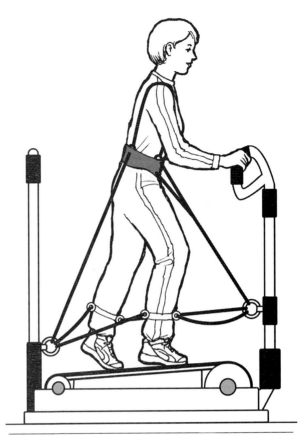

Figure 12.16   Tethered treadmill walking in microgravity. Astronauts are tethered to a treadmill using elastic resistance.

Adapted, by permission, from V.A. Convertino, 1990, "Physiological adaptations to weightlessness: Effects on exercise and work performance," *Exercise and Sports Science Reviews* 18:119-66.

Conclusion

Elastic resistance has a wide variety of applications. In addition to enhancing traditional strengthening exercise, elastic resistance is useful in assisting ROM and unloading injured tissues. Elastic resistance is also useful in measuring functional strength and ability in older adults and athletes. Elastic resistance can be integrated effectively with other types of exercise equipment to enhance strength and proprioception. Finally, its properties also make it ideal for exercise in microgravity environments. The only limitation in its use is the imagination; however, much research is needed on the effectiveness of these interventions.

References

Behm, D.G. 1988. "Surgical Tubing for Sport and Velocity Specific Training." *National Strength and Conditioning Association Journal* 10(4): 66-70.

Convertino, V.A. 1990. "Physiological Adaptations to Weightlessness: Effects on Exercise and Work Performance." *Exercise and Sport Sciences Reviews* 18: 119-66.

Jayaprakash, S., and M.B. Geiser. 1993. "A New Method of Rehabilitation to Improve Shoulder Range of Motion in Failed Shoulders." Presented at American Congress of Rehabilitation Medicine, June 1993, Denver, CO.

Lephart, S.M., D.H. Perrin, F.H. Fu, and K. Minger. 1991. "Functional Performance Tests for the Anterior Cruciate Insufficient Athlete." *Athletic Training* 26(1): 44-50.

Mikesky, A., R. Topp, A. Meyer, and K. Thompson. 1996. "Reliability of Ten Tests for Assessing Functional Performance and Strength in Older Adults" (Abstract). *Medicine and Science in Sports and Exercise* 28(5) (Suppl.): S11.

Thein, J.M., and L.T. Brody. 1998. "Aquatic-Based Rehabilitation and Training for the Elite Athlete." *Journal of Orthopaedic and Sports Physical Therapy* 27(1): 32-41.

Thein, J.M., and L.T. Brody. 2000. "Aquatic-Based Rehabilitation and Training for the Shoulder." *Journal of Athletic Training* 35(3): 382-9.

Thorton, W.E., and J.A. Rummel. 1977. "Muscular Deconditioning and Its Prevention in Space Flight." Pp. 191-197 in *Biomedical Results from Skylab*, ed. R.S. Johnson and L.F. Dietlein. NASA SP-377, Washington DC.

Topp, R.A., A. Mikesky, and K. Thompson. 1998. "Determinants of Four Functional Tasks Among Older Adults: An Exploratory Regression Analysis." *Journal of Orthopaedic and Sports Physical Therapy* 27(2): 144-53.

PART IV

SPORT-SPECIFIC APPLICATIONS

Perhaps no other application of elastic resistance is more popular than its use for sport-specific activity. Because of the portability and convenience of elastic resistance, athletes can use it as part of a rehabilitation or maintenance program. Elastic resistance offers another advantage of allowing sport-specific patterns to be strengthened throughout the movement. The following chapters describe the use of elastic resistance in 10 common sports.

CHAPTER 13

Sport-Specific Training for Football

• • • • •

Timothy F. Tyler, MS, PT, ATC
The Nicholas Institute of Sports Medicine and Athletic Trauma

Malachy P. McHugh, PhD
The Nicholas Institute of Sports Medicine and Athletic Trauma

Football has been classified not as a contact sport but as a collision sport. The physical nature of the game along with the increasing size of its competitors carries an obvious risk for injury. Many injuries occur as a result of direct player-to-player contact. Additionally, football injuries may be caused by player-to-ground contact, overuse, or intrinsic overload from ground reaction forces resulting in a noncontact injury (Fochios and Nicholas 1995). Regardless of the position an athlete plays, physiological factors contribute to performance and may play a role in preventing on-field injuries. The physical demands of the game include speed, strength, agility, quickness, power, and endurance (Pincivero and Bompa 1997). These performance factors are the focus of strength and conditioning coaches across the National Football League (Ebben and Blackard 2001) as well as successful high school football players in the United States (Williford et al. 1994). Elastic resistance exercises can provide a unique approach to developing specific performance factors as part of a training program or during rehabilitation from injury. This chapter provides an overview of the primary physical performance factors for U.S. football and the most commonly occurring injuries. The focus of this chapter is on the use of elastic resistance exercises for individual position training and during rehabilitation of football-specific injuries.

Football Performance Factors

The performance demands of specific sports have been categorized according to neuromuscular and physical factors, mental and psychometric factors, and environmental factors (Nicholas 1975). Within each category, specific performance factors have been identified. The neuromuscular and physical factors are strength, endurance, body type, flexibility, balance, agility, speed, and coordination; the mental and psychometric factors are intelligence, creativity, alertness, motivation, and discipline; and the environmental factors are playing conditions, equipment, and practice. The goal of a physical conditioning program is to train specific neuromuscular and physical performance factors so the athlete can meet the demands of the sport. Strength, body type, balance, agility, and speed have been identified as the primary factors involved in football (Nicholas 1975). The stop-and-start nature of football, where extreme physical exertion occurs during single plays lasting seconds rather than minutes, means that football players rely primarily on anaerobic energy sources (Gleim, Witman, and Nicholas 1981; Pincivero and Bompa 1997). The starting position for the majority of football players is the three-point stance, and resisted starts can improve speed and power. Resisted starts are illustrated in figures 13.01 and 13.02.

In football, body types vary considerably by position; linemen[1] are the tallest and heaviest and have the most body fat, whereas wide receivers and defensive backs are lightest and have the least body fat. Accordingly, linemen have the highest absolute upper and lower body strength, whereas wide receivers and defensive backs have the fastest 40-yd sprint times (Gleim, Witman, and Nicholas 1981). Regardless of their position, football players need to perform most movements in an explosive fashion. This involves a combination of strength and speed—that is, power. The total body extension

exercise against elastic resistance can be used to develop explosive power for the lineman. Total body extension exercises are shown in figures 13.03 and 13.04. In addition, for linemen, upper extremity power is essential and can be developed with task-specific exercises such as the pass-blocking exercise (see figure 13.05) for offensive linemen and the rip exercise (see figure 13.06) for defensive linemen. Lower extremity power is more important for wide receivers, defensive backs, and running backs and can be developed with the resisted backward run (see figure 13.07) for defensive backs and the resisted forward run (see figure 13.08) for wide receivers and running backs. These elastic resistance exercises provide the added components of agility and balance that are not ordinarily involved in task-specific power exercises. Additionally, the changing elastic resistance in an exercise such as the diagonal hops (see figures 13.09 and 13.10) provides a training stimulus for the neuromuscular system that is important in the development of agility and balance.

The balance and agility requirements for defensive backs, wide receivers, and running backs primarily involve dynamic high-speed movements. By contrast, quarterbacks function from a fixed base

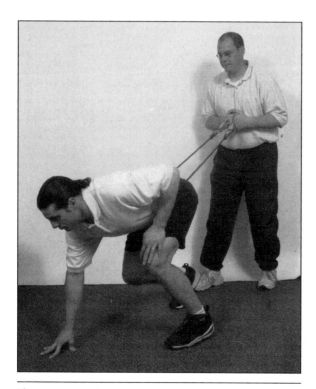

Figure 13.01 Three-point stance starts (start position).

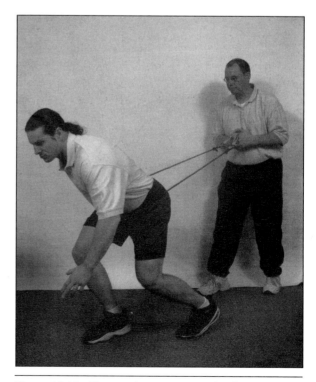

Figure 13.02 Three-point stance starts (end position).

[1]In football, *lineman* is the generic term for a player who starts from a stance position and blocks, rushes, or tackles during play.

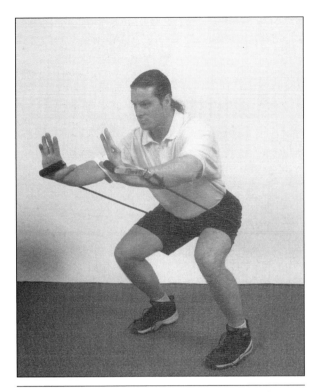

Figure 13.03 Total body extensions (start position).

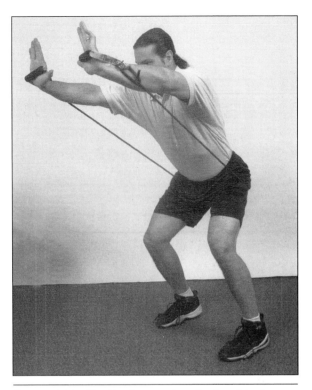

Figure 13.04 Total body extensions (end position).

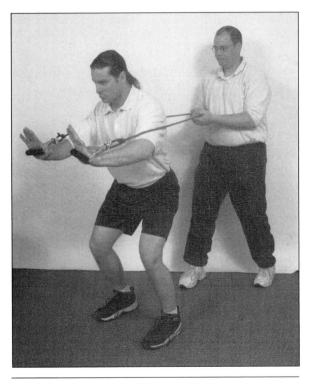

Figure 13.05 Pass blocking.

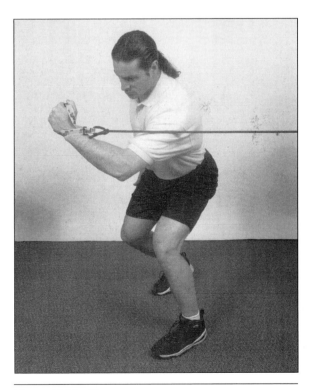

Figure 13.06 Rip.

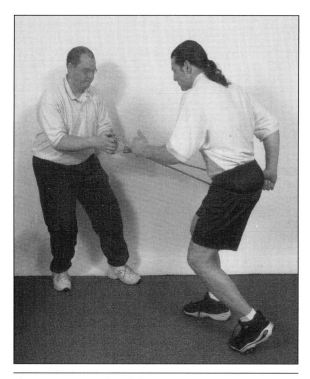

Figure 13.07   Back pedaling.

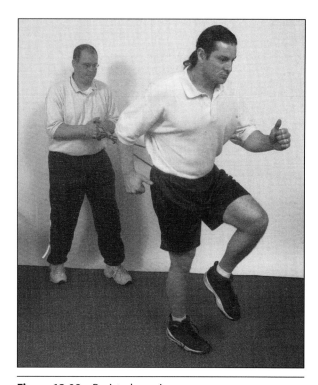

Figure 13.08   Resisted running.

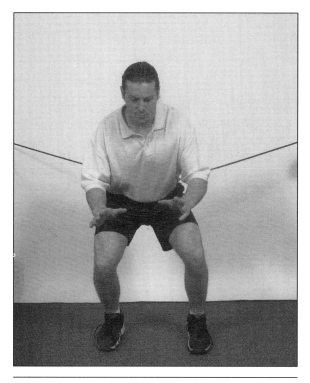

Figure 13.09   Diagonal hops (start position).

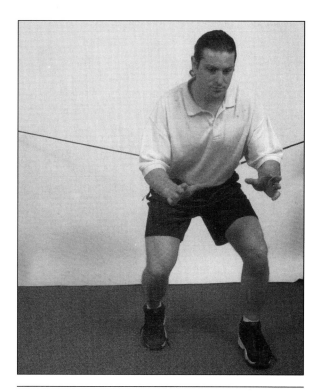

Figure 13.10   Diagonal hops (mid-movement).

of support when throwing the ball. Finely tuned balance adjustments allow the quarterback to quickly reset the base of support and maintain passing accuracy. Proprioceptive exercises with elastic resistance such as those outlined in chapter 5 (see single-leg stance with resisted contralateral limb hip abduction/adduction/flexion/extension, pp. 92) and pictured in figure 13.11 can be used to train balance and improve the quarterback's base of support. However, maintaining rotator cuff strength of the throwing shoulder should not be overlooked (see external rotation exercise at 90° of abduction in chapter 4, p. 55 and 57).

Etiology of Football Injuries

In football, injuries often are considered to be part of the game. Quantification of injury rate in football varies with the definition of an injury. Some players elect to play with minor injuries and do not seek treatment, whereas other players may hold themselves out of competition. Therefore, football injuries have been classified into categories of severity based on the number of games missed. Nicholas, Roesenthal, and Gliem (1988) defined a mild or

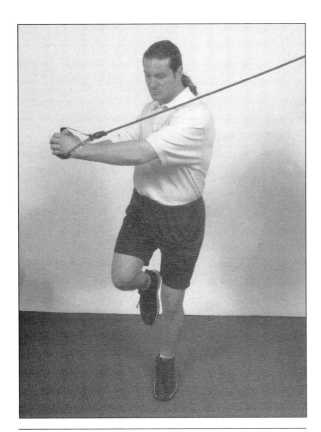

Figure 13.11 Single-leg torso rotations.

minor injury as one that caused the player to miss a single professional football game. A moderate or significant injury was described as one that caused the player to miss two games or more. A major injury was defined as one that caused the player to miss eight or more games or an injury that required surgery. In contrast, Canale et al. (1981) defined a major or severe injury as one that caused the player to miss three or more intercollegiate football games. Regardless of definition, the most severe football injuries for both professional and intercollegiate athletes occur at similar locations. Knee injuries accounted for 24% of all injuries in intercollegiate football players and 58% of major injuries in professional players. The knee, ankle, hamstring, and neck are among the most common injury sites for both levels of competition. Specific performance enhancement programs targeted at these areas may provide the dynamic stability and muscular balance required for injury prevention.

Injury rates have been reported to differ between positions. One study found that defensive ends and running backs were among the most injured, whereas linebackers and offensive lineman were the least injured (Canale et al. 1981). However, this study did not stipulate whether these injuries occurred on offensive, defensive, or special teams. Nicholas, Roesenthal, and Gliem (1988) did report a significantly higher number of major injuries on special teams during an 8-year period.

Knee Injuries

The knee joint is the most often injured part of a football player's body (Saal 1991). The knee experiences forces in three planes: flexion-extension, varus-valgus, and internal-external rotation (Fochios and Nicholas 1995). An injury to a knee ligament may change joint kinematics and create abnormal forces throughout the knee. Ligamentous knee injuries are among the most common and can be career threatening if severe (Nicholas, Roesenthal, and Gliem 1988). The anterior cruciate ligament (ACL) is frequently torn during the course of a play. Karpakka (1993) found the ACL to be the most commonly torn knee ligament in U.S. football players. Whether the ligamentous injury is treated conservatively or surgically reconstructed, restoring dynamic stability is critical to recovery (Colby et al. 1999). Closed kinetic-chain strengthening and reactive neuromuscular training have been shown to be beneficial for the patient with an ACL injury (Cook, Burton, and Fields 1999; Swanik et al. 1999).

Thus, the use of elastic resistance on the uninvolved lower extremity can provide an excellent external force for the athlete to stabilize against while standing on the involved leg for both of these techniques (see chapter 5, unilateral stance exercises, p. 92).

Cervical Spine Injuries

Cervical spine injuries can be catastrophic; however, the majority are not severe injuries. Canale et al. (1981) found that of the 16 neck injuries reported by an intercollegiate football team over the course of five seasons, only 2 were severe injuries. One player had a brachial plexus injury and the other a spinal cord injury. Cervical spine injuries can include stingers, cervical spine strains, neurologic injuries, intervertebral disk herniations, or fracture. The muscles surrounding the cervical spine provide support and protection. These muscles are short intrinsic muscles located along the cervical spine. Although individually these small muscles have poor strength, as a group they can restrict motion and potentially prevent injury if trained properly (Fochios and Nicholas 1995). In fact, when National Football League strength and conditioning coaches were asked to rank in order of importance the five most important exercises, neck strengthening was at the top of the list (Ebben and Blackard 2001). Elastic tubing can be an excellent source of isotonic resistance for strengthening the muscles surrounding the cervical spine (see figure 13.12).

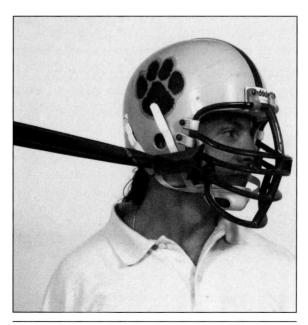

Figure 13.12   Neck rotations.

Ankle Sprains

Ankle sprains are among the most common injuries in all sports, and football is no exception (Canale et al. 1981). The typical ankle sprain is an inversion injury where the lateral ligamentous structures are disrupted. However, a significant number of injuries that might initially present as typical ankle sprains are syndesmotic sprains that will require prolonged rehabilitation (Boytim, Fischer, and Neumann 1991). The recovery period may be prolonged further by failure to recognize the injury initially. Players with syndesmotic sprains, referred to as "high ankle sprains," may continue to have symptoms for 4 to 6 weeks (Boytim, Fischer, and Neumann 1991).

The phase of ankle rehabilitation in which the player returns to sport involves strengthening exercises for the intrinsic muscles of the foot and ankle, the ankle invertors and evertors, and the proximal hip musculature as well as proprioceptive balance training. Elastic resistance exercises can be used to train these areas concurrently. Standing hip adduction, abduction, flexion, and extension with elastic resistance (see chapter 5, p. 92) simultaneously involve contralateral proprioceptive balance training. Similarly, trunk rotations against elastic resistance performed in single-limb stance (see figure 13.11) are effective proprioception exercises.

Hamstring Strains

Hamstring strains are inherent to high-speed sports involving intermittent sprinting. In football, the hamstring is the most commonly injured muscle group and overall was reported as the third most common injury, after knee and ankle injuries (Canale et al. 1981). As many as one third of hamstring strains are recurrent injuries (Seward et al. 1993). Inadequate rehabilitation of strength and flexibility has been cited as a primary factor in the recurrence of hamstring strains (Jonhagen, Nemeth, and Eriksson 1994). However, tissue repair may be incomplete despite normal clinical tests of strength and flexibility. In an animal model, Nikolaou et al. (1987) demonstrated that contractile force production was restored 7 days after experimentally induced strain injury, but significant localized fibrosis and scar tissue formation were evident at the site of injury. These findings are supported by radiographic imaging studies of muscle strains showing dystrophic calcification of hamstring muscle tissue (Garrett et al. 1989; Speer, Lohnes, and Garrett 1993).

Hamstring weakness has been shown to be a risk factor for subsequent strains (Orchard et al. 1997). Preseason hamstring strengthening may help reduce risk and can be incorporated into the elastic resistance exercise program (see chapter 5, hamstrings curls, figure 5.22). Additionally, isometric knee flexion contractions with elastic resistance can be performed early in rehabilitation of hamstring strains. The contralateral leg or the arms can be used to set the isometric angle, and isometric contractions can be performed throughout the range of motion, gradually increasing the stretch on the muscle. After isotonic contractions are added to the rehabilitation program, slow release of the elastic resistance can be incorporated to increase the eccentric phase of the contraction (figure 5.24). The elastic tubing also can be used to stretch the hamstrings muscle group in the straight leg raise position (figure 11.08).

Conclusion

The sport-specific demands of football and common injury patterns are presented in this chapter to provide both background information and rationale for the use and application of elastic resistance exercises for football. Sport-specific exercises presented in this chapter can help prevent injury and enhance performance for football players using the unique benefits and inherent characteristics of elastic resistance.

This chapter is dedicated to the late Guy F. Borreli, who served as the Washington Redskins Football Club strength and conditioning coach in 1978.

References

Boytim, M.J., D.A. Fischer, and L. Neumann. 1991. "Syndesmotic Ankle Sprains." *American Journal of Sports Medicine* 19: 294-8.

Canale, S.T., E.D. Cantler, T.D. Sisk, and B.L. Freeman. 1981. "A Chronicle of Injuries of an American Intercollegiate Football Team." *American Journal of Sports Medicine* 9(6): 384-9.

Colby, S.M., R.A. Hintermeister, M.R. Torry, and J.R. Steadman. 1999. "Lower Limb Stability With ACL Impairment." *Journal of Orthopaedic and Sports Physical Therapy* 29(8): 444-54.

Cook, G., L. Burton, and K. Fields. 1999. "Reactive Neuromuscular Training for the Anterior Cruciate Ligament-Deficient Knee: A Case Report." *Journal of Athletic Training* 34(2): 194-201.

Ebben, W.P., and D.O. Blackard. 2001. "Strength and Conditioning Practices of National Football League Strength and Conditioning Coaches." *Journal of Strength and Conditioning* 15(1): 48-58.

Fochios, D., and J.A. Nicholas. 1995. "Football Injuries." In *The Lower Extremity and Spine in Sports Medicine*, ed. J.A. Nicholas and E.B. Hershman. 2nd ed. St. Louis: Mosby.

Garrett, W.E., R. Rich, P.K. Nikolaou, and J.B. Vogler. 1989. "Computed Tomography of Hamstring Muscle Strains." *Medicine and Science in Sports and Exercise* 21: 506-14.

Gleim, G.W., P.A. Witman, and J.A. Nicholas. 1981. "Indirect Assessment of Cardiovascular 'Demands' Using Telemetry on Professional Football Players." *American Journal of Sports Medicine* 9: 178-83.

Jonhagen, S., G. Nemeth, and E. Eriksson. 1994. "Hamstring Injuries in Sprinters: The Role of Concentric and Eccentric Hamstring Strength and Flexibility." *American Journal of Sports Medicine* 22: 262-6.

Karpakka, J. 1993. "American football injuries in Finland." *British Journal of Sports Medicine* 27(2).

Nicholas, J.A., P.P. Roesenthal, and G.W. Gliem. 1988. "A Historical Perspective of Injuries in Professional Football. Twenty-Six Years of Game-Related Events." *Journal of the American Medical Association* 260(7): 939-44.

Nicholas, J.S. 1975. "Risk Factors, Sports Medicine and the Orthopaedic System: An Overview." *Journal of Sports Medicine* 3: 243-59.

Nikolao, P.K., B.L. MacDonald, R.L. Glisson, A.V. Seaber, W.E. Garrett. 1987. "Biomechanical and histological evaluation of muscle after controlled strain injury." *American Journal of Sports Medicine* 15.

Orchard, J., J. Marsden, S. Lord, and D. Garlick. 1997. "Preseason Hamstring Muscle Weakness Associated With Hamstring Muscle Injury in Australian Footballers." *American Journal of Sports Medicine* 25(1) (January-February): 81-5.

Pincivero, D.M., and T.O. Bompa. 1997. "A Physiological Review of American Football." *Sports Medicine* 23(4): 247-60.

Saal, J.A. 1991. "Common American Football Injuries." *Sports Medicine* 12(2): 132-47.

Seward, H., J. Orchard, H. Hazard, and D. Collinson. 1993. "Football Injuries in Australia at the Elite Level." *The Medical Journal of Australia* 159: 298-301.

Speer, K.P., J. Lohnes, and W.E. Garrett. 1993. "Radiographic Imaging of Muscle Strain Injury." *American Journal of Sports Medicine* 21: 89-96.

Swanik, C.B., S.M. Lephart, J.L. Giraldo, R.G. DeMont, and F.H. Fu. 1999. "Reactive Muscle Firing of Anterior Cruciate Ligament-Injured Females During Functional Activities." *Journal of Athletic Training* 34(2): 121-9.

Williford, H.N., J. Kirkpatrick, M. Scharff-Olson, D.L. Blessing, N.Z. Wang. 1994. *American Journal of Sports Medicine* 22(6): 859-62.

CHAPTER 14

Sport-Specific Training for Baseball

• • • • •

Phillip Page, MS, PT, ATC, CSCS
Benchmark Physical Therapy, Baton Rouge, LA
The Hygenic Corporation

Baseball is a complex sport that involves four basic fundamental movements: throwing, hitting, catching, and running. Virtually every position in baseball requires these simple movements to some degree; therefore, each position places unique demands of each body part. For example, a pitcher throws a ball much differently than an infielder, although the basic movement is a throwing motion. In terms of sport-specific exercises for baseball, this chapter focuses on the two most common sport-specific skills: pitching and hitting. Most of this chapter focuses on baseball pitching because of the vast amount of literature on the skill; however, the following principles of kinetic chains and of muscular coordination and balance can be applied to any position or sport.

Kinetic Chains

All functional movement involves the interaction of a biomechanical kinetic chain where larger base segments pass momentum to smaller adjacent segments (Welch et al. 1995). These adjacent segments are accelerated or decelerated through muscular force. Kibler (1998) described a "summation of forces" for the swinging or throwing mechanism. Figure 14.01 demonstrates that as the movement progresses over time, segments from the base of the kinetic chain (legs) transfer force and motion through the body to the distal segments (hands and wrist).

Any disruption in the timing or coordination of this linked system will affect overall performance (Kibler 1998); therefore, the individual links within the system must be addressed as well as the entire system. Weak links within the chain will be compensated for elsewhere in the chain. For example, rotator cuff weakness may be compensated for by additional trunk rotation during throwing, thus disrupting the timing of the entire kinetic chain. If a link within the kinetic chain is found to be weak, that link should be strengthened individually, and the athlete should work on restoring the strength of the entire kinetic chain through more dynamic and functional strengthening exercises.

Throwing Mechanism

The fundamental movement of throwing is a component of two major skills of baseball: pitching and

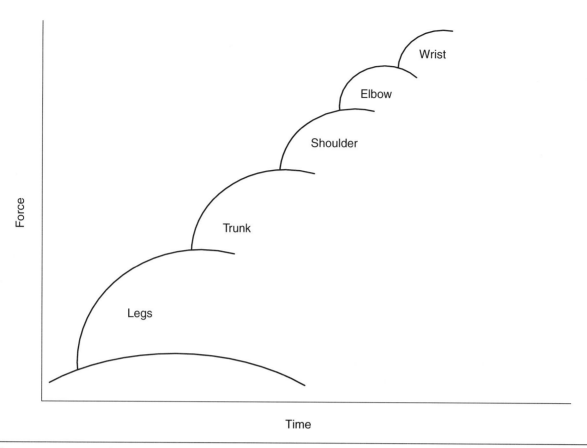

Figure 14.01   Kinetic chain summation of forces: throwing activity.

Reprinted, by permission, from W.B. Kibler, 1998, "Determining the extent of the functional deficit." In *Functional rehabilitation of sports and musculoskeletal injuries,* edited by W.B. Kibler, S.A. Herring, J.M. Press, and P.A. Lee (Gaithersburg, MD: Aspen), 16-19.

fielding. This discussion on throwing focuses on pitching specifically because of the large amount of biomechanical data available on baseball pitching. Pitching a baseball is one of the most highly dynamic skills in sports (Dillman, Fleisig, and Andrews 1993). Although most biomechanical analysis focuses on the shoulder mechanics, it is crucial to remember that the legs, hips, and trunk contribute significantly to the pitching motion, consistent with the kinetic chain theory.

The pitching mechanism has been evaluated biomechanically (Dillman, Fleisig, and Andrews 1993; Fleisig et al. 1995) and through electromyography (DiGiovine et al. 1992; Gowan et al. 1987; Jobe et al. 1983, 1984). Baseball pitching can be divided into six phases: wind-up, stride, arm cocking, arm acceleration, arm deceleration, and follow-through (Dillman, Fleisig, and Andrews 1993). Dillman, Fleisig, and Andrews (1993) noted peak angular velocities of near 7,000°/s, making baseball pitching one of the fastest skills in sports.

The wind-up and stride phases do not involve much shoulder muscular activity (Jobe et al. 1983,

1984). Jobe et al. (1983) noted sequential firing of the deltoid and rotator cuff during the early to late cocking phase. The rotator cuff is thought to be a "fine-tuner" of the glenohumeral joint rather than a primary mover (Jobe et al. 1984). The pectoralis major and latissimus dorsi are important internal rotators, providing power during the acceleration phase (Jobe et al. 1984). The biceps and triceps are used to control elbow motion; the triceps propels the forearm forward during acceleration, and the biceps eccentrically decelerates the forearm after ball release. The serratus anterior is also active throughout the cocking, acceleration, and follow-through phases, providing a stable base at the glenoid for the humerus to rotate around (Jobe et al. 1984).

Shoulder Injury

The pitching mechanism itself may be responsible for many injuries in pitchers. Pitching injuries, which are similar to overuse syndromes that result from accumulated microtrauma, usually are caused by large forces and torque exerted during pitching (Fleisig et al. 1995). In a kinetic analysis of the baseball pitch, Fleisig et al. (1995) described the pathomechanics of common upper extremity injuries in pitchers. Valgus forces about the elbow may cause ulnar collateral sprain or "valgus extension overload." The authors also noted the biomechanical implications for rotator cuff tears, impingement, and SLAP (superior labrum, anterior-posterior) lesions. Fatigue of the rotator cuff or serratus anterior may be a predisposing factor for shoulder injury in throwing athletes (Andrews and Wilk 1994; Jobe et al. 1983, 1984). In addition to excessive throwing, other causes of shoulder injuries in pitchers include lack of flexibility, muscle imbalances, and improper mechanics (Walk, Clark, and Seefeldt 1996).

The most significant and potentially dangerous phase within the pitching mechanism is deceleration. McLeod (1985) stated that deceleration forces are twice as great as acceleration forces and act for a much shorter time, with peak torque in the shoulder reaching 300 ft-lb. The angular velocities of 7,000°/s must be slowed to 0°/s within milliseconds. This places significant demands on the decelerators of the shoulder that are contracting eccentrically, in particular the posterior rotator cuff and scapular stabilizers (DiGiovine et al. 1992; Jobe et al. 1984). Scoville and colleagues (1997) reported that a deceleration force double the concentric force may be needed to maintain glenohumeral stability. Obviously, the physical demands on the shoulder necessitate a specialized exercise program specifically for pitchers to prevent injury and improve performance.

Muscular Coordination and Balance

Two important factors to consider in developing an exercise program for throwing athletes are muscular coordination and balance with other muscle groups. Functionally, muscles work as movers or stabilizers, varying contraction types from concentric to eccentric to isometric. The timing, coordination, and synchrony of muscle firing are vital for force production, optimal performance, and injury prevention. Kronberg, Nemeth, and Brostrom (1990) demonstrated the synergistic work of the shoulder musculature. They reported that coordination of muscle contraction (particularly the rotator cuff) plays a significant role in stabilizing the shoulder joint. It also has been shown that the quality of baseball pitching is determined by the selective use of

certain muscles to throw a baseball. Gowan et al. (1987) compared electromyographic activity of professional and amateur pitchers. They found that professional pitchers used the shoulder muscles more efficiently than amateurs did, and the professionals were able to achieve greater pitching velocities.

Because the throwing mechanism involves so much internal rotation, the anterior muscles of the shoulder are typically stronger than the posterior musculature. This creates muscle imbalances of the pitching shoulder between the internal and external rotators, ultimately leading to injury. Cook et al. (1987) reported muscle imbalances in the rotator cuff of baseball players. Several studies have evaluated the ratio of external rotation to internal rotation (ER/IR) strength in baseball pitchers, noting ER/IR ratios from .61 to .71 on the dominant (throwing) extremity (Alderink and Kuck 1986; Cook et al. 1987; Day, Moore, and Patterson 1987; Hinton 1988; Ivey et al. 1985; Wilk, Andrews, et al. 1993). Davies and Dickoff-Hoffman (1993) recommended a 3:4 ER/IR ratio for shoulder rehabilitation to create a "posterior-biased dominant shoulder." Pedegana et al. (1982) reported a relationship between pitching velocity and strength of the external rotators. Obviously, exercises must be prescribed specifically to strengthen the posterior shoulder and scapular stabilizers. Figures 14.02 through 14.08 provide exercises with elastic resistance for strengthening these areas.

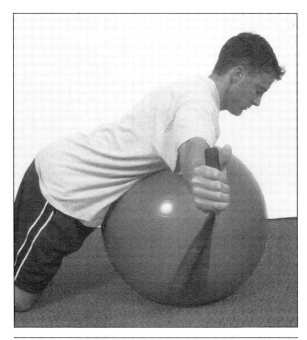

Figure 14.02 Posterior rotator cuff and scapular stabilizer strengthening: prone horizontal abduction with external rotation.

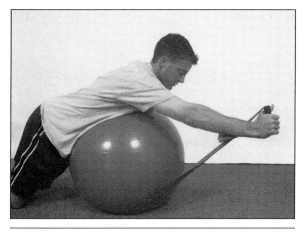

Figure 14.03 Posterior rotator cuff and scapular stabilizer strengthening: prone flexion.

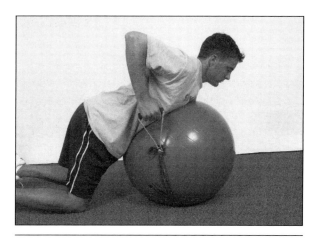

Figure 14.04 Posterior rotator cuff and scapular stabilizer strengthening: prone rowing.

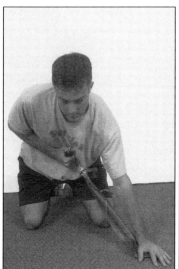 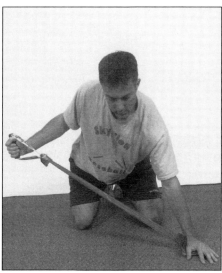 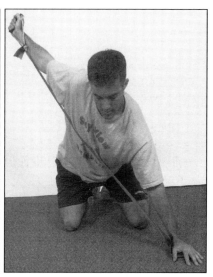

Figure 14.05-14.07 Posterior rotator cuff and scapular stabilizer strengthening: Linton external rotation (start position, mid-movement, and end position).

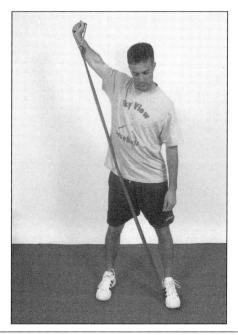

Figure 14.08 Posterior rotator cuff and scapular stabilizer strengthening: D2 flexion/extension.

Exercises for Baseball Pitchers

Baseball pitching velocity is correlated with anaerobic power (Pottieger and Wilson 1989); therefore, training should emphasize high-intensity activities over short periods of time rather than long aerobic activities. Because baseball pitching is essentially a kinetic-chain system, a general strengthening program should be performed for the entire body, including the upper and lower extremities and the trunk. Performing compound exercises for large muscle groups will provide an important base strength for the kinetic system. Because of the tremendous demands on the shoulder complex, specific exercises for the shoulder should be included as part of a preseason and in-season maintenance program. Wooden et al. (1992) reported that baseball players improved their pitching velocity following a 5-week shoulder-strengthening program.

Several studies have evaluated the electromyography of isotonic exercises used in shoulder rehabilitation programs (Moseley et al. 1992; Townsend et al. 1991). The most effective exercises to strengthen the glenohumeral joint are elevation in the scapular plane with the thumbs down (scaption or "empty can raise"), flexion, horizontal abduction with arms externally rotated, and press-up (Townsend et al. 1991). Exercises effective for the scapular stabilizers include scaption, rowing, push-up with a plus, and press-up (Moseley et al. 1992). Other studies have quantified exercises that use elastic resistance for the upper extremity, noting the shrug and forward-punch exercises as being the most effective at activating shoulder muscles (Hintermeister et al. 1998). Decker et al. (1999) found that a "dynamic hug" exercise with elastic resistance was very effective at eliciting serratus anterior activity. (See chapter 4 for a more detailed explanation and figures for these exercises.)

Elastic resistance is ideal for strengthening the pitching mechanism because the resistance is not limited by gravity. Isotonic weights offer resistance in only one plane and direction. Elastic resistance can be provided in multiple planes and motions, including diagonal patterns similar to the pitching mechanism. Elastic resistance also allows concentric, eccentric, isometric, and plyometric strengthening. Finally, the portability of elastic resistance allows training on the road or in the dugout.

Several authors have described the use of elastic resistance for baseball pitchers (Carson 1989; Davies and Dickoff-Hoffman 1993; Kelley 1995; Litchfield et al. 1993; Page et al. 1993; Pezzullo, Karas, and Irrgang 1995; Powers 1998; Scheib 1990; Wilk, Voight, et al. 1993, Williams and Kelley 2000). Although elastic resistance training is a very common and popular method of training for baseball pitchers, few clinical trials in the literature have evaluated the effectiveness of elastic resistance exercise in baseball pitchers (Page et al. 1993). Page et al. (1993) used elastic resistance to eccentrically strengthen pitchers' shoulders in a diagonal pattern, simulating the deceleration phase (figure 14.08). They found a significant increase in eccentric strength of the posterior shoulder (20%) after 6 weeks of training.

Because of the demands of the deceleration phase mentioned previously, eccentric exercise has been advocated for pitchers. When elastic resistance is used, a controlled eccentric component is inherent from the onset of training (Hintermeister et al. 1998). Carson (1989) recommended using elastic resistance for the throwing shoulder specifically for eccentric strengthening exercises.

Plyometric exercises with elastic tubing have been recommended for throwing athletes (Davies and Dickoff-Hoffman 1993; Pezzullo, Karas, and Irrgang 1995; Wilk, Voight, et al. 1993). The pitching mechanism involves a quick stretch and rapidly successive shortening of the shoulder muscles. Plyometrics are thought to enhance this stretch-shortening cycle through specialized resistance training involving rapid eccentric and concentric muscle contractions. (See chapter 7 for more details on plyometric exercise.) Elastic resistance is ideal for plyometric exercise because of its ability to provide resistance through the range of motion at high training speeds. Shoulder external rotation and biceps flexion with the shoulder elevated to 90° (figures 14.09-14.12) provide a functional positioning for plyometric exercises for pitchers.

Although each pitcher's exercise prescription should be individualized to his or her needs, a core program of exercises should be included in any thrower's routine. These exercises are based on the biomechanical demands on the shoulder as well as the electromyographic analysis of common shoulder exercises. Exercises can be added or removed depending on the individual's weaknesses or strength imbalances. The following elastic resistance exercise program should be used as an adjunct to an overall body strengthening program. Because of the repetitive nature of pitching, these exercises should be performed with higher repetitions, typically 2 to 3 sets of 20 to 25RM.

- Prone horizontal abduction on ball (figure 14.02)
- Prone flexion on ball (Figure 14.03)
- Prone row on ball (figure 14.04)
- Linton external rotation (figure 14.05)
- Forearm eccentric pronation with FlexBar (figure 14.10)
- Triceps extension at 90° shoulder flexion (figure 15.03)
- Scaption (figure 4.30)
- Dynamic hug (figure 4.01)
- Push-ups plus (figure 4.09)
- Press-ups (figure 4.10)
- Shoulder external rotation at 90° abduction (figure 4.22)
- Shoulder internal rotation at 90° abduction (figure 4.24)
- Diagonal pattern D2 flexion/extension (figure 14.08)
- Plyometric external rotation at 90° (figures 14.09-14.10)
- Biceps plyometric curls at 90° shoulder flexion (figure 14.11-14.12)
- Forearm eccentric pronation with FlexBar (figure 14.14)

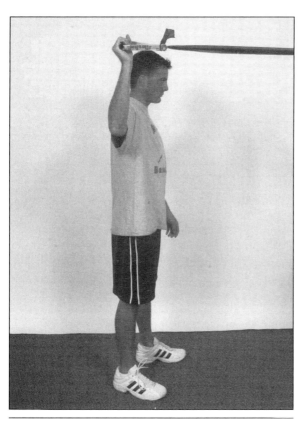

Figure 14.09 Shoulder external rotation plyometric at 90° shoulder abduction (start/end position).

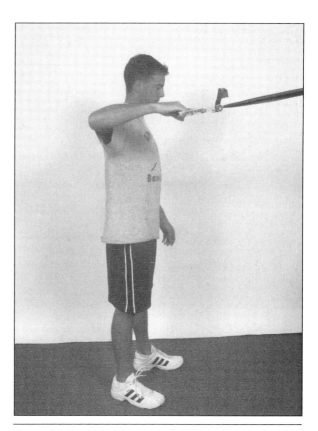

Figure 14.10 Shoulder external rotation plyometric at 90° shoulder abduction (midmovement/amortization).

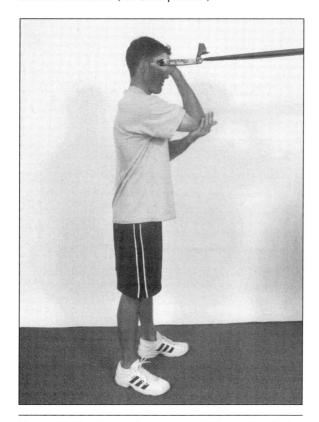

Figure 14.11 Biceps plyometrics at 90° shoulder flexion (start/end position).

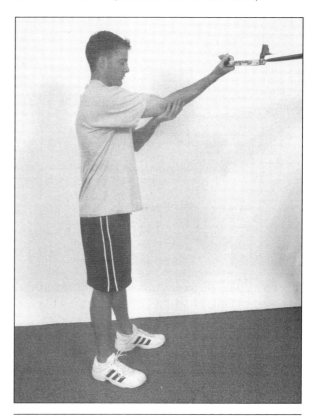

Figure 14.12 Biceps plyometrics at 90° shoulder flexion (midmovement/amortization).

Baseball Hitting Mechanism

Compared with the pitching mechanism, the baseball swing has received little biomechanical evaluation in the literature. The average hitter may only swing at a pitched ball 12 to 20 times a game; therefore, injuries are not as commonly related to the baseball swing as to pitching. However, strength and coordination are vital components of hitting a baseball. Any weakness within the kinetic chain can be detrimental to power and performance.

Welch et al. (1995) described hitting a baseball from a biomechanical perspective. During the motion, segmental rotation around the axis of the trunk was quantified at the hips, shoulders, and arms. In addition, the researchers found that the timing of each segment was crucial to facilitate successively higher rotational velocities throughout the kinetic chain, which produced bat speed and power, consistent with the kinetic-chain theory.

The baseball swing can be divided into three phases: stride, swing, and follow-through (Hay 1993). During the stride phase, the foot is lifted and advanced toward the pitcher. During the swing phase, the sequential rotation of the hips and shoulders occurs. Once the hips and shoulders are aligned, the arm swing is initiated. Finally, the wrists are "uncocked" or straightened out (ulnar deviation) as the ball contacts the bat. During the follow-through, the wrists roll over as a protective mechanism, with the back-side forearm pronating and front-side forearm supinating. (The front-side represents the side of the body closest to the pitcher.) Therefore, the hitter should also perform the strengthening exercises for ulnar deviation, pronation, and supination (figures 14.13-14.15)

Shaffer et al. (1993) evaluated the baseball swing mechanism with electromyographic analysis of the lower extremity, trunk, and upper extremity. They also noted a sequence of coordinated muscle activity from the hips, trunk, and arms. The authors advocated strengthening exercise for the hips and trunk based on these electromyographic results.

Unfortunately, no studies exist regarding the use of elastic resistance to strengthen baseball hitters. A strengthening program to enhance performance or return to activity after injury should be based on the biomechanics of the swing. Because of the kinetic chain involved in hitting, the legs, trunk, and arms all should be strengthened. Because baseball hitting is a two-handed skill, each side of the body

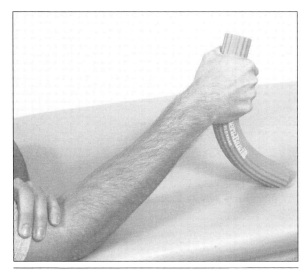

Figure 14.13 Ulnar deviation with FlexBar.

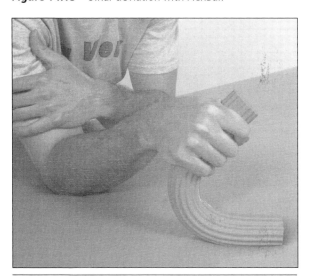

Figure 14.14 Pronation with FlexBar.

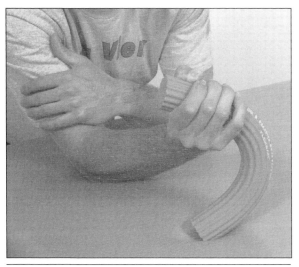

Figure 14.15 Supination with FlexBar.

may be strengthened differently according to its specific function.

A general strengthening program should be complemented by specific exercises to improve specific components of the baseball swing. Isolated components of the swing can be strengthened first, such as front-side extension (figures 14.16 and 14.17) and back-side follow-through (figures 14.18 and 14.19). The entire swing then can be integrated (figures 14.20 and 14.21) and simulated functionally with a baseball bat (figure 14.22). Following is a list of exercises for hitters:

- Ulnar deviation (figure 14.13)
- Pronation, back-side (figure 14.14)
- Supination, front-side (figure 14.15)
- Elbow extension (figure 4.32)
- D1 extension, front side (figure 4.18)
- Trunk rotation (figures 6.23 and 6.24)
- Front-side extension (figures 14.16 and 14.17)
- Back-side follow-through (figure 14.18 and 14.19)
- Swing simulation (figures 14.20 and 14.21)
- Bat simulation (figure 14.22)

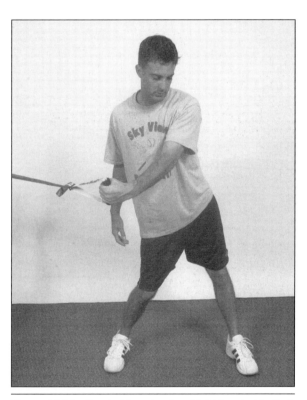

Figure 14.16 Front-side extension (right-handed batter): start position.

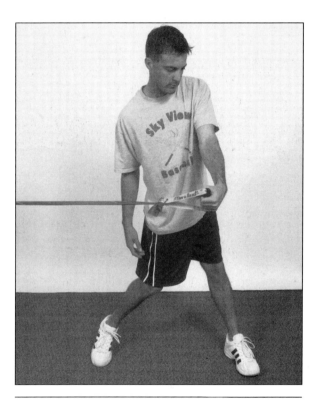

Figure 14.17 Front-side extension (right-handed batter): end position.

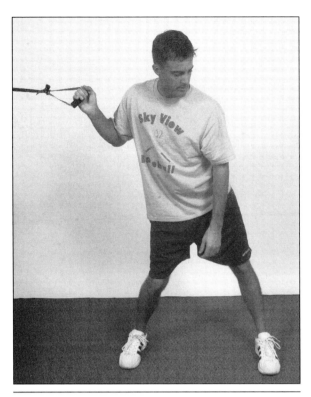

Figure 14.18 Back-side follow-through (right-handed batter): start position.

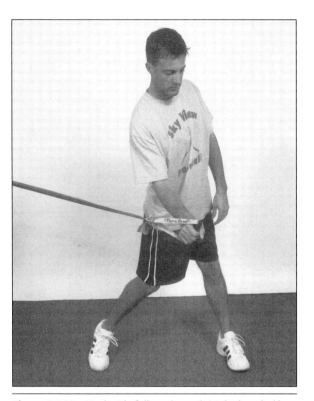

Figure 14.19 Back-side follow-through (right-handed batter): end position.

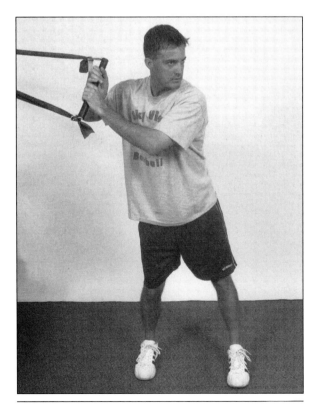

Figure 14.20 Swing simulation: start position.

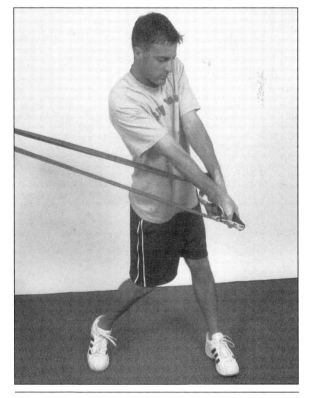

Figure 14.21 Swing simulation: end position.

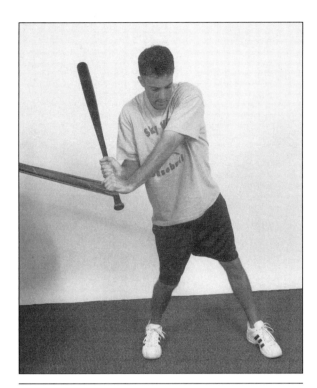

Figure 14.22 Baseball bat swing.

Conclusion

Baseball involves a variety of positional demands. Each position has component skills and fundamental movements such as hitting or throwing. Regardless of the skill, the kinetic chain passes momentum between segments from the legs to the hands. Muscle balance and coordination are vital for this kinetic chain to function properly. A scientifically based, individualized exercise program with skill-specific components is essential for optimal performance and injury prevention. This chapter has described the specific components of such a program for baseball players using elastic resistance. Much needs to be done to demonstrate the efficacy of these interventions in preventing injury and improving performance.

References

Alderink, G.J., and D.J. Kuck. 1986. "Isokinetic Shoulder Strength of High School and College-Aged Pitchers." *Journal of Orthopaedic and Sports Physical Therapy* 7: 163-72.

Andrews, J.A., and K.E. Wilk. 1994. "Shoulder Injuries in Baseball." Pp. 369-89 in *The Athlete's Shoulder*, ed. J.R. Andrews and K.E. Wilk. New York: Churchill Livingstone.

Carson, W.G. 1989. "Rehabilitation of the Throwing Shoulder." *Clinics in Sports Medicine* 8(4): 657-89.

Cook, E.E, V.L. Gray, E. Savinar-Nogue, and J. Medeiros. 1987. "Shoulder Antagonistic Strength Ratios: A Comparison Between College-Level Baseball Pitchers and Non-Pitchers." *Journal of Orthopaedic and Sports Physical Therapy* 8: 451-61.

Davies, G.J., and S. Dickoff-Hoffman. 1993. "Neuromuscular Testing and Rehabilitation of the Shoulder Complex." *Journal of Orthopaedic and Sports Physical Therapy* 13(2): 449-58.

Day, R.W., R.J. Moore, and P. Patterson. 1987. "Isokinetic Torque Production of the Shoulder in a Functional Movement Pattern." *Athletic Training* 23: 333-8.

Decker, M.J., R.A. Hintermeister, K. Faber, and R.J. Hawkins. 1999. "Serratus Anterior Muscle Activity During Selected Rehabilitation Exercises." *American Journal of Sports Medicine* 27(6): 784-91.

DiGiovine, N.M., F.W. Jobe, M. Pink, and J. Perry. 1992. "An Electromyographic Analysis of the Upper Extremity in Pitching." *Journal of Shoulder and Elbow Surgery* 1: 15-25.

Dillman, C.J., G.S. Fleisig, and J.R. Andrews. 1993. "Biomechanics of Pitching With Emphasis Upon Shoulder Kinematics." *Journal of Orthopaedic and Sports Physical Therapy* 18(2): 402-8.

Fleisig, F.G., J.R. Andrews, C.J. Dillman, and R.F. Escamilla. 1995. "Kinetics of Baseball Pitching With Implications About Injury Mechanisms." *American Journal of Sports Medicine* 23(2): 233-9.

Gowan, I.D., F.W. Jobe, J.E. Tibone, J. Perry, and D.R. Moynes. 1987. "A Comparative Electromyographic Analysis of the Shoulder During Pitching." *American Journal of Sports Medicine* 15(6): 586-90.

Hay, J.G. 1993. *The Biomechanics of Sports Techniques*. 4th ed. Englewood Cliffs, NJ: Prentice-Hall.

Hintermeister, R.A., G.W. Lange, J.M. Schultheis, M.J. Bey, and R.J. Hawkins. 1998. "Electromyographic Activity and Applied Load During Shoulder Rehabilitation Exercises Using Elastic Resistance." *American Journal of Sports Medicine* 26(2): 210-20.

Hinton, R.Y. 1988. "Isokinetic Evaluation of Shoulder Rotational Strength in High School Baseball Pitchers." *American Journal of Sports Medicine* 16: 274-9.

Ivey, F.M., J.H. Calhoun, K. Rusche, and J. Bierschenk. 1985. "Isokinetic Testing of Shoulder Strength: Normal Values." *Archives of Physical Medicine and Rehabilitation* 66: 384-6.

Jobe, F.W., D. Radovich, J.E. Tibone, and J. Perry. 1984. "An EMG Analysis of the Shoulder in Pitching. A Second Report." *American Journal of Sports Medicine* 12(3): 218-20.

Jobe, F.W., J.E. Tibone, J. Perry, and D. Moynes. 1983. "An EMG Analysis of the Shoulder in Throwing and Pitching. A Preliminary Report." *American Journal of Sports Medicine* 11(1): 3-5.

Kelley, M.J. 1995. "Anatomic and Biomechanical Rationale for Rehabilitation of the Athlete's Shoulder." *Journal of Sport Rehabilitation* 4: 122-54.

Kibler, W.B. 1998. "Determining the Extent of the Functional Deficit." Pp. 16-19 in *Functional Rehabilitation of Sports and Musculoskeletal Injuries*, ed. W.B. Kibler, S.A. Herring, J.M. Press, and P.A. Lee. Gaithersburg, MD: Aspen.

Kronberg, M., G. Nemeth, and L. Brostrom. 1990. "Muscle Activity and Coordination in the Normal Shoulder. An Electromyographic Study." *Clinical Orthopaedics and Related Research* 257: 76-85.

Litchfield, R., R. Hawkins, C.J. Dillman, J. Atkins, and G. Hagerman. 1993. "Rehabilitation of the Overhead Athlete." *Journal of Orthopaedic and Sports Physical Therapy* 18(2): 433-41.

McCleod, W.D. 1985. "The Pitching Mechanism." Pp. 22-28 in *Injuries to the Throwing Arm*, ed. B. Zairns, J.R. Andrews, and W.G. Carson. Philadelphia: Saunders.

Moseley, J.B., F.W. Jobe, M. Pink, J. Perry, and J. Tibone. 1992. "EMG Analysis of the Scapular Muscles During a Shoulder Rehabilitation Program." *American Journal of Sports Medicine* 20(2): 128-34.

Page, P.A., J. Lamberth, B. Abadie, R. Boling, R. Collins, and R. Linton. 1993. "Posterior Rotator Cuff Strengthening Using Thera-Band" in a Functional Diagonal Pattern in Collegiate Baseball Pitchers." *Journal of Athletic Training* 28(4): 346-54.

Pedegana, L.R., R.C. Elsner, D. Roberts, J. Lang, and V. Farewell. 1982. "The Relationship of Upper Extremity Strength to Throwing Speed." *American Journal of Sports Medicine* 10: 352-4.

Pezzullo, D.J., S. Karas, and J.J. Irrgang. 1995. "Functional Plyometric Exercises for the Throwing Athlete." *Journal of Athletic Training* 30(1): 22-6.

Pottieger, J.A., and G.D. Wilson. 1989. "Training the Pitcher: A Physiological Perspective." *National Strength and Conditioning Association Journal* 11(3): 24-6.

Powers, M.E. 1998. "Rotator Cuff Training for Pitchers." *Journal of Sport Rehabilitation* 7: 285-99.

Scheib, J.S. 1990. "Diagnosis and Rehabilitation of the Shoulder Impingement Syndrome in the Overhand and Throwing Athlete." *Rheumatic Disease Clinics of North America* 16(4): 971-88.

Scoville, C.R., R.A. Arciero, D.C. Taylor, and P.D. Stoneman. 1997. "End Range Eccentric Antagonist/Concentric Agonist Strength Ratios: A New Perspective in Shoulder Strength Assessment." *Journal of Orthopaedic and Sports Physical Therapy* 25(3): 203-7.

Shaffer, B., F.W. Jobe, M. Pink, and J. Perry. 1993. "Baseball Batting. An Electromyographic Study." *Clinical Orthopaedics* 292: 285-93.

Townsend, H., F.W. Jobe, M. Pink, and J. Perry. 1991. "Electromyographic Analysis of the Glenohumeral Muscles During a Baseball Rehabilitation Program." *American Journal of Sports Medicine* 19(3): 264-72.

Walk, S., M.A. Clark, and V. Seefeldt. 1996. "Baseball and Softball." Pp. 63-85 in *Epidemiology of Sports Injuries*, ed. D.J. Caine, C.G. Caine, and K.J. Linder. Champaign IL: Human Kinetics.

Welch, C.M., S.A. Banks, F.F. Cook, and P. Dravotich. 1995. "Hitting a Baseball: A Biomechanical Description." *Journal of Orthopaedic and Sports Physical Therapy* 22(5): 193-201.

Wilk, K.E., J.R. Andrews, C.A. Arrigo, M.A. Keirns, and D.J. Erber. 1993. "The Strength Characteristics of Internal and External Rotator Muscles in Professional Baseball Pitchers." *American Journal of Sports Medicine* 21: 61-6.

Wilk, K.E., W.L. Voight, M.A. Keirns, V. Gambetta, J.R. Andrews, and C.J. Dillman. 1993. "Stretch-Shortening Drills for the Upper Extremities: Theory and Clinical Application." *Journal of Orthopaedic and Sports Physical Therapy* 17(5): 225-39.

Williams, G.R., and M. Kelley. 2000. "Management of Rotator Cuff and Impingement Injuries in the Athlete." *Journal of Athletic Training* 35(3): 300-15.

Wooden, M.J., B. Greenfield, M. Johanson, L. Litzelman, M. Mundrane, and R.A. Donatelli. 1992. "Effects of Strength Training on Throwing Velocity and Shoulder Muscle Performance in Teenage Baseball Players." *Journal of Orthopaedic and Sports Physical Therapy* 15(5): 223-8.

CHAPTER 15

Sport-Specific Training for Tennis

• • • • •

Todd S. Ellenbecker, MS, PT, SCS, OCS, CSCS
Physiotherapy Associates, Scottsdale Sports Clinic, Scottsdale, Arizona

E. Paul Roetert, PhD, FACSM
USA Tennis High Performance, Key Biscayne, Florida

Tennis places repetitive demands on the human body that can lead to injury and jeopardize performance. Tennis match analyses indicate that more than 300 to 500 bursts of energy are required during of a tennis match between skilled players (Deutsch, Deutsch, and Douglas 1988). Characteristic adaptations in the tennis player's body, in response to these stresses, can lead to the development of muscular imbalances that can be addressed through exercise programs, both to prevent injury and to enhance performance (Ellenbecker 1995). Because tennis players travel extensively during tournaments and training, and because elastic resistance is portable, it is a useful part of training programs for healthy and injured tennis players. In this chapter we provide an overview of the common biomechanical stresses inherent in tennis play and discuss the most common injuries evaluated in tennis players. Finally, we present specific strategies for using elastic resistance to address the muscular imbalances commonly found in tennis players.

Biomechanics of Tennis

In addition to the highly repetitive demands inherent in tennis play, specific biomechanical stresses are encountered by the human body during successful execution of stroke mechanics and tennis-specific on-court movement patterns. Tennis involves both concentric and eccentric muscular contractions to accelerate, decelerate, and stabilize the body (Roetert and Ellenbecker 1998). Examples of the muscle groups commonly used during tennis strokes are presented in tables 15.01 through 15.03. Elastic resistance can be applied to these muscle groups because of its ability to provide resistance during both concentric and eccentric muscular contractions.

Serve

Internal rotation speeds of the shoulder during the service motion have been measured at more than 1,500°/s during the acceleration phase, with elbow

Table 15.01   Muscular Activity During the Forehand Groundstroke

Action	Muscles used
Acceleration phase	
Lower body push-off	Gastrocnemius/soleus, quadriceps, gluteals (concentric)
Trunk rotation	Obliques, abdominals, back extensors (concentric/eccentric)
Forward swing	Anterior deltoid, subscapularis (rotator cuff), biceps, serratus anterior, pectoralis major, wrist flexors, forearm pronators (concentric)
Follow-through phase	
Lower body	Gastrocnemius/soleus, quadriceps, gluteals (eccentric)
Trunk rotation	Obliques, back extensors, abdominals (concentric/eccentric)
Arm deceleration	Infraspinatus/teres minor (rotator cuff), triceps, serratus anterior, rhomboids, trapezius, wrist extensors, forearm supinators (eccentric)

Table 15.02   Muscular Activity During the One-Handed Backhand Groundstroke

Action	Muscles used
Acceleration phase	
Lower body push-off	Gastrocnemius/soleus, quadriceps, gluteals (concentric)
Trunk rotation	Obliques, abdominals, back extensors (concentric/eccentric)
Arm forward swing	Infraspinatus/teres minor (rotator cuff), posterior deltoid, rhomboid, serratus anterior, trapezius, triceps, wrist extensors (concentric)
Follow-through phase	
Trunk rotation	Obliques, back extensors, abdominals (concentric/eccentric)
Arm deceleration	Subscapularis (rotator cuff), pectoralis major, biceps, wrist flexors (eccentric)

extension velocities peaking at velocities of up to 2,500°/s (Dillman 1991; Elliot, Marsh, and Blanksby 1986). This rotation occurs with the shoulder abducted at approximately 90 to 100°. The apparent "overhead" position of the arm during the serve is achieved through both lateral flexion of the trunk and scapulothoracic upward rotation (Roetert and Ellenbecker 1998). These contributions from the scapula and trunk illustrate the use of the kinetic-chain concept during tennis-specific movement patterns. Extensive eccentric loading of the rotator cuff occurs during the follow-through of the serve and overhead, as the powerful internal rotation used to generate racket speed is dissipated after ball impact (Rhu et al. 1988).

Groundstrokes

Development of power during all strokes in tennis occurs secondary to sequential segmental rotation. This segmental rotation, often referred to as the *kinetic link principle*, involves the summation of rotational forces that start in the lower extremities, travel through the trunk, and ultimately are transferred to the upper extremity. Recent changes in the game of tennis, particularly in the last decade, have produced more powerful groundstrokes generated with different stances. Traditionally, tennis groundstrokes have been executed with square stances. Square stances involve a sideways orientation of the feet and body (body facing sideways to

Table 15.03 Muscular Activity During the Serve and Overhead

Action	Muscles used
Preparation phase	
Lower body	Gastrocnemius/soleus, quadriceps, gluteals (eccentric)
Trunk rotation	Obliques, abdominals, trunk extensors (concentric/eccentric)
Cocking phase	
Trunk extension & rotation	Back extensors (concentric), obliques (concentric/eccentric), abdominals (eccentric)
Arm motion	Infraspinatus/teres minor, supraspinatus (rotator cuff), biceps, serratus anterior, wrist extensors (concentric), subscapularis (rotator cuff), pectoralis major (eccentric)
Acceleration phase	
Lower body	Gastrocnemius/soleus, gluteals, quadriceps (concentric), hamstrings (eccentric)
Trunk rotation	Abdominals, obliques (concentric), back extensors (eccentric)
Arm motion	Subscapularis (rotator cuff), pectoralis major, serratus anterior, triceps, wrist flexors, forearm, pronators (concentric), biceps (eccentric)
Follow-through phase	
Lower body	Gastrocnemius/soleus, quadriceps, gluteals (eccentric)
Trunk rotation	Back extensors (eccentric), obliques, abdominals (concentric/eccentric)
Arm deceleration	Infraspinatus/teres minor (rotator cuff), serratus, trapezius, rhomboids, wrist extensors, forearm, supinators (eccentric)

the net). More recently, forehand groundstrokes and even two-handed backhand groundstrokes have been executed with an open lower body stance (body facing the net). This open stance forehand has allowed a greater amount of power generation from angular momentum and highlights the important transfer of power from the lower body and trunk to the upper extremity, to execute the shot. These open stances require even greater trunk rotation and trunk dynamic control (Roetert et al. 1997).

Morris et al. (1989) published an electromyographic analysis of the elbow and forearm muscles in tennis players. They found very high wrist extensor activity during the serve and tennis groundstrokes. Kelley et al. (1994) studied the extensor carpi radialis longus and brevis, flexor carpi radialis, and pronator teres in players with and without tennis elbow. They found significantly greater muscular activation in the wrist extensors of the players with tennis elbow compared with the uninjured players. In addition to finding greater activation levels, Kelley et al. (1994) found longer periods of muscular activation in these muscles in the injured group leading to premature muscular fatigue and injury. Therefore, electromyographic research shows substantial activation of the wrist and forearm musculature even in uninjured players but greater and longer activation in players with either improper technique or more novice levels of skill.

Movement Patterns

Tennis-specific on-court movement patterns reveal a great deal about the stresses incurred by the tennis player's body. Average points in tennis last less than 10 s. There are on average 4.2 directional changes in a point, and less than 20 yd is ever run in any one direction during a point. The work/rest ratios in tennis are formulated by estimating that points in tennis last less than 10 s, and rest periods between points cannot be greater than 25 s, according to the United States Tennis Association (USTA) and international rules governing the sport of tennis. This produces an approximate 1:3 work/rest cycle and places a large demand on both anaerobic power during points and the aerobic system during recovery between points and games (Roetert and Ellenbecker 1998).

Thus, training for tennis involves training the entire body to improve muscular strength, power, and endurance, in addition to performing specific exercises to enhance trunk and scapular stabilization, rotator cuff strength, and wrist and forearm strength. Although the force-velocity relationships inherent in elastic resistance may differ from actual tennis strokes, exercises with elastic resistance can be used to prevent injury and improve performance. The kinetic chain or link system, clearly evident in analysis of tennis movement patterns discussed in this section, forms the groundwork for this whole-body training approach.

Tennis Injury Epidemiology

Because of the whole-body demands of tennis, musculoskeletal injuries in elite performers are reported in nearly all areas of the body. A recent survey conducted by the USTA Player Development Department regarding the location of tennis injuries in its elite national junior team revealed incidences of low back, shoulder, elbow, knee, and ankle injuries. Injuries are of the overuse type and affect the upper and lower body as well as the trunk. Table 15.04 summarizes some of the available research on upper extremity injuries in tennis. Injuries to the shoulder and elbow are quite common, with the incidence of shoulder injuries among elite junior performers reported at 10% to as much as 30% (Kibler, McQueen, and Uhl 1988; Reece, Fricker, and Maguire 1986).

Of particular interest is the high association between elbow and shoulder injuries. Priest and Nagel (1976) studied 84 world-class professional tennis players and found that 74% of men and 60% of women had a history of shoulder or elbow injury in the dominant arm, which affected play. Injuries to both the shoulder and elbow of the dominant arm were reported in 21% of men and 23% of women. This finding indicates the need for total arm strength rehabilitation and training programs that integrate shoulder and scapular exercise for players with elbow injuries and elbow and forearm strengthening for players with shoulder injuries (Ellenbecker and Mattalino 1996).

Injuries to the low back are also quite common among tennis players. Marks, Haas, and Weisel (1988) found that 38% of 148 male professional tennis players have missed at least one tournament because of low back problems. According to Hainline (1995), tennis players may develop low back problems because of the large repetitive momentum in axial rotation coupled with hyperextension generated during play.

Finally, lower body injuries also are reported among tennis players. Reece, Fricker, and Maguire (1986) studied 66 elite junior tennis players at the Australian Institute of Sport, monitoring the players over a 4-year period for injury prevalence. Sixty percent of the injuries that occurred were classified as overuse injuries. Of those injuries, 59% were to the lower extremities, 21% to the trunk, and 20% to the upper extremities. In a similar epidemiological study, Winge, Jorgensen, and Nielsen (1989) studied elite adult players and found that 39% of all injuries

Table 15.04   Epidemiology of Upper Extremity Overuse Injuries in Tennis Players

Population	Age (years)	Sample (N)	Incidence (%)	Source
Shoulder				
Elite juniors	11-14	97	14	Kibler, McQueen, and Uhl 1988
Elite juniors	16-20	66	8	Reece, Fricker, and Maguire 1986
Elite juniors	14-17	24	30	United States Tennis Association 1991
Professional	14-48	104	17	Winge, Jorgensen, and Nielsen 1989
Recreational	25-55	2,633	7	Priest et al. 1990
Elbow				
Recreational	25-55	231	47	Priest, Jones, and Tichenor 1977
Professional	14-48	104	11	Winge, Jorgensen, and Nielsen 1989

over a 1-year period in 108 players were in the lower extremity. Injuries specifically documented in the knee joint in tennis players range in incidence from 7.5% in professionals (Winge, Jorgensen, and Nielsen 1989) to 15% in the United States Junior National Team (USTA 1991).

Use of Elastic Resistance in Tennis

When tennis players use elastic resistance, they can apply several rehabilitation and training concepts by using the specificity principle. These concepts are listed below. Recent research by Kraemer et al. (2000) demonstrated improvements in muscular strength and tennis-specific performance parameters after a multiple-set training program in female collegiate tennis players. Specific applications to the shoulder, elbow and forearm, trunk, and lower body are discussed next.

Shoulder

Research on the muscular strength relationships in the dominant shoulder of the tennis player consistently has demonstrated significantly greater dominant arm internal rotation strength, with either no significant difference between arms in external rotation or weaker dominant arm external rotation relative to the nondominant arm (Chandler et al., 1992; Ellenbecker 1991, 1992). This creates an imbalance between the external and internal rotators in the dominant shoulder and has been implicated in increasing injury risk and decreasing performance (Davies 1992; Ellenbecker 1995). Additionally, isokinetic research has demonstrated that the external rotators in the shoulder fatigue more rapidly during maximal-effort concentric muscle performance than the internal rotators in elite tennis players (Ellenbecker and Roetert 1999).

Finally, research on elite female college tennis players showed that a 4-month season of college tennis did not increase shoulder internal and external rotation strength or grip strength (Ellenbecker and Roetert 2002). Treiber et al. (1998) studied the effects of a 4-week elastic resistance training program for the shoulder internal and external rotators in college tennis players. Their results showed significant improvements in shoulder internal and external rotation strength as well as improvements in serving velocity.

These research studies indicate that training programs for tennis players should aim to normalize muscular strength relationships by focusing on the external rotators via supplemental exercises, using a low resistance and high repetition. The exercises listed for promoting shoulder external rotation and scapular strengthening are based on electromyographic research (Ballantyne et al. 1993; Blackburn et al. 1990; Decker et al. 1999; Hintermeister et al. 1998; Moesley et al. 1992; Townsend et al. 1991). These exercises include external rotation in neutral (chapter 4, p. 55), external rotation at 90° abduction with and without an oscillating device (figure 15.01), prone horizontal abduction (chapter 4, p. 50), seated rowing (chapter 4, p. 44), serratus punches (chapter 4, p. 46), and the dynamic hug (chapter 4, p. 44). Although many other exercises can be used, these exercises specifically target the muscles with noted weakness in elite tennis players, which are muscles with important functional implications in tennis-specific movement patterns (Morris et al. 1989; Rhu et al. 1988). Elastic resistance exercises that recruit muscles in tennis-specific movement patterns include the high backhand exercise (figure 15.02) for the posterior shoulder and scapular musculature at 90° of shoulder elevation. A low-resistance/high-repetition format is recommended with 3 sets of 15 repetitions typically applied to improve strength and local muscular endurance.

CONCEPTS FOR APPLICATION OF ELASTIC RESISTANCE FOR TENNIS PLAYERS

Use low-resistance/high-repetition format to match the demand of the sport.

Emphasize weak muscle groups to address sport-specific muscular imbalances.

Emphasize both concentric and eccentric muscular contractions.

Use lower extremity patterns that emphasize directional change.

Include trunk rotation whenever possible.

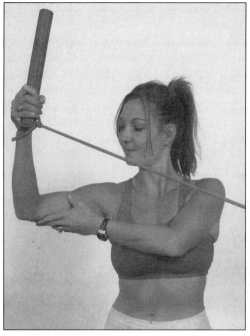

Figure 15.01 External rotation oscillation exercise with 90° of elevation in the scapular plane using the Flex-Bar (Statue of Liberty).

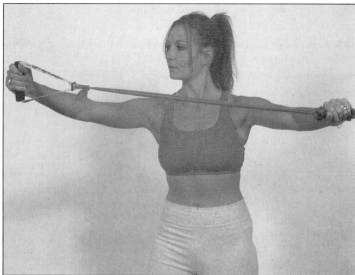

Figure 15.02 High backhand exercise.

Elbow

Research on elite tennis players again can be used to provide rationale for including elastic resistance exercise in training and rehabilitation programs for tennis players. Isokinetic testing has shown that dominant arm elbow extension, wrist flexion and extension, and forearm pronation all are greater in the dominant arm compared with the nondominant arm (Ellenbecker 1991; Ellenbecker and Roetert 2001). Forearm supination is not typically stronger on the dominant arm.

The use of elastic resistance exercise to increase strength and muscular endurance is recommended in tennis players to prevent tennis elbow and to guard against local muscular fatigue in these muscles, which would jeopardize performance. Morris et al. (1989) documented high levels of wrist extension activation in electromyographic research of tennis strokes. Exercises such as wrist flexion/ extension with elastic tubing (chapter 4, page 61), as well as forearm pronation/supination and wrist radial/ulnar deviation with a tennis handle or 12-in. long stick (chapter 4, pages 62-63), are recommended. An elbow extension exercise to strengthen the triceps in a position specific to the acceleration phase of the tennis serve is shown in figure 15.03. Again, a low-resistance/high-repetition format is recommended, with 3 sets of 15 repetitions typically used.

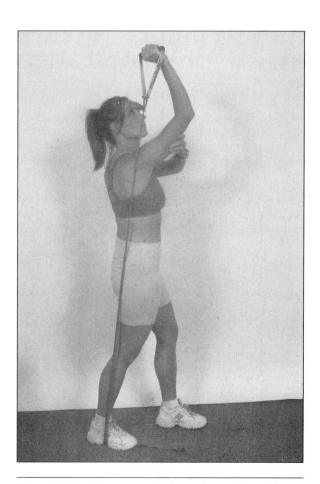

Figure 15.03 Elbow extension in serving position with supported elbow.

Trunk

Roetert et al. (1996) studied trunk strength in elite junior tennis players. Isokinetic trunk flexion and extension strength was measured in 60 elite junior players. Results showed stronger abdominals (trunk flexors) compared with gluteals and erector spinae (trunk extensors) in the tennis players. This is in contrast to testing performed in the normal population, where trunk extension is greater than trunk flexion (Timm 1995). Therefore, again, specific adaptations occur in the tennis players' body, most likely attributable to the high activation levels of the abdominal musculature during the service motion (Quinn 1986). This finding has led sports scientists to recommend exercises for the back extensors, to provide muscular balance, in addition to the traditional abdominal exercises. Exercises for the tennis player's trunk include back extension and hip extension to activate the gluteals and hip extensors in addition to rotational exercises to recruit the obliques (see figure 15.04).

Lower Body

Tennis players can perform many typical lower body exercises using elastic resistance. One specific application of tennis movement patterns to elastic resistance exercises is demonstrated in this chapter. By tying a piece of elastic band around the feet as pictured in figure 15.05, the athlete can resist 45° angled steps and side-stepping. This exercise can be made more challenging by having the player hold a medicine ball and mimic forehand and backhand stroke patterns, rotating the trunk and shoulders while moving the lower body in 45° angles or side-stepping patterns. This specific training drill, combined with quarter squats and hip abduction/adduction and flexion/extension training, can provide the tennis player with an excellent strength training stimulus to increase performance. The drill pictured in figure 15.06 reflects the challenges imparted to the trunk and lower body in the modern game of tennis. The open-stance forehand technique used by most players today has increased the amount

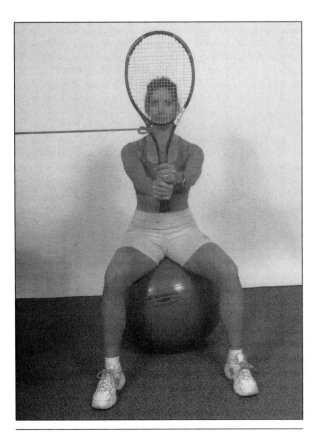

Figure 15.04 Seated trunk rotation on Swiss ball with racquet.

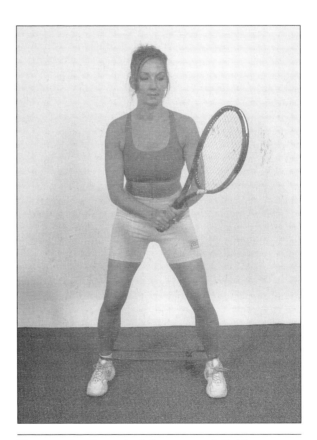

Figure 15.05 Lower body "monster walks" with racquet.

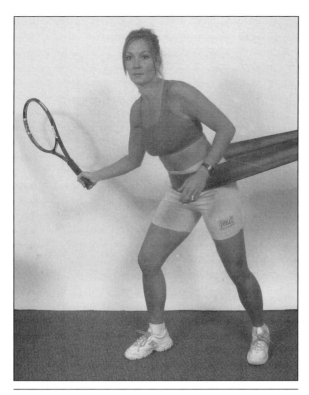

Figure 15.06 Open stance forehand preparation drill with racket.

of trunk rotation and angular momentum generated during the stroke. This drill involves resisting the first lateral step (right foot side-step for a right-handed player's forehand) with a piece of elastic resistance while rotating the shoulders with the racket to prepare for hitting an open-stance forehand.

Conclusion

Elastic resistance can provide specific training stimuli to address muscular imbalances in tennis players. The available research indicates that tennis-specific elastic resistance exercise can be applied to improve muscular strength, endurance, and balance; to treat and prevent injury; and to enhance performance.

References

Ballantyne, B.T., S.J. O'Hare, J.L. Paschall, M.M. Pavia-Smith, A.M. Pitz, J.F. Gillon, and G.L. Soderberg. 1993. "Electromyographic Activity of Selected Shoulder Muscles in Commonly Used Therapeutic Exercises." *Physical Therapy* 73: 668-82.

Blackburn, T.A., W.E. McLeod, B. White, and L. Wofford. 1990. "EMG Analysis of Posterior Rotator Cuff Exercises." *Athletic Training* 25:40-5.

Chandler, T.J., W.B. Kibler, E.C. Stracener, A.K. Ziegler, and B. Pace. 1992. "Shoulder Strength, Power and Endurance in College Tennis Players." *American Journal of Sports Medicine* 20: 455-8.

Davies, G.J. 1992. *A Compendium of Isokinetics in Clinical Usage.* LaCrosse, WI: S & S.

Decker, M.J., R.A. Hintermeister, K.J. Faber, and R.J. Hawkins. 1999. "Serratus Anterior Muscle Activity During Selected Rehabilitation Exercises." *American Journal of Sports Medicine* 27(6): 784-91.

Deutsch, E., S. Deutsch, and P. Douglas. 1988. "Exercise Training for Competitive Tennis." *Clinics in Sports Medicine* 7: 417-27.

Dillman, C.J. 1991. "The Upper Extremity in Tennis and Throwing Athletes." Presented at the United States Tennis Association Annual Meeting, March, 1991, Tucson, AZ.

Ellenbecker, T.S. 1991. "A Total Arm Strength Isokinetic Profile of Highly Skilled Tennis Players." *Isokinetics and Exercise Science* 1: 9-21.

Ellenbecker, T.S. 1992. "Shoulder Internal and External Rotation Strength and Range of Motion of Highly Skilled Junior Tennis Players." *Isokinetics and Exercise Science* 2: 1-8.

Ellenbecker, T.S. 1995. "Rehabilitation of Shoulder and Elbow Injuries in Tennis Players." *Clinics in Sports Medicine* 14(1): 87-110.

Ellenbecker, T.S., and A.J. Mattalino. 1996. *The Elbow in Sport.* Champaign, IL: Human Kinetics.

Ellenbecker, T.S., and E.P. Roetert. 1999. "Testing Isokinetic Muscular Fatigue of Shoulder Internal and External Rotation in Elite Junior Tennis Players." *Journal of Orthopaedic and Sports Physical Therapy* 29(5): 275-81.

Ellenbecker, T.S., and E.P. Roetert. 2001. "Isokinetic Profile of Elbow Flexion/Extension Strength in Elite Junior Tennis Players." Unpublished manuscript.

Ellenbecker, T.S., and E.P. Roetert. 2002. "The Effects of a Four Month Season on Glenohumeral Joint Rotational Strength and Range of Motion in Female Collegiate Tennis Players." *J Strength and Conditioning Research* 16:92-96.

Elliot, B., T. Marsh, and B. Blanksby. 1986. "A Three Dimensional Cinematographic Analysis of the Tennis Serve." *International Journal of Sport Biomechanics* 2: 260-71.

Hainline, B. 1995. "Low Back Injury." *Clinics in Sports Medicine* 14: 241-65.

Hintermeister, R.A., G.W. Lange, J.M. Schultheis, M.J. Bey, and R.G. Hawkins. 1998. "Electromyographic Activity and Applied Load During Shoulder Rehabilitation Exercises Using Elastic Resistance." *American Journal of Sports Medicine* 26(2): 210-20.

Kelley, J.D., S.J. Lombardo, M. Pink, J. Perry, and C.E. Giangarra. 1994. "Electromyographic and Cinematographic Analysis of Elbow Function in Tennis Players With Lateral Epicondylitis." *American Journal of Sports Medicine* 22: 359-63.

Kibler, W.B., C. McQueen, and T. Uhl. 1988. "Fitness Evaluation and Fitness Findings in Competitive Junior Tennis Players." *Clinics in Sports Medicine* 7: 403-16.

Kraemer, W.J., N. Ratamess, A.C. Fry, T. Triplett-McBride, P. Koziris, J.A. Bauer, J.M. Lynch, and S.J. Fleck. 2000. "Influence of Resistance Training Volume and Periodization on Physiological and Performance Adaptations in Collegiate Women Tennis Players." *American Journal of Sports Medicine* 28(5): 626-33.

Marks, M., S. Haas, and S. Weisel. 1988. "Low Back Pain in the Competitive Tennis Player." *Clinics in Sports Medicine* 7: 277-87.

Moesley, J.B., F.W. Jobe, M. Pink, J. Perry, and J. Tibone. 1992. "EMG Analysis of the Scapular Muscles During a Shoulder Rehabilitation Program." *American Journal of Sports Medicine* 20(2): 128-34.

Morris, M., F.W. Jobe, J. Perry, M. Pink, and B.S. Healy. 1989. "Electromyographic Analysis of Elbow Function in Tennis Players." *American Journal of Sports Medicine* 17: 241-7.

Priest, J.D., H.H. Jones, C.J.C. Tichenor, et al. 1977. "Arm and Elbow Changes in Expert Tennis Players." *Minnesota Medicine* 60: 399-404.

Priest, J.D., and D.A. Nagel. 1976. "Tennis Shoulder." *American Journal of Sports Medicine* 4: 28-42.

Quinn, A. 1986. "Abdominal and Lower Back Muscle Involvement in Selected Tennis Strokes." Unpublished master's thesis, University of Illinois.

Reece, L.A., P.A. Fricker, and K.F. Maguire. 1986. "Injuries to Elite Young Tennis Players at the Australian Institute of Sport." *Australian Journal of Science and Medicine in Sport* 18: 11-5.

Rhu, K.N., J. McCormick, F.W. Jobe, D.R. Moynes, and D.J. Antonelli. 1988. "An Electromyographic Analysis of Shoulder Function in Tennis Players." *American Journal of Sports Medicine* 16: 481-5.

Roetert, E.P., and T.S. Ellenbecker. 1998. *Complete Conditioning for Tennis*. Champaign, IL: Human Kinetics.

Roetert, E.P., T.S. Ellenbecker, D.A. Chu, and B.S. Bugg. 1997. "Tennis-Specific Shoulder and Trunk Strength Training." *Journal of Strength and Conditioning* 19(3): 31-9.

Roetert, E.P., T. McCormick, S. Brown, and T.S. Ellenbecker. 1996. "Relationship Between Isokinetic and Functional Trunk Strength in Elite Junior Tennis Players." *Isokinetics and Exercise Science* 6: 15-30.

Timm, K.E. 1995. "Clinical Applications of a Normative Database for the Cybex TEF and TORSO Spinal Isokinetic Dynamometers." *Isokinetics and Exercise Science* 5:43-9.

Townsend, H., F.W. Jobe, M. Pink, and J. Perry. 1991. "Electromyographic Analysis of the Glenohumeral Muscles During a Baseball Rehabilitation Program." *American Journal of Sports Medicine* 19: 264-72.

Treiber, F.A., J. Lott, J. Duncan, G. Slavens, and H. Davis. 1998. "Effects of TheraBand and Lightweight Dumbbell Training on Shoulder Rotation Torque and Serve Performance in College Tennis Players." *American Journal of Sports Medicine* 26(4): 510-5.

United States Tennis Association. 1991. Unpublished data on injury epidemiology in elite national team players.

Winge, S., U. Jorgensen, and A.L. Nielsen. 1989. "Epidemiology of Injuries in Danish Championship Tennis." *International Journal of Sports Medicine* 10: 368-71.

CHAPTER 16

Sport-Specific Training for Golf

● ● ● ● ●

Andre Labbe, PT, MOMT

Advantage Physical Therapy, New Orleans, Louisiana

Golf has become one of the most popular recreational sports in the United States and the world over the past 10 years and has seen an explosion in popularity over the past 3 years. It is one of the few games that allow players with different athletic backgrounds and skill levels to compete, which means the sport has a wide variety of participants. A major misconception about golf is that anyone can take up the game because of its minimal physical requirements. It is one of the few sports in which speed, strength, and flexibility are not perceived to be requirements.

With the increase in popularity of the sport, golf-related injuries have increased. These injuries have been reported primarily in the professional ranks, but as more people take up the game, more golf-related injuries are seen in the general public. The most frequently injured area of the professional golfer is the wrist and hand (Batt 1992). Because of the tremendous amount of time professionals spend practicing and playing, they tend to have wrist and hand pathologies related to impact. The spine is the second most injured area of the professional golfer and is the most injured area of the amateur golfer (Batt 1992). The effect of the golf swing on the untrained spine is tremendous, because the swing it-

self is a mechanism for injury in the lumbar spine. The rotation and side-bending that occur during the swing can cause excessive stress to the articular and ligamentous structures of the spine (Hosea et al. 1990).

This chapter highlights proper biomechanics of the golf swing and relates it to common pathologies and physiological requirements of the body. Finally, the chapter discusses common exercises with elastic resistance for the treatment and prevention of golf-related injuries.

The advantage of using elastic resistance is the creativity and versatility that it affords. It also allows the golfer to take his or her exercise equipment to the golf course and allows for proper warm-up and pregame strengthening. Elastic resistance also gives constant proprioceptive feedback to the golfer throughout the swing. This feedback can be used by the clinician and teaching professional to promote proper position and movement within the swing.

Biomechanics of the Golf Swing

Before treating the injured golfer, clinicians must understand the basic mechanics of the swing phases and the stresses that each phase places on the body. The swing can be broken down into four basic parts: setup, take-away/backswing, acceleration to impact, and follow-through.

There is no such thing as the ideal swing. The perfect swing is one that allows the body to get out of the way of the path of the club. This varies from person to person, club to club, and situation to situation. A golfer 5 ft 2 in. who weighs 200 lb will have a different swing than someone 6 ft 4 in. who weighs 170 lb. Even though their swings may look completely different, they both can exhibit the fundamentals of good golf mechanics.

Setup

The setup position is the most important aspect of the swing mechanics. Unlike most sports, in golf, the starting position has a great impact on the end result. The setup position also has great impact on the stresses placed on the body throughout the swing. Many times the most significant changes to a swing are made just in the setup position. In addition, most swing faults are seen in the setup position.

Flexion at the hip is probably the most important aspect of the setup, because a proper hip hinge is essential for the spine to remain in a relatively safe and neutral position throughout the swing (Cochran and Stobbs 1968; Hogan and Wind 1957). The spine is angled forward 45° from the hip hinge position. This angle of forward flexion (at the hips) is called the *primary spine angle* (Cochran and Stobbs 1968). Figure 16.01 shows the primary spine angle formed with the forward hip hinge position. This forms a 45° angle of forward inclination. Excessive thoracic flexion at setup is the most common fault among amateurs. Spinal flexion automatically limits some segments of the spine from rotating, and it changes the golfer's center of gravity by moving it posterior to the midline.

Another aspect of the spine is the *secondary spine angle*, which is formed when one hand is lower than the other on the club (Cochran and Stobbs 1968; figure 16.02). In a right-handed golfer, the secondary spine angle would be 5 to 7° to the right. This spine angle is also important for maintaining a neutral spine during the swing.

In general, the setup should look and feel like any other balanced and athletic position. An easy way to test a player's setup position is to challenge his or her balance while maintaining the setup position. If the player is easily knocked off balance, there is usually some fault within the setup.

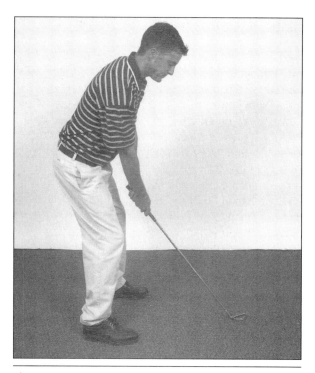

Figure 16.01   Set-up (side view).

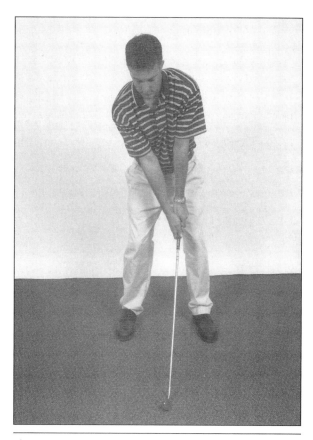

Figure 16.02   Set-up (frontal view).

Take-Away and Backswing

The second phase of the swing is the take-away and backswing. It is the beginning of the swing and is usually a mirror image of the follow-through. The take-away begins with rotation of the trunk away from the target (Hogan and Wind 1957). During the backswing, the shoulders must be able to assume positions that allow for the club to be brought to the top of the swing. The front-side shoulder must have good posterior capsular flexibility as well as good stabilization of the posterior rotator cuff musculature. This is important because the front-side shoulder assumes an extreme position of horizontal adduction at the top of the swing. In contrast, the back-side shoulder must be able to assume a position of external rotation of 15 to 35° (Cochran and Stobbs 1968; Hogan and Wind 1957). In total, the shoulders rotate 90° in relation to the setup position of the feet.

The hips are an important part of the backswing because they allow for full trunk rotation when the front-side hip externally rotates and the back-side hip internally rotates. The back-side hip and associated external rotators increase in tension and eccentrically load at the top of swing. This load is a form of stored energy that the body uses to accelerate from the top of the swing. In a 90° shoulder turn, 30 to 45° of motion comes from hip mobility, and 40 to 50° of motion comes from spinal mobility (Cochran and Stobbs 1968).

Acceleration

From the position at the top of the swing, the player begins to uncoil the "spring" that has been loaded. The hips begin to come back to neutral, followed by the lumbar and thoracic spine, while the player maintains the primary (hip flexion) and secondary (lateral side-bending) spine angles. The shoulders then begin to return to the impact position, followed by the wrist and hands moving from a radially deviated position to neutral.

Impact/Deceleration and Follow-Through

At impact, the body has shifted most of the weight back to the front foot at the same time that the club head has reached impact. At the impact position, the left shoulder, arm, wrist, and hand form a straight line to the ball. At impact, the primary spine angle is close to its original position during setup, with an increase in the secondary spine angle formed when more lateral flexion is required to transfer the force to the ball. After impact, the body begins to decelerate during the follow-through phase of the swing. Body weight shifts to the front-side leg.

During deceleration, many muscles begin to act eccentrically. The left-hip external rotators contract to slow the body and absorb some of the momentum gained throughout the swing. The back-side shoulder muscles also decelerate the swing. The largest energy-absorbing aspect of the swing is the eccentric load of the spinal paravertebrals and the abdominals. They originally are used to begin and increase rotational speed, but after impact they quickly reverse their roles and become decelerators. If the golf swing were a top spinning on a pivot point, then the abdominals and paravertebrals would control the center or axis of rotation around the spine.

After deceleration, the body ends in the follow-through position. This is a position of balance with the body weight shifted to the front-side lower extremity and the shoulders turned toward the target line. The front-side hip is internally rotated and the back-side hip is slightly externally rotated.

There are many keys to an efficient swing. It is essential for the player to realize his or her limitations and play within them. As stated earlier, all golfers have a swing that fits their body type, and they should not attempt to learn a swing that their bodies can't perform correctly. Golf-specific exercises should help adapt the body to the swing to prevent injury and promote better mechanics. At no time should a clinician teach the swing unless he or she has had extensive training from a licensed professional as well as experience of playing the game.

Exercises for the Golf Swing

When choosing from the variety of exercise tools for a certain sport, the clinician must use something that will be easy and accommodating to the golfer. It also must be versatile enough to address the different skills needed to be trained for golf (Jobe, Moynes, and Antonelli 1986). Elastic resistance seems to address all the needs of the golfer. It provides resistance in all phases of the swing and allows the golfer to work specific body parts for strength and endurance, including the lower extremity, spine, and upper extremity.

The most important aspect of the golf swing is balance (Hogan and Wind 1957). The balance and postural stability of the golfer at setup and throughout the swing can be the origin of many swing faults that cause injury. The foot and ankle are important for balance. They undergo the general stresses of supination/pronation during the swing and can cause stresses throughout the kinetic chain (Cochran and Stobbs 1968). The player's ability to train balance while maintaining a functional play position is important. This training can be accomplished with exercise balls or foam balance pads that will train proper balance and stability. The key for proper swing technique is the ability of the individual's postural stability to translate to the swing. Balance training can be addressed at all positions of the swing and can be carried over onto the course relatively quickly (figure 16.03).

Knee

The lower extremity is one of the least injured areas of the body related to the golf swing (Batt 1992; Duda 1987). There have been some instances of meniscal tears from the rotation of the femur on the tibia attributable to overcompensation with knee torsion to achieve a full backswing (Batt 1992; Duda

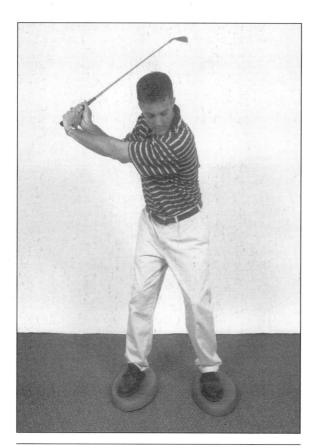

Figure 16.03 Golf swing while balance training.

1987). Of particular concern to the knee is the tension that may be placed on a postoperative anterior cruciate ligament (ACL). The closed-chain rotation that occurs at the knee during the swing can mimic the mechanism of injury for the ACL.

With the increase in the aging population, there is also an increase in golfers with total knee arthroplasties (total knee replacements). These individuals may want to return to golf and usually can as long as their swing does not generate any excessive torque to the knee. This is usually not a problem with aging, because the swing becomes more compact and inherently produces less lower extremity motion in older golfers (Cochran and Stobbs 1968). Also, by the time the patient has had the knee replacement, he or she probably has decreased the knee action in the golf swing out of necessity. General exercises to improve the lower extremity strength should be included, such as a lunge, squat, or leg extension.

The Hip

The hip undergoes excessive stress because it is a transitional zone between the movement of the spine and the stability of the lower extremity. The hip also absorbs energy during the backswing and follow-through (Cochran and Stobbs 1968). A lack of external rotation strength and a decrease in hip mobility can lead to poor osteo- and arthrokinematics at the hip. Exercises must be specific to the hip to maintain good hip motion and to strengthen the rotational muscles of the hip. This will allow the hip to withstand the stresses throughout the swing and lessen the chance of early degenerative changes to the joints. Elastic resistance can be used to strengthen the hip in many different planes with varying resistance and little equipment. General strengthening of the hip against resistance in cardinal planes (such as flexion, extension, abduction, and adduction) is important for hip stability. Hip rotational strengthening addresses the acceleration and deceleration needs of the hip throughout the swing (figures 16.04-16.06).

The Lumbar Spine

The lumbar spine is the most commonly injured area of the body in amateur golfers (Batt 1992; Duda 1987; Hosea et al. 1990; McCarroll and Gioe 1982). The swing, even at its best, causes excessive stresses to the spine. Professional golfers, even with their perfect mechanics and highly trained bodies, also have lumbar pain related to the game. In 1990, 24%

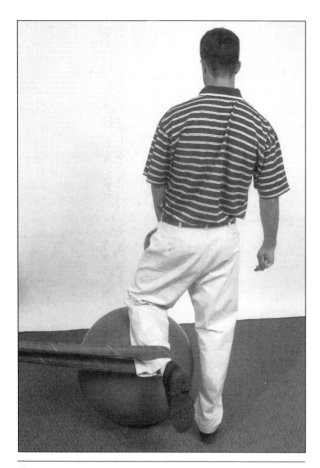

Figure 16.04   Hip external rotation.

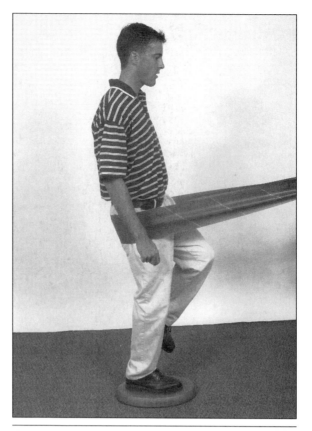

Figure 16.05   Closed-chain hip external rotation (start position).

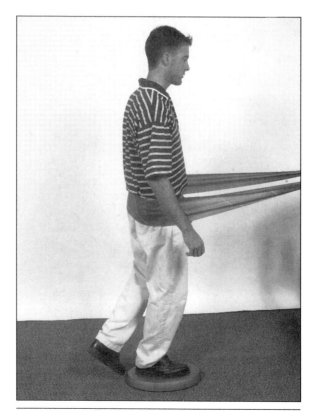

Figure 16.06   Closed-chain hip external rotation (end position).

of the professionals on the Professional Golfers' Association of America (PGA) tour had some form of lumbar pain (McCarroll and Gioe 1982).

Strength and stability of the abdominals and lumbar paravertebrals are necessary to control the rotary motion of the swing. The athlete can perform abdominal strengthening exercises using elastic resistance or an exercise ball. In particular, the abdominal obliques and lumbar paravertebrals can be trained in the diagonal and rotary planes that dominate their function during the swing (figure 16.07). Fatigue of these muscles will cause excessive stresses to the lumbar facets and intervertebral discs, which can lead to degenerative changes within the spine (Hosea et al. 1990; Pink, Perry, and Jobe 1993). The obliques are also the prime trunk accelerator during the swing (Hosea et al. 1990, Pink, Perry, and Jobe 1993). Enhancing their strength will assist in injury prevention and promote more acceleration throughout the swing. More acceleration translates into more clubhead speed and enhanced performance.

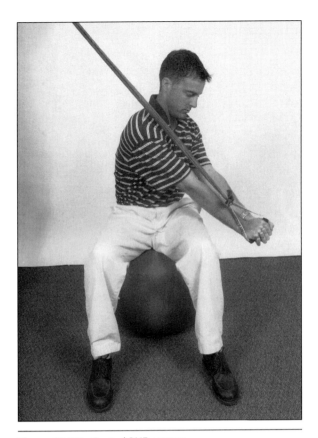

Figure 16.07 Seated PNF pattern.

The Shoulders

The shoulders also undergo a large amount of stress during the golf swing. Primarily, the front-side shoulder has excessive posterior rotator cuff stress attributable to repeated horizontal adduction at the top of the backswing. This repeated stretch of the posterior capsule can lead to subtle instability and weakness (Jobe, Moynes, and Antonelli 1986). In addition, at impact, the front-side shoulder undergoes a fast eccentric load to the posterior cuff while it is in a lengthened position. This may be a mechanism for rotator cuff tears or posterior rotator cuff impingement. The front-side rotator cuff should be strengthened with external rotation (see external rotation exercises, chapter 4).

The back-side shoulder must undergo the stress of external rotation (10-45°) at the top of the back swing (Cochran and Stobbs 1968; Jobe, Moynes, and Antonelli 1986). This constant stretching can compromise the anterior shoulder, thus causing anterior rotator cuff pathology or injury. This should be considered in patients with anterior instability as well as patients who plan to return to play postoperatively. Internal rotation exercises should be em-

phasized on the back-side shoulder (see chapter 4). Certain shoulder surgeries will limit the amount of rotation and therefore change the swing mechanics. The clinician should take this into account when suggesting that a player return to activity. In some cases this motion could compromise the integrity of a rotator cuff repair.

The swing mechanism during acceleration and impact can be trained with elastic resistance. Figures 16.08 and 16.09 demonstrate the proper exercises for each side of the body during a golf swing.

Forearm, Wrist, and Hands

Although often overlooked, the wrist and hands are a vital link in the golf swing. Holding the club throughout the swing is difficult enough without the added stresses of ball impact. At impact, the stress to the hands can be enough to cause fractures, muscle tears, and ligament damage.

The repetitive stress to the hands and forearm may lead to flexor tendinosis (golfer's elbow) and extensor tendinosis (tennis elbow). Both are caused by repetitive action of the wrist and hand and the constant stresses caused by impact of the club with the ball, as well as contact with the hitting surface.

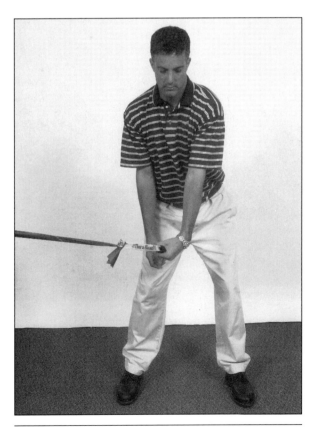

Figure 16.08 Shoulder strengthening at impact position.

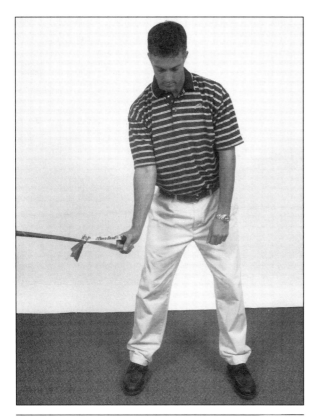

Figure 16.09 Back-side shoulder internal rotation strengthening at impact.

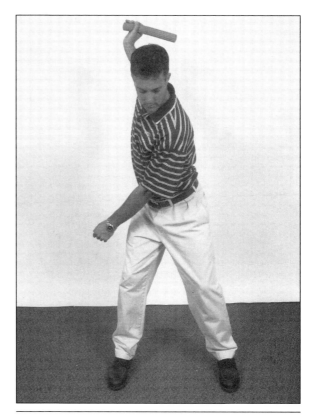

Figure 16.10 Unilateral oscillation with FlexBar.

A "fat" shot (when the club head contacts the ground before the ball) causes a substantial increase in torque and load to the wrist and hands and is often the origin of trauma to the involved musculature.

Preventive strengthening is an effective and efficient way to avoid forearm, wrist, and hand trauma. The Thera-Band FlexBar is an elastic resistance device for the hand and wrist that offers an easy way to perform all the basic exercises for the golfer. Figures 4.39 through 4.44 in chapter 4 demonstrate various wrist and hand strengthening with the FlexBar to mimic ulnar and radial deviation. Figures 16.10 and 16.11 demonstrate oscillatory training for general hand and wrist stability.

The best part about using elastic resistance with any sport is that the clinician and patient can use the elastic resistance in ways that are similar to the natural motion of the activity. The next two figures show some golf-specific and swing-specific activities that can be performed with elastic resistance. Figure 16.12 shows elastic resistance training at different points in the golf swing, whereas figure 16.13 shows elastic resistance used to resist the impact

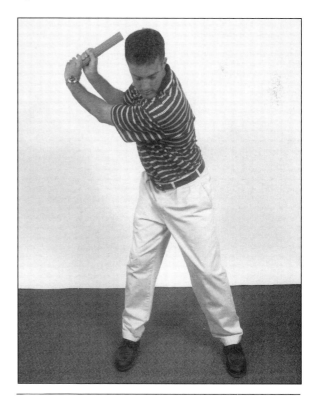

Figure 16.11 Bilateral oscillation with FlexBar.

position. This allows the patient to return to some sport-specific activity while still using safe and documented methods of resistance.

Conclusion

This is only a brief overview of some golf-specific injuries and the exercises that can be used to prevent and rehabilitate them. The key is prevention through proper biomechanics and exercise. The player must assume a proper setup position and maintain good balance and coordination throughout a movement that requires side-bending and rotation of the spine while the upper and lower extremities work in opposite directions. Obviously, the golf swing can be detrimental to the body, and proper strength and endurance are necessary to prevent injury.

References

Batt, M.E. 1992. "A Survey of Golf Injuries in Amateur Golfers." *British Journal of Sports Medicine* 26(1): 63-5.

Cochran, A., and J. Stobbs. 1968. *The Search for the Perfect Swing*. Philadelphia: Lippincott.

Duda, M. 1987. "Golf Injuries: They Really Happen." *The Physician and Sportsmedicine* 15(7): 191-6.

Hogan, B., and W.H. Wind. 1957. *The Modern Fundamentals of Golf*. New York: Simon & Schuster.

Hosea, T.M., C.J. Gatt, N.A. Langrana, and J.P. Zawadsky. 1990. "Biomechanical Analysis of the Golfer's Back." In *Science and Golf*, ed. A.J. Cochran. London: Chapman & Hall.

Jobe, F.W., D.R. Moynes, and J.E. Antonelli. 1986. "Rotator Cuff Function During a Golf Swing." *American Journal of Sports Medicine* 14(5): 388-92.

McCarroll, J.R., and T.J. Gioe. 1982. "Professional Golfers and the Price They Pay." *The Physician and Sportsmedicine* 10(7): 64-70.

Pink, M., J. Perry, and F.W. Jobe. 1993. "Electromyographic Analysis of the Trunk in Golfers." *American Journal of Sports Medicine* 21(3): 385-8.

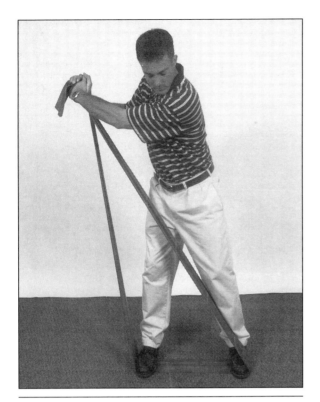

Figure 16.12 Resisted golf swing.

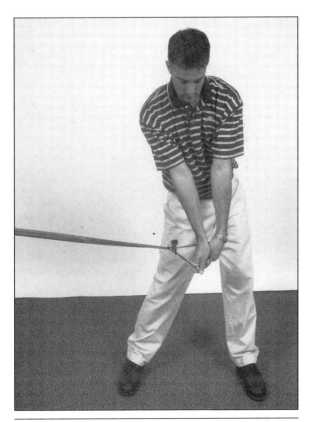

Figure 16.13 Resisted golf swing to impact.

CHAPTER 17

Sport-Specific Training for Soccer

• • • • •

Robert Wood, Chartered Physiotherapist
Active Life Therapy Center, Norfolk, United Kingdom

A s with training for most team field sports, soccer training once revolved around general cardiovascular conditioning, sprint work, and game skills practice. However, we now see a much broader scope of training techniques used at both elite and amateur levels. This has filtered down to soccer injury rehabilitation, with functional and sport-specific rehabilitation techniques now the preferred option. Elastic resistance training is still a relatively new concept within soccer and initially was used with basic rehabilitation exercises before it found favor within standard training activities. Its use is largely confined to either the clinical rehabilitation setting or training programs to enhance ballistic and multidirectional explosive performance (often called "speed, agility, and quickness" sessions).

Soccer is a game of unique physical dynamics. It is a team game of two 45-min halves, each half having no time-outs other than the short breaks attributable to normal game stoppages. The outfield players are in almost constant motion as the game ebbs between offensive and defensive action. There is clearly a strong endurance aspect to the game, with most of the gross activity being made up of sprint-recover demand; however, the fundamentals of soc-

cer skills are the control, distribution, and competition for a single ball, with 95% of ball contact being made with the foot. Essentially this is a high-velocity running game where the free running element is destabilized by the unpredictable ballistic demands of kicking, ball control, dribbling, tackling, jumping, and marking. The gross movement patterns that we associate with a soccer player in a game are of an oblique and rotary short-duration explosive nature. No other sport puts quite the same demands on total lower limb ballistic and dynamic control.

Lower limb injuries are by far the most common injuries sustained in soccer, with also a small but significant percentage of lumbar and pelvic injuries. A study of four English league professional clubs (Hawkins and Fuller 1999) found that during a competitive season, 83% of injuries sustained were to the lower extremity, with injuries to the thigh, ankle, and knee accounting for 54% of injuries sustained. The same study also cataloged the mechanism of these injuries and found that 56% of the injuries sustained occurred during tackling or running.

The incidence of injury is high, with a professional club expecting to see 10% of its players unavailable for match selection because of injury at any one time during the season. Soccer players are known to suffer relatively high rates of injury when compared with participants of other sports (Albert 1983; Ekstrand 1982; Nielsen and Yde 1989). When soccer playing is considered on an occupational basis, the level of injury to professional soccer players is approximately 1,000 times higher than that found in industrial occupations more traditionally regarded as high risk (Hawkins and Fuller 1999).

Clinical or Rehabilitation Applications

When elastic resistance is part of the overall rehabilitation strategy, it is used through early, intermediate, and late-stage rehabilitation, with a progressive integration of functional training activities and eventual crossover into pure performance enhancement protocols. As with most rehabilitation regimes, many of the activities used within soccer rehabilitation will be of a proven generic nature, as discussed in previous chapters; however, there are certain potential applications of elastic resistance training that lend themselves to soccer.

Although movement qualities during soccer are unpredictable, we can isolate recognizable movement patterns and kinetic chains and introduce these as patterning activities during all stages of rehabilitation.

When we consider movement as a chain, many soccer injuries of the "strain" nature occur during the eccentric decelerative component of the movement pattern, or at the point of transition between concentric and eccentric activity. This has particular relevance when we look at the actions of kicking, tackling, and directional cutting within soccer. Elastic resistance techniques can be applied to develop eccentric power and also eccentric fine motor control.

On the topic of movement patterns and chains, it is accepted that the gross kinetic range of movement of these patterns usually stays within the confines of the player's structural build, muscular flexibility, and joint range. It is also accepted that if the demands of the game situation suddenly dictate an excursion out of this "envelope" of kinetic performance, then injury is more likely to occur. Within soccer we see this during lunging tackles, "reaching" for the ball, and evasive actions. Elastic resistance techniques can be devised to load an activity throughout and, more importantly, at the extreme outer range of that activity's kinetic envelope. A controlled challenge of structures at their outer range is a prime example of applying a more functional approach to rehabilitation.

To deliver the free foot to the ball during the dribble, tackle, or shot, the soccer player relies heavily on a stable, secure, and strong weight-bearing limb—a dynamic base of support. As the player is doing this, he or she may be under challenge from an opponent, who, by the physical contact nature of the sport, is trying to destabilize this action. This lower limb duel is further fuelled by the torsional conflict between body momentum and playing surface grip and is the perfect recipe for twisting and gapping joint injury. The recovering limb will have to return to this exact activity, and elastic resistance techniques offer the most versatile and effective way of redeveloping and improving both peripheral and core stability. Challenging the limb and the trunk in positions of controlled destabilization forces will prepare the structures to resist these forces when they are encountered again in the game situation.

Performance Enhancement Applications

Training for soccer is not just about aerobic and anaerobic conditioning. We also need to increase functional strength, but at the same time, we should be working to improve range of motion (helping to prevent injury) and to improve ballistic movement. Elastic resistance techniques and equipment are being integrated into training sessions and can be seen in three main areas.

Explosive ballistic movement requires impulse and power (speed); it requires flexibility, adaptability, and control of directional change (agility); and it requires rapid, yet "light" foot movement with cadence variation and control (quickness). Because raw speed is of little value to the soccer player unless it is combined with agility and quickness, ballistic training sessions are concentrating on all three of these areas. The physically nonintrusive nature and portability of elastic equipment offers an ideal option to provide the resistance element within these drills.

Static stretching of muscle traditionally has been a staple component of soccer conditioning; however, when we start to look at the sport as a biomechanical flow of movement, we find that the extreme stretch end-range positions occur while the player is moving, usually at high speed. This has spurred the development of a more sport-specific functional approach toward stretching, with "stretch and move" or "dynamic flexibility" now being preferred.

Examples of Elastic Resistance Exercises

Exercise 1

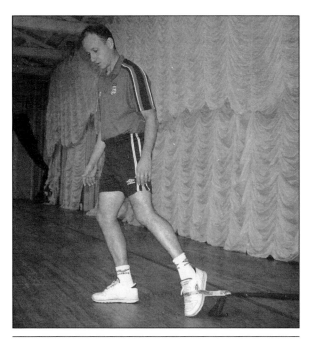

Figure 17.01   Basic kicking pattern: Start position.

This exercise shows the basic kicking pattern (figures 17.01 and 17.02). It is essentially open-chain resisted for the non-weight-bearing kicking leg. Notice the transition of the leg from external rotation to internal rotation and adduction at the end position, almost following a proprioceptive neuromuscular facilitation pattern. Stop-and-starts can be introduced and also a degree of eccentric control on the return to the starting position. This exercise provides useful early stage and patterning activity, but also progressions can be made toward power work by following "strength $\times$ speed" protocols into more ballistic movements.

Exercise 2

The open-chain kicking pattern can be destabilized to challenge the athlete's core stability by using a Swiss ball as a support surface (figure 17.03). Particular attention should be paid to pelvic girdle control and maintaining lower limb internal rotation at the end-range of the kick.

Exercise 3

This exercise uses the classic progression of using the kicking pattern but with the weight-bearing leg as the object side (figure 17.04). Initially, a firm base of support and small range kicking excursion are progressed to an unstable base (foam block/wobble board) and a larger excursion of movement. Different directions and angle of kick are also used,

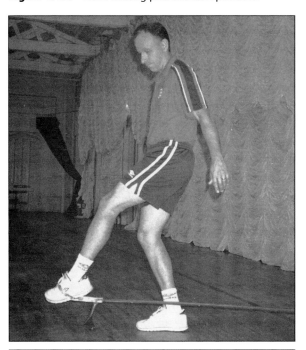

Figure 17.02   Basic kicking pattern: End position.

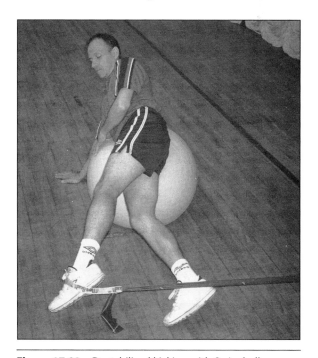

Figure 17.03   Destabilized kicking with Swiss ball.

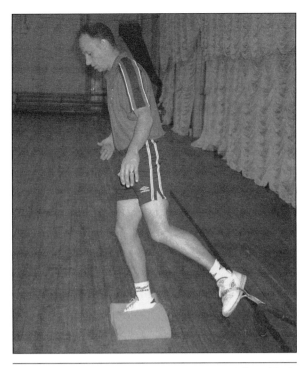

Figure 17.04   Destabilized kicking pattern with foam block.

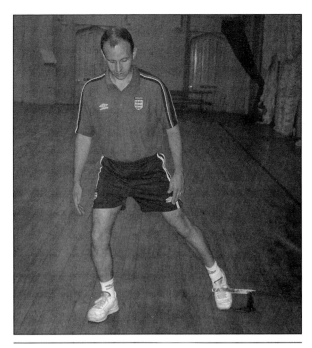

Figure 17.05   Adductor pattern: internal rotation and abduction (start position).

producing a rotational and lateral stress around the weight-bearing leg.

Exercise 4

This exercise works the adductor pattern, an essential functional pattern within soccer (figures 17.05 and 17.06). Note the reversal of the rotational component as internal rotation flows into external rotation as the movement pattern progresses. Progressions and applications are similar to the kicking pattern, apart from the introduction of the adduction pattern fixed in hip flexion.

Exercise 5

This exercise promotes hamstring deceleration control; the athlete mainly works on controlled eccentric lengthening into hip flexion (figures 17.07-17.09). This is a useful early-stage rehabilitation activity that can be progressed to include a core-stability component with use of a Swiss ball and then can be progressed further into standing as a deceleration component of the kicking pattern.

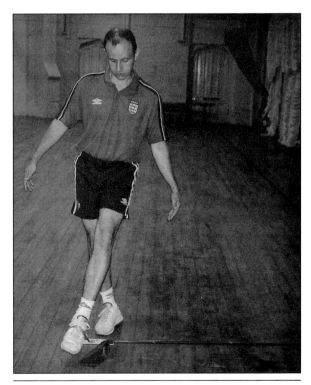

Figure 17.06   Adductor pattern: external rotation and adduction (end position).

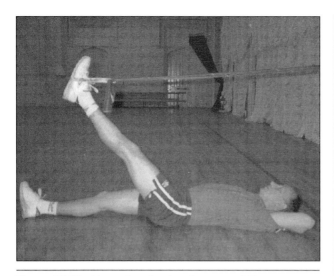

Figure 17.07 Hamstring deceleration control: Floor.

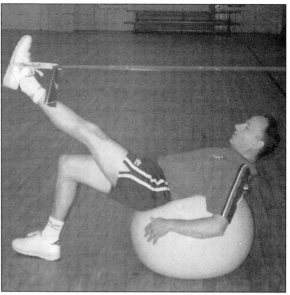

Figure 17.08 Hamstring deceleration control: Exercise ball.

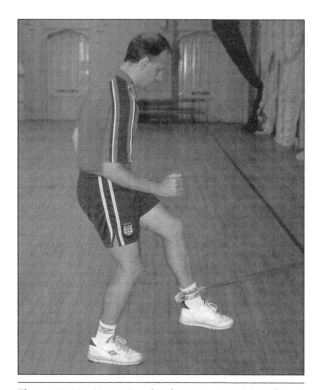

Figure 17.09 Hamstring deceleration control: Standing.

Exercise 6

This exercise involves the abduction/lunge pattern (figures 17.10 and 17.11). It is most useful when exercised as a dynamic functional movement with ankle cuffs and tubing. Initially the athlete works on range of movement and control, moving onto precision by using a floor grid, and then progressing to ball work to emphasize unpredictability and ballistic movement.

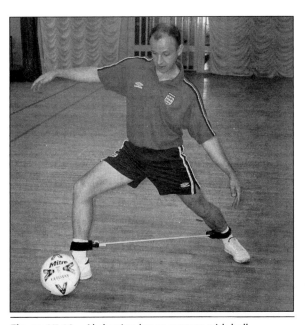

Figure 17.10 Abduction lunge pattern with ball.

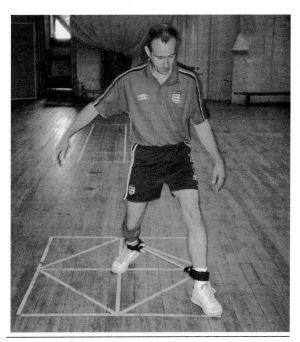

Figure 17.11 Trunk and lower limb combined control.

Exercise 7

This exercise challenges lower limb and trunk control (figure 17.12). Elastic cord is used with various body fixation points as the athlete goes through basic kicking or lunging patterns. The athlete is required to maintain control of the weight-bearing leg and also optimum pelvic girdle position. Relatively light resistance is used as controlled instability is used to promote functional stability.

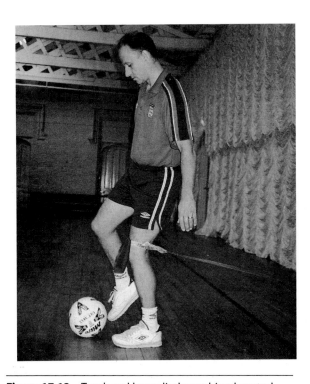

Figure 17.12 Trunk and lower limb combined control.

Exercises Used in Performance Enhancement Training Sessions

Exercise 1

This exercise involves lateral movement/cutting and burst acceleration (figure 17.13). Resistance is provided by two belt-fixed elastic cords at roughly a 45° angle. An initial 10-yd maximum acceleration sprint is combined with a cutting side-step. Variations of this activity include straight sprinting and repeated cutting (with the anchor players following to maintain a resistance).

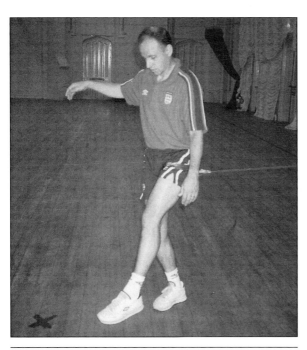

Figure 17.13   Lateral agility/cutting.

Exercise 2

Game skills can be introduced to the explosive sprinting drills such as heading or kicking (figure 17.14). With these activities, an in-line resistance is advised to reduce unnecessary destabilization forces, and the athlete is asked to perform the skill at one half to three fourths of the resistance range and to sprint through and past the skill to end-range. This maintains a more functional fluidity to the kinetic chain.

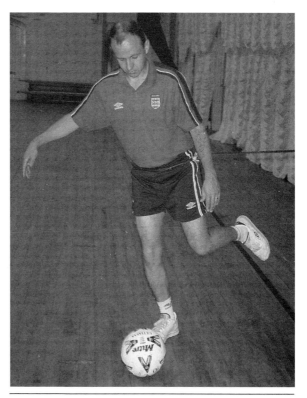

Figure 17.14   Functional game skills with elastic resistance.

CASE HISTORY

Patient F sustained a lunging groin injury while making a tackle.

- Day 1: Diagnosed as an adductor musculotendinous strain.
- Days 2 and 3: 48 hr of relative rest/immobilization and ice application.
- Day 4: Begin modalities along with local soft tissue work and controlled assisted stretching.
- Day 5: Light elastic resistance quads, hamstrings, and abductor open-chain patterns.
- Day 7: Begin elastic resistance kicking pattern for affected leg, including unaffected leg balances.
- Day 9: Begin light elastic resistance adductor patterns, with the hip "fixed" in flexion. Progress kicking pattern to use the affected leg for balance. Increase resistance in all other activities.

- Day 11: Introduce basic core stability challenges (exercise ball and band) and light jogging. Progress and destabilize balance work on affected leg.
- Day 14: Start "cuff and cord" lunging exercises. Begin standard light training activities. Controlled introduction of side-foot kicking and "blocking" can be preempted by using elastic resistance in these patterns.
- Day 18: Heavy resistance adductor work, kicking patterns destabilized by elastic resistance fixation at hip/thigh/waist. Three-fourths pace speed work, changes of direction, easy cutting, stop-and-start.
- Day 21: Elastic cord and harness with sprints, cutting, and jumps. Join in full training session.
- Day 25: Fitness test, back-to-game scenario.

Conclusion

Elastic resistance allows the freedom necessary to provide sport-specific movement patterns during exercise. This chapter provides background information about the sport of soccer and describes soccer-specific exercises with elastic resistance. These exercises can help to provide strength and endurance training to prevent injury and enhance performance.

References

Albert, M. 1983. "Descriptive 3 Year Data Study of Outdoor and Indoor Professional Soccer Injuries." *Athletic Training* 18: 218-20.

Ekstrand, J. 1982. "Soccer Injuries and Their Prevention." Linkoping, Sweden: Linkoping University Medical Dissertations, No. 130.

Hawkins, R., and C. Fuller. 1999. "A Prospective Epidemiological Study of Injuries in Four English Professional Football Clubs." *British Journal of Sports Medicine* 33: 196-203.

Nielsen, A.B., and J. Yde. 1989. "Epidemiology and Traumatology of Injuries in Soccer." *American Journal Sports Medicine* 17: 803-7.

Thanks to:

Alan Hodson, Head of Sports Medicine, The English Football Association, Sports Medicine Centre, Lilleshall, Shropshire, UK

Andrew Thomas, Deputy Head of Sports Medicine, The English Football Association, Sports Medicine Centre, Lilleshall, Shropshire, UK

Richard Hawkins, Medical Research and Physiological Research Coordinator, The English Football Association, Sports Medicine Centre, Lilleshall, Shropshire, UK

John Larner, Academy Physiotherapist, Norwich City F.C., UK

Alan Pearson, SAQ International, UK

CHAPTER 18

Sport-Specific Training for Swimming

• • • • •

Timothy C. Murphy, MA, PT, ATC
Concorde Therapy Group, Canton, Ohio

S wimmers compete in four strokes (Colwin 1992; Costill, Maglischo, and Richardson 1992; Councilman 1968; Maglischo 1982). The freestyle stroke is the most widely used and preferred stroke. It is characterized by alternating overhead stroking of the arms with alternating (flutter) kicking of the legs. The backstroke is similar to freestyle but is performed with the swimmer on his or her back. The breaststroke is performed by symmetrical movements of the arms and legs without breaking the plane of the water. The butterfly, which is the most demanding of the four, involves the simultaneous movement of the arms over the water, accompanied by concurrent kicking of the legs (dolphin kick).

The elite competitive swimmer can look forward to training 10 to 11 months per year in a competitive career that may last more than 15 years. Many swimmers practice twice a day and may average, at the elite high school and collegiate levels, as high as 8,000 to 20,000 yd (11.4 miles!) per day. Based on an average of 6 to 10 stroke cycles per 25-yd pool length, a swimmer completing a 10,000-yd freestyle workout performs 2,400 to 4,000 overhead strokes per arm per session. This figure does not account for the fact that the swimmer, as he or she fatigues and as stroke efficiency declines, must take additional strokes to complete each pool length.

Shoulder and knee complaints are the most frequently encountered orthopedic problems in this population (Johnson, Sim, and Scott 1987; Kennedy, Craig, and Schneider 1985; Kennedy, Hawkins, and Krissoff 1978). Knee pain may be experienced by up to 25% of competitive swimmers, the vast majority of which are breaststrokers. These problems usually are related to some combination of inadequate preparation, aggressive (inappropriate) training increases, and faulty technique.

When surveyed for past shoulder pain, 47% of 13- to 14-year-olds, 66% of 15- to 16-year-olds, and 73% of elite college swimmers reported positive histories (McMaster and Troup 1993). Interestingly, this applies to swimmers regardless of stroke preference or specialty, presumably because of the predominance of freestyle as a training stroke. Nonfreestylers may swim as much as 60 to 90% of their workouts in freestyle, depending on either the nature of their training or the relative fatigue of their primary stroke (such as butterfly). For this reason, most shoulder problems manifest themselves during the freestyle stroke.

Technique Fundamentals

The single most important factor in training the competitive swimmer is technique (Colwin 1992; Costill, Maglischo, and Richardson 1992; Councilman 1968; Maglischo 1982). Although we generally assume that the elite swimmer demonstrates good fundamental technique, muscular fatigue may be a factor in the deterioration of stroke mechanics over the course of a long workout. In other words, a swimmer with excellent technique but with poor local muscular endurance may become a swimmer with compromised technique (and attendant biomechanical overuse stresses) as specific areas of weakness develop during a fatiguing workout.

The Kick

The kick is unquestionably an important component in the overall propulsive force of the swimming stroke, although it is secondary by far to the arm force in all of the competitive strokes (Colwin 1992; Costill, Maglischo, and Richardson 1992; Richardson 1986). The kick also smoothes out the intermittent surges of the arms during both alternating and symmetrical upper extremity stroke patterns.

The kicking movements in freestyle and backstroke (alternating) and butterfly (symmetrical) involve hip and knee flexion/extension in the sagittal plane. Breaststroke involves a whiplike kick in the frontal and sagittal planes (figures 18.01-18.03), which begins with active knee flexion (along with hip flexion which is passive), then progresses to abduction followed by a forceful whip of hip and knee extension followed by hip adduction (Colwin 1992; Costill, Maglischo, and Richardson 1992).

In addition to having a propulsive role, the kick creates a lift that raises the body into a horizontal position, minimizing cross-sectional drag in the water (Colwin 1992; Costill, Maglischo, and Richardson 1992; Councilman 1968; Maglischo 1982). This elimination of drag not only improves speed through the water but significantly reduces

fatigue with time. Unfortunately, as leg fatigue reduces this lift, the drag that results will accelerate arm fatigue and attendant stroke deterioration.

The Arm Stroke

Upper extremity propulsive force in the primary competitive strokes comes about specifically by some combination of shoulder extension, adduction, and internal rotation (figures 18.04-18.07) during the pull phase in the water (Colwin 1992; Costill, Maglischo, and Richardson 1992; Councilman 1968; Maglischo 1982; Richardson 1986). The swimmer attempts to pull him- or herself past a given point in the water rather than simply moving the arms through the water. As the hand enters the water at the beginning of the pull phase (the catch), the swimmer sets the hand to "grasp" the water. The swimmer then pulls the hand past the body using a sculling motion that combines movements of the shoulder, elbow, wrist, and hand. This pull-through phase makes up about 65% of the swimming stroke (both arms are actually in the water at the same time for about one third of the cycle) and is the major emphasis of muscular strength and muscular endurance training for most swimmers.

The remaining 35% of the stroke cycle consists of the recovery phase, which returns the arm to the starting position for the next pull-through. Although recovery is not a productive part of the stroke in terms of propulsion, many coaches and sports medicine professionals are interested in the recovery as a potential contributor to many of the overuse problems associated with swimming (Aronen 1985; Cuillo 1986; Falkel 1990; Falkel and Murphy 1988; Johnson, Sim, and Scott 1987; Pettrone 1985). For the swimmer's arm to provide consistent power over many repetitions, the recovery must continue to place the arm in an optimal position for initiating the pull-through phase time after time. The muscles that perform the recovery generally do not hold the highest priority in most training programs, because of the heavy emphasis on the pull-phase muscles. It is fairly predictable then, that a break-

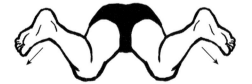  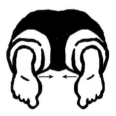

Figure 18.01-18.03 The whip phase of the breaststroke kick initially involves knee extension, followed by combined knee extension and hip adduction, and finally hip adduction with full knee extension. During combined knee extension and hip adduction, significant valgus stress may be placed on the knee.

Reprinted, by permission, from J.E. Cousilman, 1968, *The Science of Swimming* (Englewood Cliffs, NJ: Prentice Hall).

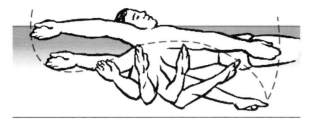

Figure 18.04   Phases of pull for the backstroke.

Reprinted, by permission, from J.E. Cousilman, 1968, *The Science of Swimming* (Englewood Cliffs, NJ: Prentice Hall).

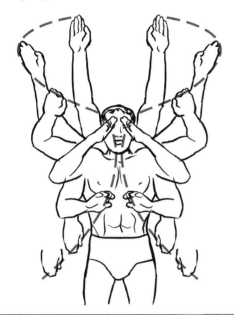

Figure 18.06   Phases of pull for the butterfly.

Reprinted, by permission, from J.E. Cousilman, 1968, *The Science of Swimming* (Englewood Cliffs, NJ: Prentice Hall).

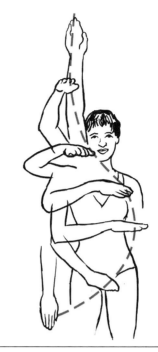

Figure 18.05   Phases of pull for the freestyle.

Reprinted, by permission, from J.E. Cousilman, 1968, *The Science of Swimming* (Englewood Cliffs, NJ: Prentice Hall).

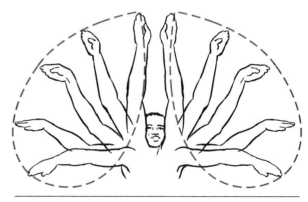

Figure 18.07   Phases of pull for the breaststroke.

Reprinted, by permission, from J.E. Cousilman, 1968, *The Science of Swimming* (Englewood Cliffs, NJ: Prentice Hall).

down in the mechanics of stroke recovery is one of the first observable fatigue-related changes in the stroke during a long workout (figures 18.08-18.09).

Dryland Training for the Competitive Swimmer

The open-chain, concentric nature of swimming simplifies the choice of dryland training options for the swimmer based on training specificity. There are few if any truly eccentric loads in swimming, and the only closed-chain activities of any significance are starts and turns (legs). Although there are relatively few of these types of loads, the cross-training benefits of eccentric and closed-chain exercise have been well documented (Fleck and Kraemer 1987).

Lower extremity exercise in the swimmer is focused on both hip and knee function. The primary effort in performing the flutter kick for freestyle and backstroke, as well as the dolphin kick for butter-

fly, comes from repetitive hip flexion and hip and knee extension (Colwin 1992; Costill, Maglischo, and Richardson 1992), areas overlooked in most dryland training programs. Additional emphasis may be placed on the explosive push-off needed during starts and turns, which suggests the use of closed-chain plyometric exercises.

Dryland training for the shoulder should be as sport-specific as possible, incorporating resisted training of the power stroke (extension, adduction, and internal rotation) as well as the recovery phase (external rotation, abduction, and horizontal abduction). Because the dynamics of all of the swimming strokes cross both the frontal and sagittal planes (sometimes concurrently), functional strength

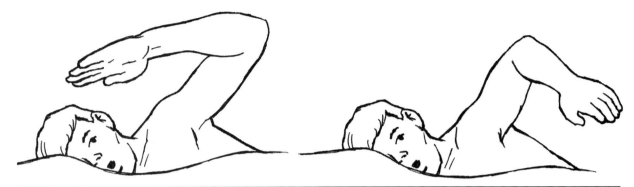

Figure 18.08-18.09 External rotation during freestyle recovery (18.08). Fatigue-related external rotation failure (18.09) is a factor in subacromial impingement.

Adapted, by permission, from J.E. Falkel and T.C. Murphy, 1988, "Case principles: The swimmer's shoulders." In *Shoulder injuries—sports injury management*, edited by T.R. Malone (Philadelphia, PA: Lippincott, Williams, and Wilkins), 115.

training is best accomplished through the use of stretch cords, free weights, and, to a lesser degree, manual resistance. Isokinetic and machine resistance methods primarily involve isolation and "guided" movements, which may contribute more to basic conditioning than to sport-specific training.

In-Season Management Considerations

Historically, swimmers' injuries have been difficult to manage in the face of continued training and competition (Greipp 1985; Russ 1997). Frequently, swimmers are able to modify technique for temporary symptomatic relief but end up in treatment when they run out of "compensations." It has been common for the swimmer to receive "damage control" treatment until the end of the swimming season, when it was hoped that the swimmer would cooperate and reduce training. For many swimmers, with competitive training lasting 10 to 11 months per year, this is clearly an unrealistic expectation.

Management generally has consisted of therapeutic modalities, medication, and rest, with occasional attempts at management through steroid injection or surgical decompression (Falkel and Murphy 1988; Murphy 1994; Murphy and Riester 1988; Penny and Smith 1980; Russ 1997). Unfortunately, the swimmer usually experiences recurrence of the problem shortly after returning to training, attributable to renewal of the abnormal or excessive behaviors and physical stresses that initiated the problem (Falkel and Murphy 1988; Johnson, Sim, and Scott 1987; Kennedy, Craig, and Schneider 1985; Penny and Smith 1980).

My colleagues and I advise the injured swimmer to continue swimming to whatever extent is asymptomatic and progress in a controlled fashion back to regular levels (Murphy 1994; Murphy and Riester 1988). Concurrently, the swimmer performs a series of remedial exercises, primarily using elastic resistance, in an effort to establish necessary strength and endurance to allow for successful pain-free resumption of unrestricted swim training. These exercises are performed 1 to 2 times per day. In addition, they frequently are repeated between workout sets to break up the swimming routine. In many cases, it may be possible to allow the swimmer to compete without restrictions during this management regimen while still curtailing the extent of "fatiguable" training.

There is generally no need for the health care provider to attempt to change the swimmer's stroke pattern in an effort to avoid the stresses discussed here. The goal of rehabilitation should be to provide the swimmer with the ammunition to combat overuse by maintaining good mechanics rather than manipulating the basic techniques of the sport.

Elastic Resistance Exercise Applications to Swim Training

Table 18.01 summarizes some important exercises and their applications to swimming.

Tubing Low Row

The swimmer starts with arms 30° forward (with light tension on cords; figures 18.10 and 18.11). Shoulders are extended until hands are next to hips while shoulder blades are pinched together in back.

Tubing Middle Row

The swimmer starts with arms 30° forward (with light tension on cords; figure 18.12). The swimmer

Table 18.01 Applications to Swim Training

Exercise	Swimming application	Muscle actions
Tubing low row (figures 18.10 and 18.11)	Late pull and early recovery	Scapular retraction Shoulder extension
Tubing middle row (figure 18.12)	Late pull and early recovery	Scapular retraction Shoulder extension Shoulder horizontal abduction
Tubing high row (figure 18.13)	Recovery	Scapular retraction Shoulder horizontal abduction Shoulder external rotation
Tubing press (figures 18.14 and 18.15)	Recovery	Shoulder elevation
Tubing shrugs and backward circles (figures 18.16 and 18.17)	Pull and recovery	Scapular elevation Scapular retraction
Tubing pull-through (figures 18.18 and 18.19)	Pull	Scapular retraction Shoulder extension
Tubing high row press (figures 18.20 and 18.21)	Recovery	Scapular retraction Shoulder horizontal abduction Shoulder external rotation Shoulder elevation
Tubing 90° curl (figures 18.22 and 18.23)	Early pull	Elbow flexion
Tubing triceps finish (figures 18.24 and 18.25)	Late pull	Elbow extension
Standing hip extension (chapter 5)	Kick	Hip extension (swing leg)
Standing hip flexion (chapter 5)	Kick	Hip flexion (swing leg)
Standing hip adduction (chapter 5)	Kick (breaststroke)	Hip adduction (swing leg)

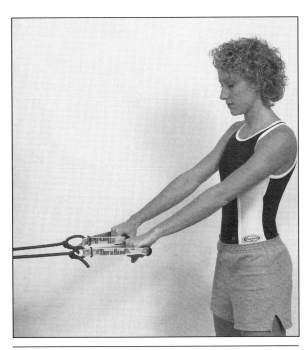

Figure 18.10 Low row (start position).

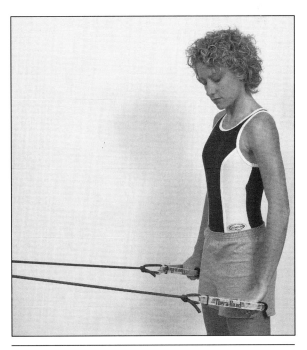

Figure 18.11 Low row (end position).

should pull hands toward chest (ending at breast level) while pinching shoulder blades together in back. Emphasize the shoulder blade component.

Tubing High Row

The swimmer starts with arms 30° forward (with light tension on cords; figure 18.13). The swimmer externally rotates shoulders while bending elbows to 90° and finishes in a position (shoulders) of about 70° elevation and thumbs pointing toward the ears. Shoulder blades should be pinched together.

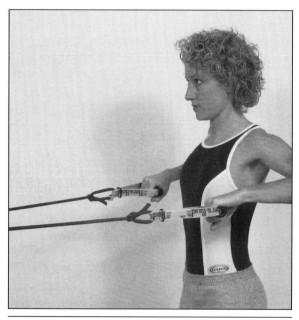

Figure 18.12 Mid row.

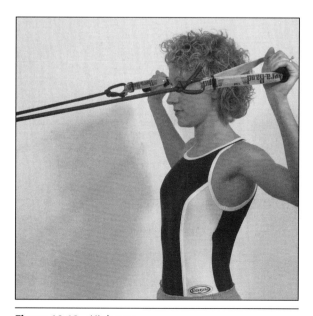

Figure 18.13 High row.

Tubing Press

The swimmer raises the hands 30 to 70° (away from the side) only (figures 18.14 and 18.15). Hands should not be raised above eye level (raising above 90° may "impinge" the shoulder). Palms are kept facing forward, and shoulder blades are pinched together.

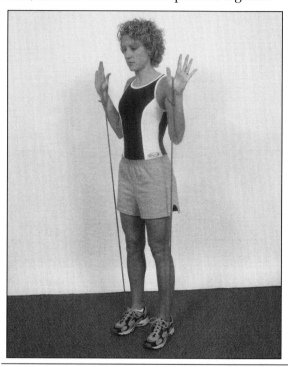

Figure 18.14 Shoulder press (start position).

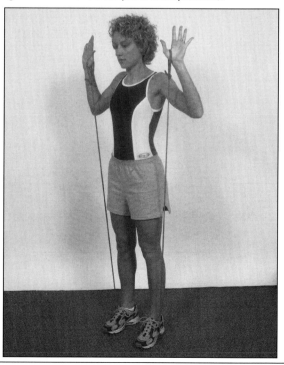

Figure 18.15 Shoulder press (end position).

Tubing Shrugs and Backward Circles

The swimmer stands on the tubing with hands grasping handles and elbows straight (figures 18.16 and 18.17). The swimmer begins the exercise by shrugging the shoulders straight up and then continues by pulling (pinching) the shoulder blades backward and lowering to the start position in a smooth motion.

Tubing Pull-Through

The swimmer bends forward at the waist and starts with the arms in an overhead position (figures 18.18 and 18.19). With the elbows straight, he or she pulls the arms through to the finish position while stabilizing the shoulder blades.

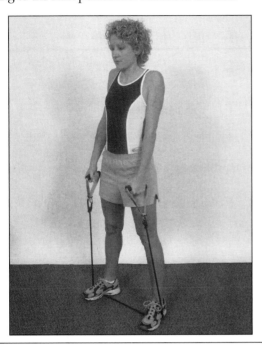

Figure 18.16 Shoulder shrugs.

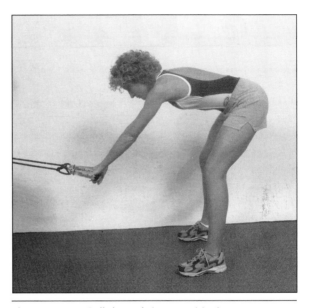

Figure 18.18 Pull-through (start position).

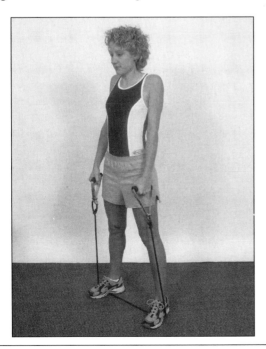

Figure 18.17 Shoulder backwards circles.

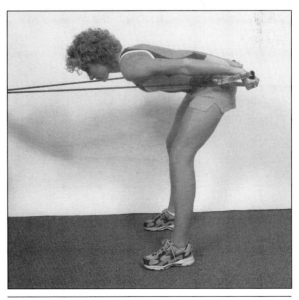

Figure 18.19 Pull-through (end position).

Tubing High Row Press

Holding the arms in the finish position of the high row (upside-down *M* position) and keeping the shoulder blades pinched together, the swimmer moves the arms up and down in a 30° arc (figures 18.20 and 18.21). The elbows should not go above shoulder height.

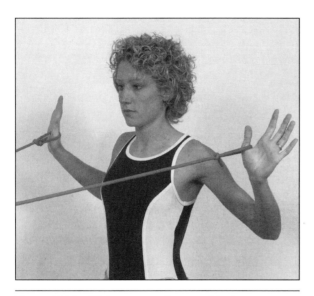

Figure 18.20   High row press (start position).

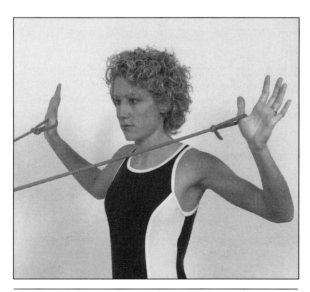

Figure 18.21   High row press (end position).

Tubing 90° Curls

Curls are performed with the shoulders flexed to 90° and the tubing going straight ahead (figures 18.22 and 18.23). Maintaining shoulder position, the swimmer performs curls by pulling hands toward the face.

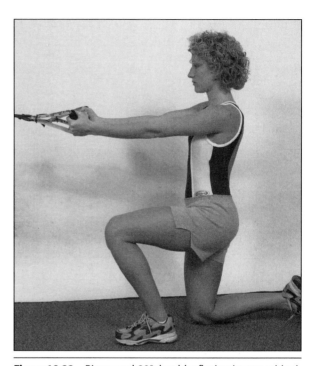

Figure 18.22   Biceps curl: 90° shoulder flexion (start position).

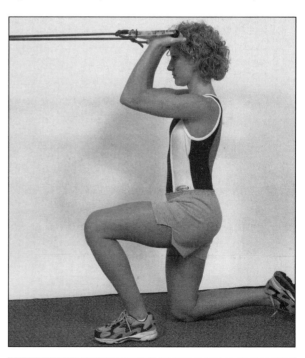

Figure 18.23   Biceps curl: 90° shoulder flexion (end position).

Tubing Triceps Finish

The swimmer starts by bending forward at the waist, with upper arms at the side and elbows flexed (figures 18.24 and 18.25). He or she performs the exercise by extending the elbows into the finish position while stabilizing the shoulder blades.

Also see chapter 5, figures 5.01, 5.10, 5.11, 5.14 through 5.17, and 5.28 through 5.30, for standing hip extension, flexion, and adduction exercises.

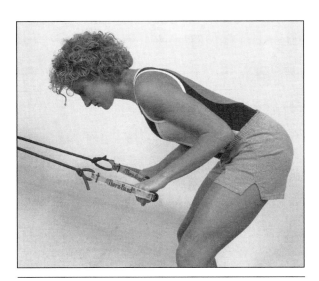

Figure 18.24 Triceps "finish" (start position).

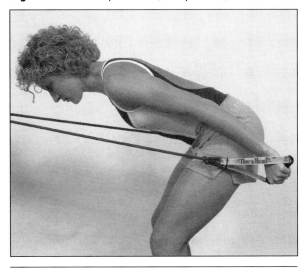

Figure 18.25 Triceps "finish" (end position).

Conclusion

The most effective approach to managing the unique orthopedic problems of the swimmer is to be aware of the stresses brought about by swimming as well as the mechanisms most likely to be responsible for such specific patterns of overuse. Managing the mechanism of the injury along with the symptoms is most likely to provide a satisfactory solution to the swimmer's problems, and incorporation of this type of program on a prophylactic basis is likely to improve performance as well as avoid injury. The clinical issues raised in this discussion are based, to a large degree, on practical experience. The relative lack of clinical research in the management of swimming injuries represents an excellent opportunity for the development of controlled clinical outcome studies.

References

Aronen, J. 1985. "Swimmer's Shoulder." *Swimming World* 25(4): 4-47.

Colwin, C.M. 1992. *Swimming Into the 21st Century.* Champaign, IL: Human Kinetics.

Costill, D.L., E.W. Maglischo, and A.B. Richardson. 1992. *Handbook of Sports Medicine and Science: Swimming.* Oxford, UK: Blackwell Scientific.

Councilman, J.G. 1968. *The Science of Swimming.* Englewood Cliffs, NJ: Prentice-Hall.

Cuillo, J.V. 1986. "Swimmer's Shoulder." *Clinics in Sports Medicine* 5: 115-37.

Falkel, J.E. 1990. "Swimming Injuries." Pp. 477-503 in *Sports Physical Therapy,* ed. B. Sanders. Norwalk, CT: Appleton & Lange.

Falkel, J.E., and T.C. Murphy. 1988. "Shoulder Injuries." In *Sports Injury Management Series,* ed. T. Malone. Baltimore: Williams & Wilkins.

Fleck, S.J., and W.J. Kraemer. 1987. *Designing Resistance Training Programs.* Champaign, IL: Human Kinetics.

Greipp, J.F. 1985. "Swimmer's Shoulder: The Influence of Flexibility and Weight Training." *The Physician and Sportsmedicine* 13(8): 92-105.

Johnson, J.E., F.H. Sim, and S.G. Scott. 1987. "Musculoskeletal Injuries in Competitive Swimmers." *Mayo Clinic Proceedings* 62: 289-304.

Kennedy, J.C., A.B. Craig, and R.C. Schneider. 1985. "Swimming." In *Sports Injuries: Mechanisms, Prevention and Treatment,* ed. R.C. Schneider, J.C. Kennedy, and M.L. Plant. Baltimore: Williams & Wilkins.

Kennedy, J.C., R. Hawkins, and W.B. Krissoff. 1978. "Orthopaedic Manifestations of Swimming." *American Journal of Sports Medicine* 6: 309-22.

Maglischo, E.W. 1982. *Swimming Faster.* Palo Alto, CA: Mayfield.

McMaster, W.C., and J. Troup. 1993. "A Survey of Interfering Shoulder Pain in United States Competitive Swimmers." *American Journal of Sports Medicine* 21: 67-70.

Murphy, T.C. 1994. "Shoulder Injuries in Swimming." In *The Athlete's Shoulder,* ed. J.R. Andrews and K.E. Wilk. New York: Churchill Livingstone.

Murphy, T.C., and J.N. Riester. 1988. "Managing the Young Swimmer: A Practical Approach to Prevention and Treatment." *The Student Athlete* 1(5): 4-8.

Penny, J.N., and C. Smith. 1980. "The Prevention and Treatment of Swimmer's Shoulder." *Canadian Journal of Applied Sport Science* 5: 195-202.

Pettrone, F.A. 1985. "Shoulder Problems in Swimmers." In *Injuries to the Throwing Arm*, ed. B. Zarins, J.R. Andrews, and W.G. Carson. Philadelphia: Saunders.

Richardson, A.B. 1986. "The Biomechanics of Swimming: The Shoulder and Knee." *Clinics in Sports Medicine* 5: 103-13.

Russ, D.W. 1997. "A Case Report: In-Season Management of Shoulder Pain in a Collegiate Swimmer—A Team Approach" (Abstract). *Journal of Orthopaedic and Sports Physical Therapy* 25(1): 86.

CHAPTER 19

Sport-Specific Training for Basketball

• • • • •

Greg Brittenham, MS

New York Knickerbockers

The numerous physiological and mechanical systems of the human body must cope continuously with a vast assortment of internal and external demands and constraints. Athletes are individuals who, through a proper, well-organized progression of training, more closely maximize their potential through a greater mastery over these demands and constraints. For thousands of years, athletes have searched for the advantage that would enable them to run faster, jump higher, and throw farther. More often than not, this search has resulted in less than acceptable outcomes. As athletic developmental specialists, we too are in search of the best way to maximize performance of our athletes. Recently, the scientific community has lent insight into some of the old tried-and-true training methods and has discovered that many are obsolete.

The challenge we face is to determine the optimum combination of traditional techniques and new methods. The continuing evolution of these new paradigms moves us closer and closer to record-breaking performances. One such practice that is becoming widely used and universally embraced is elastic resistance training, a nontraditional functional approach to rehabilitation and training. The purpose of this chapter is to discuss the use of elastic resistance training to enhance physical development and performance in basketball.

Physiological Demands of Basketball

The metabolic demands of basketball involve all three energy stages. It is not unusual for a 48-min professional game to last 2-1/2 hr. Stone and Kroll (1986) indicated that the continuous nature of the game and the constant movement required of high-caliber play make basketball a game of high endurance. Occasional bursts of fast-break basketball rely on anaerobic capacity, and this also must be considered in the conditioning program (Stone and Kroll 1986). Once the game begins, the player derives energy from all three systems (i.e., adenosine triphosphate/creatine phosphate [ATP-PC], glycolysis, and aerobic systems). The relative contribution of each system depends on the intensity and duration of the activity. Basketball is about 20% aerobic and 80% anaerobic; however, many factors influence the exact energy expenditure ratio for individual players (Brittenham 1996). For example, because of position requirements some players are on the constant move to "get open," whereas other players remain relatively stationary but are continually "fighting" in the post for position. When we examine the total energy demands for an entire 2-1/2 hr game, we find that the percentage contributions of the energy systems change continually. Therefore, assigning individual work-rest ratios is difficult. However, we can make assumptions based on a team's style of play (a fast break offense vs. half-court, a player-to-player defense vs. zone defense) and position considerations. The exact energy system training regimen depends on the team's style of play and the specific positions involved.

Strength, power, speed, quickness, agility, coordination, body control, and all other components of athleticism are of critical importance to successful basketball performance. In determining the appropriate training protocol for the team, the coach must establish an individual assessment profile for each player. Armed with this needs analysis, the coach can design a program based on the individual's metabolic and athletic needs.

Common Injuries

The most common injury experienced by high school basketball players is an ankle sprain. More than half the injuries to girls, and almost half of those to boys, are sprains (Edwards 2000). Conditioning for specific requirements of the game is essential for injury prevention and performance enhancement. A study from the Cincinnati Sports Medicine Research and Education Foundation and Deaconess Hospital indicated that female basketball players who consistently participated in some form of neuromuscular training had fewer injuries and enhanced landing characteristics (Hewett et al. 1996). There is a concomitant improvement in basketball-specific skills, athleticism, and injury severity when a player regularly undertakes functional neuromuscular training such as elastic resistance.

Primary Skills

Passing, dribbling, and shooting are the three primary basketball skills. The obvious objective of passing is to displace the ball from one player to a teammate. Dribbling is a necessary means of advancing the ball when passing is not possible or is ill advised. Shooting is similar to passing; however, the ultimate goal is displacement of the ball through the basket. In general, a player has available a large

number of muscular forces that may be used to ensure that the ball obtains a release velocity of the desired magnitude and direction for all three of these necessary skills. The primary muscles involved in the three primary basketball skills are the extensors and flexors of the wrist, elbow extensors, and the musculature of the chest and shoulder.

Muscle generates force. Motor unit recruitment, coordination and synchronization of muscle activation, neural inhibition or protective mechanisms, and cross-sectional muscle area are the primary focuses of a strength development program. Elastic resistance allows us to execute programs that go beyond the major strength issue and explore functional, multiplane, proprioceptive, balance, and coordination perspectives. Any training method must conform to the principles governing physiological adaptation. Progressive overload is a simple hypothesis which suggests that if an athlete adapts to the resistance or demand placed on the various systems, then that demand must be increased to ensure continued gains. In other words, continue to challenge the system. A coaching cue used with athletes is to train beyond the comfort zone, and that zone is ever-expanding.

Specificity Principle Applied to Basketball

Skeletal muscle possesses the intrinsic ability to adapt to the physical activity that it is required to perform. Athletes who implement training programs that closely mimic the predominant energy systems and movement patterns associated with their sport greatly increase their ability to perform that sport. Such is the concept of specificity of training. Adaptation is specific to the stress imposed. For example, in basketball, a sport that is primarily anaerobic, the player would not run long-distance aerobic workouts like the marathoner. Similarly, acceleration, deceleration, and rapid changes of direction (forward, backward, lateral, and vertical) are some of the movement variables associated with basketball. It is an explosive and quite physical sport. Adaptation to explosive exercise training results in the recruitment of more powerful motor neurons. A shift toward power activities is necessary to optimize this development. The constant resistance provided by elastic resistive devices accommodates maximal acceleration through the entire movement, as opposed to a fixed weight exercise whereby much movement is spent in deceleration. Therefore, elastic training is specific to the explosive demands and movement characteristics of basketball.

Elastic Resistance Exercises for Basketball Players

The dynamic nature of basketball suggests a specific functional approach to training. In the weight room and on the court, we constantly search for challenging ways to specifically stress the system within safe and productive parameters. Many drills too numerous to mention meet this criterion. The following are drills that typify the identifiably basketball-specific variables such as dynamic mobility, proprioception, balance, and, of course, strength.

Core Stability Training With Elastic Resistance

The main focus of this training program is the abdominals and low back, or the "center of power." All movement either originates, transfers through, or is stabilized by the center of power. Strength and toning exercises are many, but developing power in the abdominals and low back often becomes a challenge. The following are four simple exercises that will stress the core muscles involved in the movement.

For this exercise the athlete uses a dip stand/abdominal apparatus (figures 19.01 and 19.02). Re-

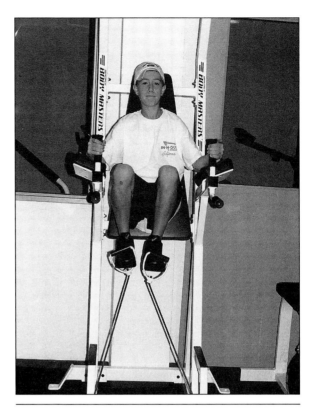

Figure 19.02 Low row (end position).

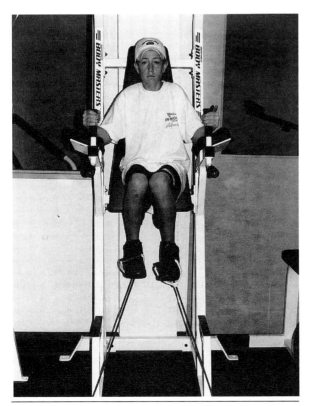

Figure 19.01 Low row (start position).

sistive bands are fixed securely to the bottom of the apparatus directly under the feet. Tension is adjusted by lengthening or shortening the bands. With the bands attached to the feet, the athlete bends the knees to 90°, keeping the chest slightly forward. The athlete lifts the legs with the lower abdominal musculature and simultaneously crunches the upper body toward the knees. The athlete returns to the starting position, without allowing the knees to drop below 90°. Repeat.

Bands are fixed to a sturdy object at approximately chest level (figures 19.03 and 19.04). Tension is adjusted by lengthening or shortening the bands. With feet perpendicular to the bands, the athlete stands tall and grasps the handles. The athlete turns slightly to the left toward where the bands are attached and then twists to the right, maintaining correct posture throughout. There is a slight pivot on the feet to avoid torque at the knee. The athlete controls the resistance and returns to the starting position. The athlete continues for the predetermined repetition range and repeats on the other side.

Bands are fixed to a sturdy structure overhead (figures 19.05 and 19.06). Tension is adjusted by lengthening or shortening the bands. The athlete kneels on the floor and holds the handles just under his or her ears. The athlete should bend forward at the hips and keep the back straight (slightly hyperextended but with caution). The athlete should

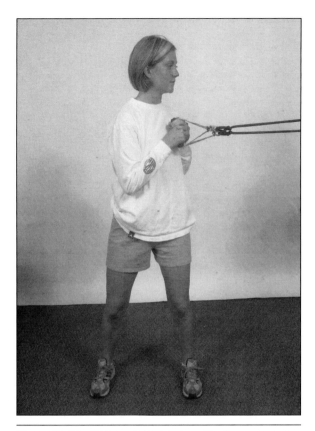

Figure 19.03   Oblique twist (start position).

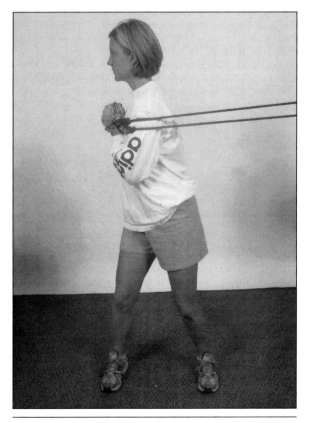

Figure 19.04   Oblique twist (end position).

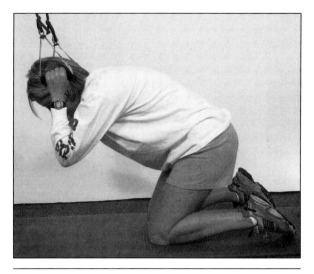

Figure 19.05   Upper ab pull-down (start position).

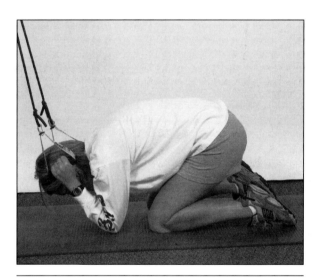

Figure 19.06   Upper ab pull-down (end position).

crunch the upper abs, "round" the back, and move the elbows toward the knees. The athlete controls the resistance, returns to the starting position, and repeats.

The exercise is performed seated on the floor with the bands around the feet (figures 19.07 and 19.08). Tension is adjusted by lengthening or shortening the bands. The athlete sits tall and perpendicular to the floor or slightly forward. Arms should be fully extended when the handles are gripped. The athlete leans back and taps the shoulder to the floor, then raises back to the starting position, and repeats.

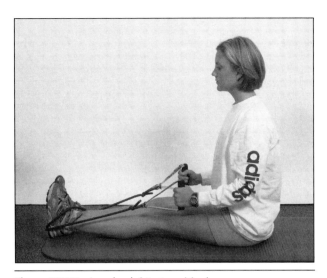

Figure 19.07   Low back (start position).

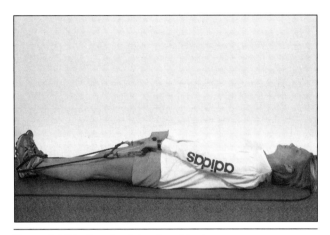

Figure 19.08   Low back (end position).

Upper and Lower Body Exercises With Elastic Resistance

Rarely in basketball does the player have the luxury of just standing still with his or her feet firmly planted on the floor. Unfortunately, most of the machines in the weight room are designed to move in one or two planes while the athlete is literally "fixed" within the apparatus. Sternum pads, thigh supports, and back supports negate the functionality of the movement. Additionally, the path of resistance on most equipment is finite and strictly dictated. This is not basketball. The next four exer-

cises can be performed on an unstable surface, thereby eliminating a stable base of support. Using an unstable surface, such as a balance board, the athlete can still build strength and power in the muscles being trained; however, because the feet are not firmly planted on the floor, the center-of-power region must act as the stabilizer. This is similar to the stabilization and balance requirements during a game of basketball, again suggesting specificity and functionality of training.

For this exercise the athlete positions the elastic bands under the feet and stands on a balance apparatus (figures 19.09 and 19.10). (Note: As with any training exercise, an element of risk is involved. The athlete may want to begin by simply standing on the floor and progressing to a balance apparatus.) Tension is adjusted by lengthening or shortening the bands. The athlete stands tall, with stabilization derived from the core. The band runs along the back.

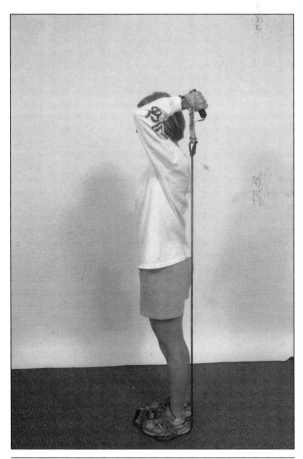

Figure 19.09   Triceps extension on a balance board (start position).

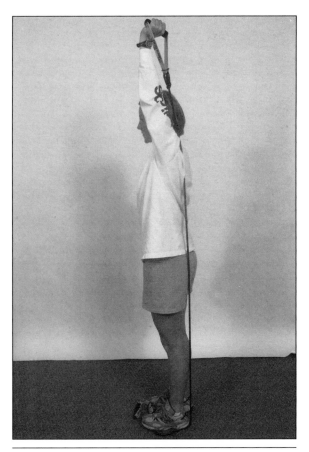

Figure 19.10 Triceps extension on a balance board (end position).

The elbow is pointed forward or slightly out. The athlete extends the elbow, controls the resistance, and returns to the starting position. After the set is completed, it is repeated on the opposite side.

Position the elastic bands under the feet and stand on a balance apparatus (figure 19.11). (Note: As with any training exercise, an element of risk is involved. The athlete may want to begin by simply standing on the floor and progressing to a balance apparatus.) Tension is adjusted by lengthening or shortening the bands. The athlete should stand tall, because stabilization comes from the core. The athlete grips the handles and keeps the elbow tight to the side. The athlete contracts the biceps and curls the hand toward the shoulder, controlling the resistance and returning to the starting position. The athlete can either alternate sides or complete the set and repeat on the opposite side.

The athlete positions the elastic bands under the feet and stands on a balance apparatus (figure 19.12). (Note: As with any training exercise, an element of risk is involved. The athlete may want to begin by simply standing on the floor and progressing to a balance apparatus.) Tension is adjusted by

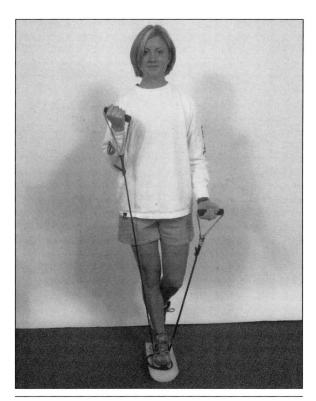

Figure 19.11 Biceps curl on a half round.

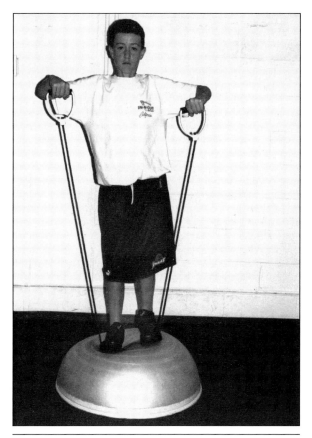

Figure 19.12 Lateral deltoid raise on a bosu ball.

lengthening or shortening the bands. The athlete should stand tall, with stabilization derived from the core. The athlete grips the handles and begins with palms together slightly below the waist. Arms are raised to a position no higher than parallel to the floor (palms down). The athlete should maintain a constant 90 to 135° angle at the elbow throughout the movement. In the "up" position, the hands should be at the same height as the elbows and the elbows should be slightly in front of the shoulder. The athlete should control the resistance, return to the starting position, and repeat.

The athlete positions the elastic bands under the feet and stands on a balance apparatus (figure 19.13). (Note: As with any training exercise, an element of risk is involved. The athlete may want to begin by simply standing on the floor and progressing to a balance apparatus.) Tension is adjusted by lengthening or shortening the bands. The athlete should stand tall, with stabilization derived from the core. The athlete grips the handles and begins with palms on the thighs. The athlete raises the right arm to a position no higher than parallel to the floor, controlling the resistance and then returning to the starting position. The athlete can either alternate sides or complete the set and repeat on the opposite side.

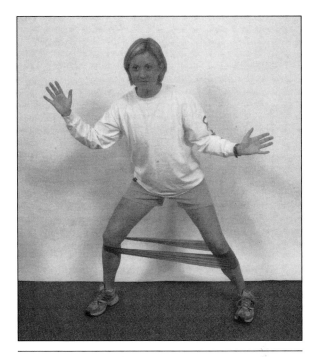

Figure 19.14 Step-slide.

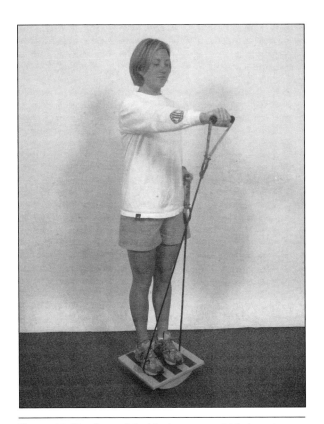

Figure 19.13 Front deltoid raise on a wobble board.

Elastic resistance can be used on the court to mimic many of the actual movements specific to basketball. For example, the resistance can be placed at the midsection and the athlete can then move forward, backward, laterally, vertically, and using combinations of movements. Or, as in the following example, the resistance can be placed other than at the midsection, such as around the ankles.

For this exercise, place a loop band around the athlete's shins (figure 19.14). The athlete should assume the proper defensive stance, with the lead foot (right) pointed at a 45° angle toward the direction of the movement. The athlete should maintain a wide base of support throughout the exercise. The athlete performs a step-slide, continuing for a predetermined number of repetitions or distance. The exercise is repeated in the opposite direction (left leg leading).

Many variations of the step-slide could be incorporated. For example, the athlete could simply slide continuously for a predetermined distance or repetitions, the coach could call out changes of direction, the player could mirror an offensive player, and so on.

Figure 19.15 demonstrates an outstanding multiple-joint, closed-chain leg exercise that requires tremendous balance and body control. Again, it is a functional exercise and is therefore a specific approach toward athletic development.

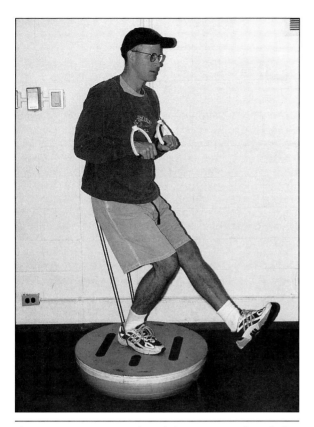

Figure 19.15 Functional single leg squat on a bosu ball.

To perform the exercise, the athlete positions the elastic bands under the right foot and stands on a balance apparatus. (Note: as with any training exercise, an element of risk is involved. The athlete may want to begin by simply standing on the floor and progressing to a balance apparatus.) Tension is adjusted by lengthening or shortening the bands. The bands will move up the back and around the shoulders. The athlete should hold the handles at approximately chest level, depending on the length of the bands at chest level. The athlete should stand tall because stabilization is derived from the core. The athlete extends the left leg forward slightly and performs a single leg squat to a position no lower than 45° at the knee (to begin, just maintaining balance might be challenge enough). The athlete should start slowly and progress gradually, always maintaining proper technique. The athlete continues for a predetermined number of repetitions and repeats on the opposite side. Note: This particular lift will require more than the 1-s time limit as mentioned in the following guidelines.

Guidelines for Training

- Determine the purpose of the exercise: Injury rehabilitation, strength training, or power development.
- Typically the athlete performs one repetition per second, but this will vary depending on the exercise (slightly faster on the "positive" phase of power development).
- Repetitions per set are high and range from between 15 and 30. Continue until the predetermined range has been met or until the repetitions drop below one per second or technique begins to falter.
- Use a multiple set approach (3-5 sets per exercise).
- In-season, the athlete should perform functional training a minimum of 2 days per week.

Safety Considerations

- Never sacrifice technique for added repetitions or sets.
- The athlete should always breathe (preferably diaphragmatic breathing).
- Instruct the athlete to maintain high intensity.
- Select a drill based on assessed needs. Always challenge the system and focus on the weakness within that system.
- Train both agonists and antagonists.
- When the athlete is using a functional apparatus, use caution and maintain proper technique.
- The athlete should always work with a partner (i.e., coach or teammate).
- The coach can adjust the tension of the rubber band to ensure that forced deceleration does not occur.

Conclusion

When assessing one's approach toward training athletes, one needs to respect the scales of development and weigh value against value. A blending of the traditional with the nontraditional training models tips the scales of productivity toward success. For example, are the benefits worth the risks? Do the results justify the time invested? What works for one athlete may in fact be deleterious to another.

In the constant search for superior training methods, we must aggressively seek new information from research, review literature from around the world, and continually assess what works and what doesn't. The functional advantages of elastic resistance exercises are that they allow both concentric and eccentric stimulation throughout the entire range of motion independent of position and within multiple planes. And the best part is that elastic resistance exercises are challenging, productive, and safe.

References

Brittenham, G. 1996. *Complete Conditioning for Basketball.* Champaign, IL: Human Kinetics.

Edwards, A.R. 2000. "Fast Facts." *Biomechanics* 7(3): 14-20.

Hewett, T.E., A.L. Stroupe, T.A. Nance, and F.R. Noyes. 1996. "Plyometric Training in Female Athletes: Decreased Impact Forces and Increased Hamstring Torques." *American Journal of Sports Medicine* 24(6): 765-73.

Stone, W.J., and W.A. Kroll. 1986. "Basketball." In *Sports Conditioning and Weight Training.* 2nd ed. Boston: Allyn & Bacon.

CHAPTER 20

Sport-Specific Training for Hockey

• • • • •

Randy Craig, MS, PT, ATC
Owner, PRORehab, PC, St. Louis, Missouri

Scott Gallant, MS, PT, ATC
Staff Physical Therapist, PRORehab, PC, St. Louis, Missouri

Ray Barile, MS, ATC, CSCS, LMT
Head Athletic Trainer, St. Louis Blues Hockey Club, St. Louis, Missouri

Hockey requires a unique combination of strength, speed, skill, power, agility, anaerobic and aerobic capacity, flexibility, balance, and proprioception. These physiological demands, coupled with a playing surface that is confined, hard, and slippery, characterize one of the most demanding of all sports. The very nature of the ice surface itself leads the hockey player to constantly vacillate from periods of control to loss of control. Kinematically, this unstable playing surface creates a tremendous eccentric load virtually unequaled in other sports. This load is especially noticeable regarding the lower extremity and trunk musculature.

These internal and external factors alone create an environment where proper conditioning is paramount and injury is common. Because participation in the sport is increasing, players are larger, hockey seasons are longer, and game pace is faster and rougher, it is easy to understand how injuries are relatively common. One study recently reported that the competitive hockey player suffers some sort of injury every 7 hr of play (Cox et al. 1995).

Countless studies have looked at injury occurrence rates in hockey, especially over the past decade. To provide a complete understanding of the rehabilitation of hockey players, we briefly review the nature and occurrence rate of these injuries.

Hockey Injuries

Recent data presented by the National Hockey League Injury Surveillance System (NHLISS) break down the proportion of game injuries by body category for the 1999-2000 NHL season (Powell 2000). It is clear from this data that the face/scalp category has the highest injury rate (31.6%), largely attributable to lacerations and contusions. This is followed by the hip/thigh/leg category (13.8%), which accounts primarily for sprains and strains of the hip and thigh musculature.

A recent study took a more in-depth look at groin and abdominal injuries in the NHL (Emery, Meeuwisse, and Powell 1999). This study analyzed more than 7,000 NHL players who played between 1991 and 1997. Some interesting findings were reported. First, the incidence rate of groin and abdominal injuries increased over 6 years of play from 12.99 injuries per 100 players per year in the 1991-92 season to 19.87 injuries per 100 players per year in the 1996-97 season. Injuries were 5 times more likely to occur in training camp versus during regular season training, raising suspicion of poor preseason conditioning. Incidence density was 6 times greater in games versus practice. The mechanism of injury recorded was noncontact in nature in greater than 90% of injuries reported. Finally, and of great importance to the sports medicine practitioner, 23.5% of the injuries reported were recurrent.

Although only a small sample of hockey injury data is available, this study alone makes it clear that proper conditioning (both in-season and off-season) and proper, thorough rehabilitation are paramount to the prevention and treatment of hockey injuries.

Skating Mechanics and Muscular Imbalances

Hockey requires several skills: shooting, passing, body checking, and, most importantly, skating. Skating is a fluid motion that when done properly looks effortless to a bystander. Skating is the result of repetitive striding. Striding has two components: the push or acceleration phase and the recovery phase. The purpose of this section is to summarize the mechanics of striding and discuss possible muscular imbalances that hockey players may acquire from this repetitive motion.

The first component of striding is the push phase, which propels the player forward. The ipsilateral gluteals, deep hip external rotators, and quadriceps work concentrically to extend and abduct the hip and knee, respectively. Eccentrically, the iliopsoas and the hip adductors control the final stages of hip extension and abduction. Simultaneously, the triceps surae work concentrically to plantar flex the ankle completing the push-off phase. During the push phase, the athlete's trunk is rotated to the contralateral side (i.e., right leg push-off occurs with left trunk rotation). This torsion is driven primarily by the obliques and upper extremity.

As the push phase propels the athlete forward, an efficient recovery phase is required for the athlete to maintain speed and save energy by using momentum to continue forward progression. Recovery begins when toe-off occurs at the end of the push phase. This phase incorporates strong eccentric and concentric components. The iliopsoas and the hip adductors initially act eccentrically to decelerate the lower extremity and then forcefully concentrically contract to return the lower extremity to neutral to prepare for push-off. Lower abdominal and obliques are recruited to derotate the trunk.

These phases of striding are performed countless times during games or practices. The repetitive nature of skating leads to muscle imbalances and overuse syndromes. Janda (1986) identified two groups of muscles. Postural muscles tend to tighten, and they include erector spinae, quadratus lumborum, iliopsoas, tensor fasciae latae, rectus femoris, and hip adductors. Phasic muscles that are inhibited and weak tend to be the rectus abdominis, obliques, gluteals, vastus medialis, and vastus lateralis.

To determine if muscle imbalances are present, the clinician must perform a thorough assessment. Assessment of standing posture, posture during skating, muscle length, strength, and activation patterns will help to determine which muscles are imbalanced (Norris 1995a). If we consider Janda's theory (1986) in conjunction with the predominant muscles used during striding, it is likely that erector spinae, iliopsoas, tensor fasciae latae, rectus femoris, and hip adductors will shorten and tighten. Hockey players often display an accentuated lordosis during skating and standing, which indicates short, strong hip flexor and low back muscles. The exaggerated lordosis contributes to many conditions for hockey players. According to the NHLISS study by Powell (2000) noted earlier, injuries to the hip, thigh, and leg accounted for 13.8% of hockey injuries over two seasons in the NHL. Trunk injuries accounted for 9.5% of injuries. Thus, 23.3% of injuries may originate from a muscle imbalance. Besides causing muscular injury related to imbalances, the lordotic posture increases the lumbosacral angle, which predisposes these athletes to lumbar rotational instability, iliolumbar ligament sprains, spondylolisthesis, disc lesions, sacroiliac (SI) joint dysfunction, and lumbar facet joint dysfunction.

In summary, because of the mechanics of striding, muscle imbalances are likely to occur. And, because of the intensity of the sport, the size and strength of players, and the relatively unforgiving nature of the ice surface, injuries are common. However, injuries can be minimized through proper preseason conditioning, stretching of postural muscles, spinal stabilization techniques (Lee 1997; Norris 1995b), and sport-specific rehabilitation.

Exercise Prescription

Before designing a therapeutic exercise program, the clinician may benefit from a brief review of exercise physiology relevant to hockey. Hockey, as stated earlier, is unique because it combines several components of fitness. Anaerobic capacity combined with aerobic power for recovery is important with respect to energy utilization. Anaerobic capacity is the ability to sustain high-intensity exercise for 30 to 60 s by using adenosine triphosphate (ATP) and adenosine triphosphate/creatine phosphate (ATP CP) stores (McArdle, Katch, and Katch 1991). Exercises prescribed should follow the overload principle, whereby specific physiological mechanisms are taxed to enhance those mechanisms, making the athlete more suited to the sport and resistant to injury. Anaerobic training and muscle reconditioning for injured hockey players should promote efficient anaerobic metabolism and muscle reeducation. Work/rest ratios as well as mode, frequency, and duration of exercises must be specific to hockey.

Elastic Resistance Exercises for Hockey Players

The following exercises are designed to assist the injured hockey player in returning to play. Because of high incidences of lower extremity overuse syndromes in hockey, we present a progression from cardinal plane movements to functional activity followed by examples of upper extremity and trunk exercises. All exercises incorporate strong concentric and eccentric components. Work/rest ratios should be sport-specific. An average hockey shift averages 20 to 40 s with 1 to 2 min rest. It seems logical that exercises should be performed according to similar guidelines.

High stepping (figure 20.01), reaching back (figures 20.02-20.04), squat walks (figures 20.05 and 20.06), and the monster walk (figures 20.07-20.09) primarily involve the hip flexors and gluteals. These straight-plane movements are helpful in early stages of rehabilitation when simple, isolated muscle strengthening is the goal. Initially, a work/rest ratio of 1:3 is appropriate, for example, 20 s of exercise followed by 60 s of rest.

A functional progression to begin simulation of the skating stride involves the addition of lateral movement exercises. Lateral stepping (figure 20.10), the skating stride (figure 20.11), and variations on the slideboard (single-leg striding, figure 20.12; double-leg striding, figure 20.13; and butterfly, figure 20.14) are excellent to regain lateral mobility and strength. Work/rest ratios can begin at 1:3 and progress to 1:2.

Rehabilitation of trunk and forearm injuries requires specific simulation for players to regain proper neural patterning (especially in the trunk) and power. Modifying a hockey stick with elastic resistance allows players to practice technique and improve quickness and power with the slap shot (figures 20.15 and 20.16) and wrist shot (figures 20.17 and 20.18) exercises. The wrist shot exercise is primarily an upper extremity exercise, whereas the slap shot exercise incorporates greater trunk rotation and lower extremity dynamic stabilization. Because power is primarily neurally driven, the work/rest cycle differs compared with previous exercises. Initially, athletes should perform 10 "shots" using good mechanics as quickly as possible. As the athlete improves, he or she should increase the number of sets, not the number of repetitions per set (e.g., 3 sets × 10 reps initially, progressing to 6 sets × 10 reps).

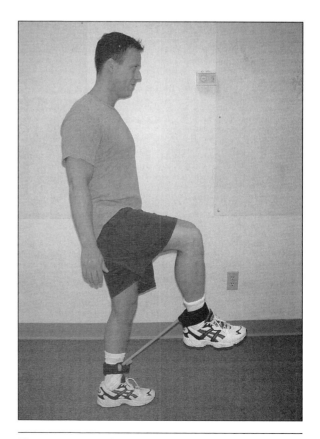

Figure 20.01 High stepping.

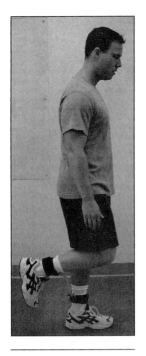 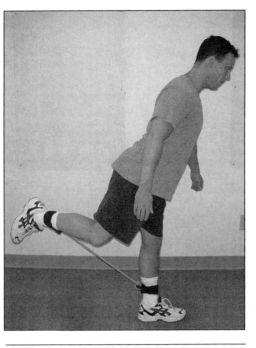 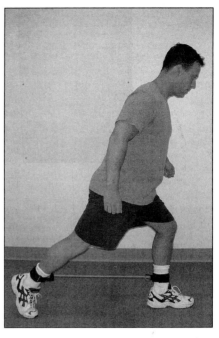

Figure 20.02 Reaching back (start position).

Figure 20.03 Reaching back (midmovement).

Figure 20.04 Reaching back (end position).

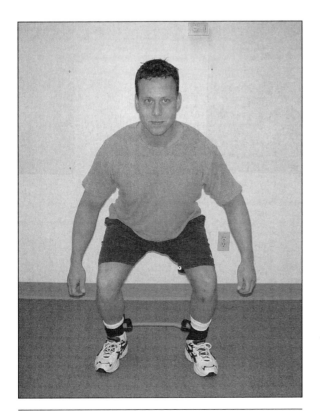 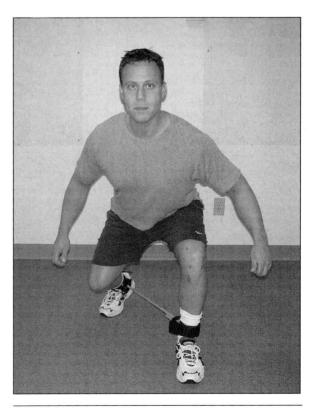

Figure 20.05 Squat walks (start position).

Figure 20.06 Squat walks (end position).

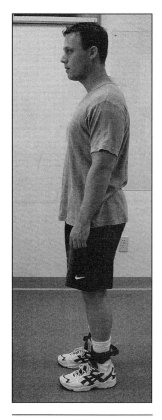 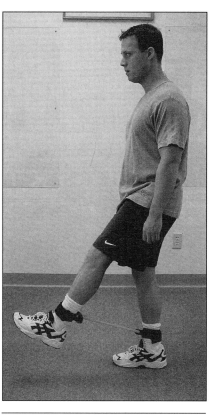 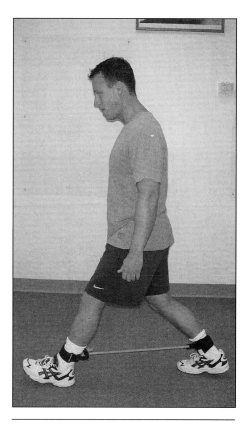

Figure 20.07 Monster walk (start position).

Figure 20.08 Monster walk (midmovement).

Figure 20.09 Monster walk (end position).

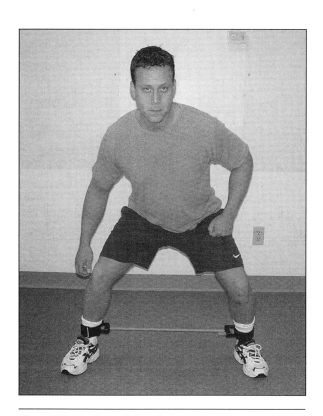 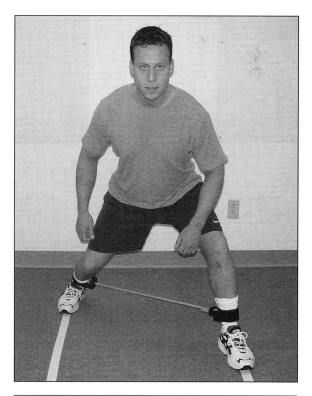

Figure 20.10 Lateral stepping.

Figure 20.11 Skating stride.

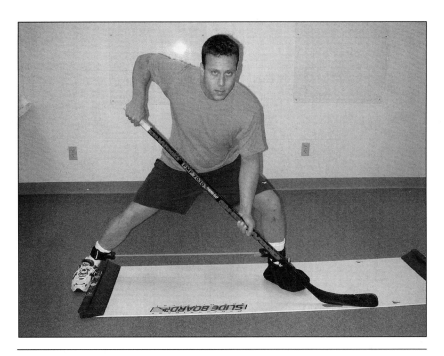

Figure 20.12 Single-leg striding.

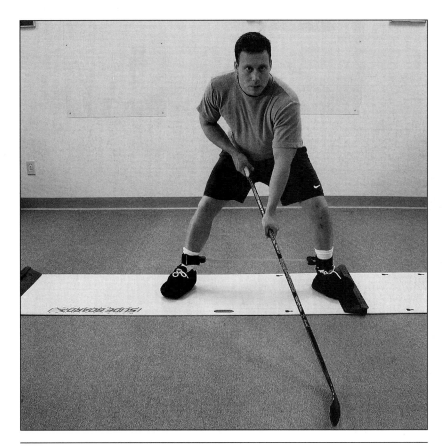

Figure 20.13 Double-leg striding.

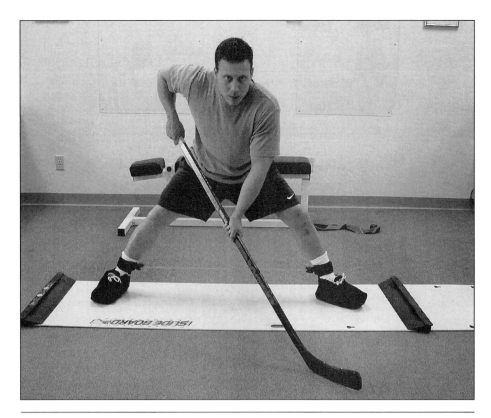

Figure 20.14 Butterfly.

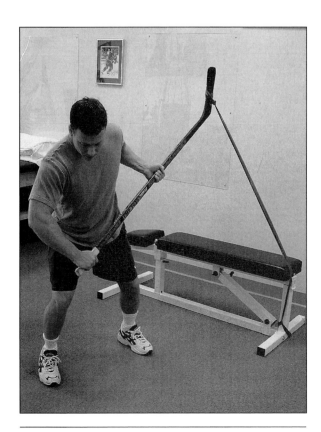

Figure 20.15 Slap shot (start position).

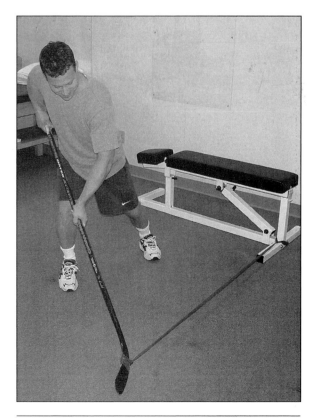

Figure 20.16 Slap shot (end position).

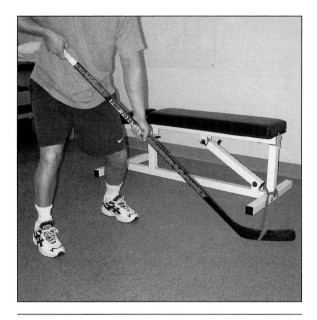

Figure 20.17 Wrist shot (start position).

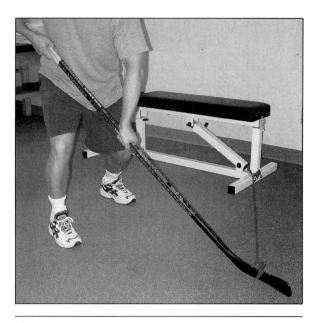

Figure 20.18 Wrist shot (end position).

Conclusion

Knowledge of the specific demands and injury patterns discussed in this chapter provides the framework for the sport-specific exercises recommended for the hockey player. The chapter highlighted elastic resistance exercise with particular emphasis on the muscles that stabilize the hips and pelvis and provide power and control during skating. Integration of the exercises in this chapter can both enhance performance and normalize muscular strength balance to prevent injury.

CASE STUDY

Greg, a 20-year-old minor league hockey player, presented in the clinic with intense pain in the left groin region. He described a mechanism whereby during a game the night before, his right skate got caught in a "rut" on the ice, forcefully abducting and externally rotating his right lower extremity. He described immediate pain and a pop in the left groin region, and he had to be helped from the ice. Immediate examination by the team physician and subsequent X-ray ruled out fracture and other hip joint pathology, and a diagnosis of second-degree strain of the adductor longus was made.

The acute phase of rehabilitation lasted for 5 days and consisted of modalities to decrease pain and swelling and to promote circulation, active range of motion (ROM) and light stretching to promote flexibility, and pain-free cardiovascular exercise (aqua jogging, light-resistance stationary cycling, and upper body ergometry) to maintain fitness.

On Day 6, Greg exhibited full hip and knee ROM, and the strength in his adductors was judged as 4 out of 5; he was deemed ready to begin resistance exercise. At this time, he was also allowed to begin light-intensity, straight-ahead skating for 20 min. As for his rehabilitation program, he began with straight sagittal plane exercises, using primarily the hip flexors and gluteals. These exercises included high stepping, reaching back, squat walks, and the monster walk. Greg initially began with a work/rest ratio of 1:3, exercising for 20 s and resting for 60 s. He began with 2 sets of each exercise, progressing to 5 sets over a 2-day period.

On Day 8 postinjury, Greg began lateral movement exercises using elastic tubing and a slide board. Stationary biking, modalities, moderate passive stretching of the adductors, proprioceptive neuromuscular facilitation manual resistance exercise, and isotonic strengthening also were incorporated during this phase. Exercises initiated that used elastic tubing on level ground were lateral stepping and the skating stride. He tolerated these exercises well, and more challenging exercises in which he used the tubing while on the slide board were initiated the following day. These exercises included single- and double-leg striding and the butterfly exercise. Initially, he began with a work/rest ratio of 1:3, exercising for 20 s and resting for 60 s for 2 sets of each exercise. These exercises were performed twice daily along with the previously noted treatment regimen. He tolerated the exercises well, and the work/rest ratio was decreased to 1:2 (20 s exercise, 40 s rest) for 5 sets of all exercises. He also began moderate-intensity skating including crossovers and footwork drills that incorporated starts, stops, and quick directional changes.

On Day 12 postinjury, Greg was re-evaluated and noted to have full ROM, no pain on palpation, 5 out of 5 strength in the adductors, and pain-free skating. The adductors were wrapped with an elastic bandage for support and he was allowed to return to competition. He incorporated the elastic tubing regimen into his conditioning program and performed these exercises 3 times per week.

References

Cox, M.H., D.S. Miles, T.J. Verde, and E.C. Rhodes. 1995. "Applied Physiology of Ice Hockey." *Sports Medicine* 19(3): 184-210.

Emery, C.A., W.H. Meeuwisse, and J.W. Powell. 1999. "Groin and Abdominal Injuries in the National Hockey League." *Clinical Journal of Sport Medicine* 9(3): 151-6.

Janda, V. 1986. "Muscle Weakness and Inhibition (Pseudoparesis) in Back Pain Syndromes." In *Modern Manual Therapy of the Vertebral Column*, ed. G. Grieve. Edinburgh, UK: Churchill Livingstone.

Lee, D. 1997. "The Treatment of Pelvic Instability." In *Movement Stability and Low Back Pain—The Essential Role of the Pelvis*, ed. A. Vleeming, V. Mooney, T. Dorman, C. Snijders, H. Stoeckart. Edinburgh, UK: Churchill Livingstone.

McArdle, W., F. Katch, and V. Katch. 1991. *Exercise Physiology: Energy, Nutrition and Human Performance*. 3rd ed. Philadelphia: Lea & Febiger.

Norris, C. 1995a. "Muscle Balance and the Low Back." *Physiotherapy* 81(3): 127-38.

Norris, C. 1995b. "An Exercise Programme to Enhance Lumbar Stabilisation." *Physiotherapy* 81(3): 138-46.

Powell, J.W. 2000. *National Hockey League Injury Surveillance System: Summary Report 1998-1999 and 1999-2000 Seasons*. New York, NY: National Hockey League.

CHAPTER 21

Sport-Specific Training for Martial Arts

● ● ● ● ●

George J. Davies, MEd, PT, ATC, SCS, CSCS
University of Wisconsin at LaCrosse

"The martial arts have evolved over millennia as a means to kill or disable. It is only in the last few decades that the martial arts have been marketed and sold as sport. It would appear that this transition to sport is incomplete"(Oler et al. 1991, p. 252). Unfortunately there are numerous examples of serious injuries (Birrer 1996; Brown 1998; Davies in press; Hirano and Seto 1973; Jaffe and Minkoff 1988; Walker 1975) or deaths resulting from martial arts (Brown 1998; Davies in press; Imamura et al. 1996; Koiwai 1981, 1987; Lannuzel et al. 1994; Owens and Ghadiali 1991; Reay and Eisle 1982; Schmidt 1975).

There has been a veritable explosion of interest and participation in the martial arts globally. It is estimated that because of commercial entrepreneurism, media promotion, the health and fitness resurgence, and international diplomacy and goodwill, the martial arts have attracted close to 100 million participants worldwide (approximately 10 million in the United States alone). Reasons for participation include self-defense; health and recreation; self-confidence; conditioning and fitness; self-discipline; social and environment support; sport competition; and psychological, philosophical, and religious transformation. In many locations the annual growth is expected to be 20 to 25% (Birrer 1996).

Seasoned practitioners can accelerate their feet from 0 to 30 mph in milliseconds and kick an opponent with a force of 675 lb/in.^{2} (Feld, McNair, and Wilk 1979). Examples of different kicks that are fast and powerful are illustrated in figures 21.01 and 21.02 of a karate front kick and side kick. If one were to add a jumping "flying kick" (figure 20.03) to the front kick, the power would increase even more.

Although there is limited information in the medical literature dealing with martial arts injuries, the following examples demonstrate the high intensity level of participating in karate. Zigun and Schneider (1988) described an example of "effort" thrombosis (Paget-Schroetter's syndrome) secondary to martial arts training. Russell and Lewis (1975) stated that myoglobinuria has occurred in other high-intensity exercise situations like in Marine Corps training, but they also recently described karate myoglobinuria in a karate practitioner after several hours of intense karate practice. I have been involved in the martial arts for more than 20 years and can relate to the efforts required in the martial arts relative to several other vigorous sports (Davies 1996).

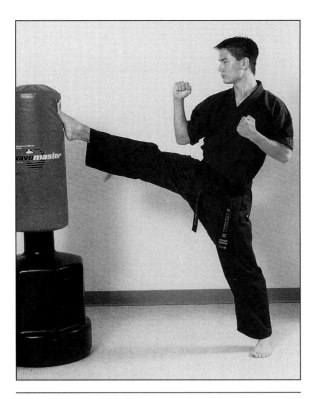

Figure 21.01   Karate front leg, front kick.

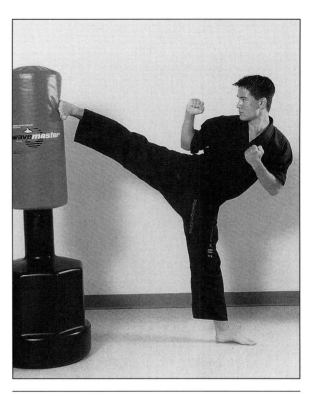

Figure 21.02   Karate side kick.

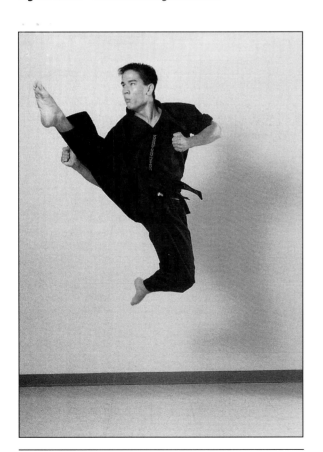

Figure 21.03   Karate flying front kick.

Historical Perspective

Throughout much of history, the martial arts have been shrouded in mystery. The term *martial arts* refers to arts concerned with the waging of war and loosely refers to any of the offensive and defensive fighting styles or systems of fighting techniques that are derived in whole or part from the Far East and that use one or more body parts. Weapons also may be incorporated in 20th-century martial arts, but martial arts are no longer practiced entirely for military purposes. Thousands of different schools, systems, and styles of martial arts exist, and most are associated with a way of life based on Eastern philosophy. *Martial disciplines* collectively refers to both the martial ways and the fighting arts. All forms have some form of achievement designation. Typically, belt or sash color is used to identify skill level (lighter colors denote less experience and darker colors are reserved for advanced levels of proficiency.) Only about 1 in 500 participants achieve the coveted black belt, which is the departure point for advanced studies (Davies, Durrall, and Fater 2001).

Martial Arts Training and Conditioning

Cavanagh and Landa (1976) wrote that the sport of karate had been somewhat neglected by sport scientists, who had directed their attention chiefly toward traumatology and conditioning of the hand. More than 25 years later, this comment still holds true.

There is limited information in the professional literature regarding training programs for martial artists. Several articles have evaluated the effects of certain martial arts activities on physiological (Brown et al. 1989; Callister et al. 1991; Francescato, Talon, and diPrampero et al. 1995; Imamura et al. 1996, 1997, 1999; Lai et al. 1995; Lan et al. 1996, 1998; Matsumoto et al. 1997; Schneider and Leung 1991; Shaw and Deutsch 1982; Stricevic et al. 1980; Wolf, Coogler and Tingsen 1997; Young et al. 1999) or biomechanical (Cavanagh and Landa 1976; Davies, Durall, and Fater 2001; Pieter and Pieter 1995; Staley 1996, 1999; Vos and Brinkhorst 1966; Wolf, Coogler and Tingsen 1997; Zehr, Sale, and Dowling 1997) characteristics. There are virtually no prospective controlled training studies that demonstrate the type of training or the efficacy of the training programs. The articles that are available are typically empirical anecdotal articles regarding particular individuals' recommended training programs (Ratamess 1998; Sanders and Antonio 1999). Furthermore, although several books are available (Kim 2000; Norris 1975; Staley 1996,1999), they are not peer-reviewed publications regarding specific quality or outcomes of performance. As with many other sports, and perhaps more so in the martial arts because of tradition, many of the training techniques are handed down from one master to the next. The philosophy is, "If it worked for me, then it should work for you." This philosophy continues to perpetuate much of the training and oftentimes is unsafe and inefficient from the biomechanical or physiological standpoint.

Motor Learning, Types of Feedback, and Practice Conditions

Before initiation of any conditioning and training program, particularly when it involves sophisticated techniques such as in most of the martial arts, it is important to also consider some of the basic aspects of motor learning. Shumway-Cook and Woollacott (1995) described the numerous factors that contribute to motor learning including the types of feedback and practice conditions. In the literature, there is really no consensus on the optimal method for practice to further improve motor learning. Various types of practice methodologies have included massed and distributed practice, variable practice, contextual interference, whole versus part training, transfer, mental practice, and guidance. All of the aforementioned techniques have their advantages as well as their disadvantages. It is because of the lack of consensus on the best way to train that so many different programs have been advocated in motor learning. Most, however, are based on experience.

Martial Arts Techniques to Improve Speed

In a classic book by Chuck Norris (of Walker, Texas Ranger fame; 1975), guidelines are provided for learning new techniques and training. However, Norris wrote about the progressive increase in producing speed during practice of various karate techniques. Norris recommended beginning with slow motion and then going on to the next speed when one can consistently perform a technique perfectly. Progression to half speed without sacrificing perfection is the next step with emphasis on rhythm, focus, and balance. After the individual is satisfied that he or she has mastered a perfect form at half speed, then Norris recommended the very same form at the fastest speed at which one is capable of performing. Norris emphasized that at this point, the tendency is to get sloppy, so particular attention must be paid to maintain perfect form without sacrificing form for speed. Further recommendations include finishing a workout with performing a technique 10 consecutive times without a mistake. Finally, the techniques need to be performed at "red-line speed." The purpose of the red-line is twofold. First, it will provide a good workout and enhance the muscular and anaerobic endurance. Second, it will push one's full speed ability to new and greater heights. Red-line calls for one to achieve a speed faster than one has ever before attained. It is an open-ended drill with the emphasis on constant attainment of more and more speed. As always, it is very important to maintain excellence in form, although some techniques may be sacrificed to increase speed training. The final phase of training Norris called the "mixing it up" phase. After one has improved the speed through the red-line drill, then mixing speeds often provides a good drill for control in rhythm, balance, and form. This is ultimately the key many times in competitive fighting (full contact or point fighting) or in a real self-defense situation. How quickly and decisively one reacts in a self-defense situation literally may mean the difference between life and death.

Techniques For Speed and Power Training

Many books (Baechle 1994; Bompa 1993, 1995; Chu 1996; Cook and Woollacott 1995; Costello and Kreis 1993; Davies 1992; Davies, Wilk, and Ellenbecker 1997; Davies, Durall, and Fater 2001; Dintiman and Ward 1988; Fleck and Kraemer 1996, 1997; Kim 2000; Norris 1975; Staley 1996, 1999; Zatsiorsky 1995) and articles (Chu and Plummer 1984; Davies and Ellenbecker 1992; Ratamess 1998; Sanders and Antonio 1999; Takahashi 1992) describe methods of training and conditioning. Therefore, many of the typical principles used for weight training also are applicable to use with a Thera-Band. Examples of principles that apply include periodization design training, overload, intensity, duration, frequency, training volume, progression, mode of muscle contraction, muscle group specificity, energy-source specificity, speed specificity, functional specificity, individuality, reversibility, and rest/recovery. Because most of these principles are commonly applied in training, conditioning, and rehabilitation, only a few are discussed in more detail.

As with most training and conditioning programs, the goal is to enhance functional specificity of sports performance, in this case, martial arts. Consequently, regardless of which type of training and conditioning program is used, it should be designed in a periodized fashion to develop a good total fitness foundation and then should progress to more specific technique training.

Fleck and Kraemer (1996, 1997) stated that most coaches and athletes maintain that some resistance training should be performed at the velocity required during the actual sporting event. For many sporting events, this means a high velocity of movement. This belief is based on the concept that resistance training produces its greatest strength gains at the velocity at which the training is performed.

Scientific evidence supports this view (Davies 1992; Davies, Wilk, and Ellenbecker 1997). Training at a fast velocity promotes gains in strength and power at a fast velocity to a slightly greater extent than does training at a slow velocity. Thus, velocity-specific training to maximize strength and power gains at a specific velocity is appropriate for athletes at some point in their training.

Techniques for Elastic Resistance Training Described in Martial Arts Literature

Kim (2000) stated that although weight lifting is a good supplement to martial arts training, many martial artists are increasingly learning the benefits of elastic resistance training. With the resistive tubing firmly in place, one can execute punches, strikes, throws, and kicks (figures 21.04-21.07) while the elastic provides resistance for the muscles. The advantage over weight training is that one directly works the muscles that are used in martial arts training, thereby guaranteeing targeted results.

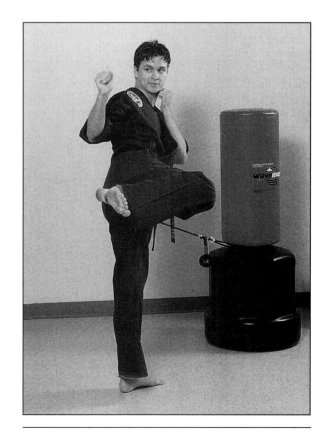

Figure 21.04 Karate side kick (chamber position).

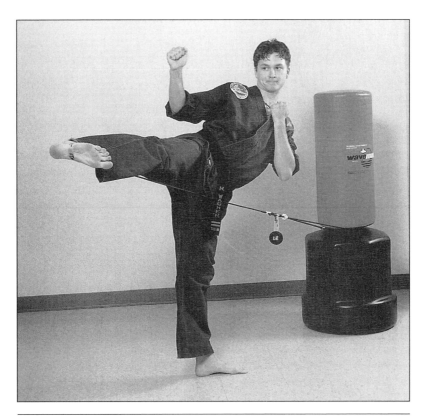

Figure 21.05   Karate side kick.

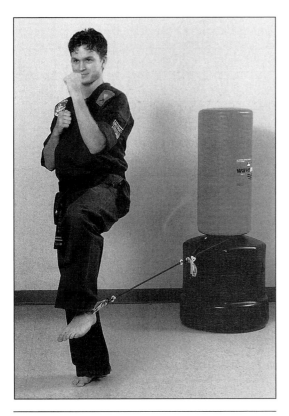

Figure 21.06   Karate front kick (chamber position).

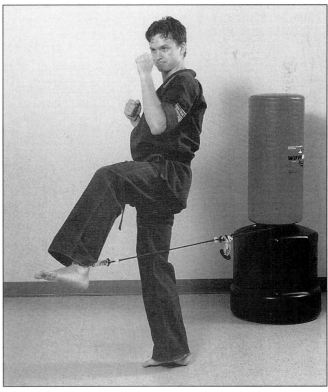

Figure 21.07   Karate front kick.

Techniques for Speed and Power Training With Elastic Resistance

Because it has been demonstrated that the angular velocities during a karate kick reach several thousand degrees per second, then obviously faster velocity training is appropriate (Chu 1996; Chu and Plummer 1984; Davies 1992; Davies, Wilk, and Ellenbecker 1997; Dintiman and Ward 1988; Fleck and Kraemer 1996, 1997; Norris 1975; Staley 1996, 1999; Takahashi 1992; Vos and Brinkhorst 1966; Zehr, Sale, and Dowling 1997). There are certainly many ways that this can be accomplished. Some examples are to train with high-speed isokinetic exercise (Davies 1992; Davies, Wilk, and Ellenbecker 1997) or to use impulse inertial exercise training. Other techniques include the use of plyometric exercises, which are one of the most effective methods of enhancing speed, power, and sports performance (Chu 1996; Chu and Plummer 1984; Davies, Durall, and Fater 2001; Fleck and Kraemer 1997; Sanders and Antonio 1999; Takahashi 1992). For the martial artist, performing the techniques as described by Norris (1975) in progressive speed training is certainly another methodology. Speed can be improved by martial arts speed drills, simulations, pad work, controlled sparring, or free sparring. The remainder of this chapter discusses and presents several examples of the empirical use of elastic resistance training for martial artists. There are no studies to date on martial artists using elastic resistance training that can be referenced to demonstrate the absolute efficacy of these techniques. However, numerous other references that involve elastic resistance have demonstrated successful improvement of functional performance in many other areas. Therefore, because there is no research, an extrapolation is probably appropriate regarding similar improvements in performance of martial artists.

Because of the controversy regarding the most effective way to increase speed, as with many other modes of training, it seems that using different stimuli to challenge the neuromusculoskeletal system would be the most effective.

Concentric Muscle Training

Elastic resistance training can be used for short arc range of motion (ROM) and full ROM training with a concentric muscle contraction for resistance. The full ROM applies the concept of specificity of training (Davies 1992). The motions are designed to replicate the actual punches or kicks performed throughout the full ROM to strengthen the muscles exactly as they are used with the martial arts activity. Consequently, the muscle is strengthened at the different biomechanical leverage angles and the different length-tension ratios with the full ROM training. This training is performed slowly with a lot of tension on the elastic band for a strengthening effect attributable to the overload principle. See figures 21.08-21.10. Additionally, the training should be performed quickly for power and speed training.

Short Arc ROM Training

Training also can be performed with short arc ROM to strengthen the muscle at the weaker points in the ROM or to actually "supercompensate" and strengthen the muscles even more at their strongest points in the ROM (Davies 1992).

Another example of performing short arc training is form training that uses the full ROM versus sparring or street-fighting situations, where speed would be more important. As illustrated in figure 21.02, this is the proper form for performing the side kick where one chambers (prepares the kick by prestretching the muscles using the stretch-shortening plyometric concept), kicks, and then rechambers the kick. The return to the rechamber position acts like a whip and is as important as the initial part of the motion to generate power as well as to prepare for a follow-up technique. In sparring or street fighting, however, one does not have the time to perform the chamber or preparation position for the kick. So a short arc of motion is performed to make the kick a faster and more practical "speed kick." Instead of bringing the leg off the ground and chambering it, the athlete brings the leg directly from the ground into the opponent and performs the second part (kicking), and then the leg returns immediately to the ground after performing the kicking motion for a base of support and for a follow-up technique. This training is performed slowly with a lot of tension on the elastic band for a strengthening effect attributable to the overload principle. Similarly, the short arc exercises to the full ROM are performed quickly for power and speed training. The full ROM and short arc exercises also can be used to facilitate hand speed and punching power as illustrated in figures 21.11-21.12.

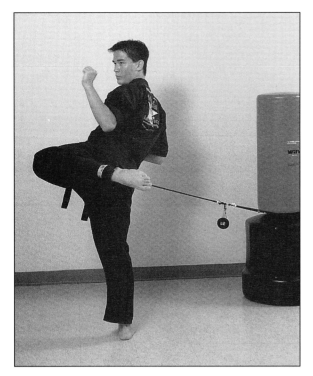

Figure 21.08 Karate round kick (chamber position).

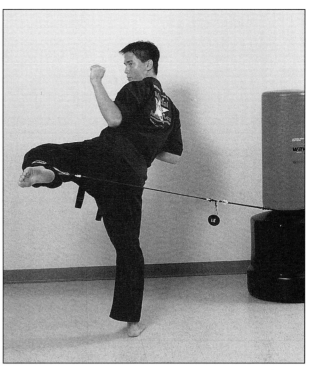

Figure 21.09 Karate round kick (mid-movement).

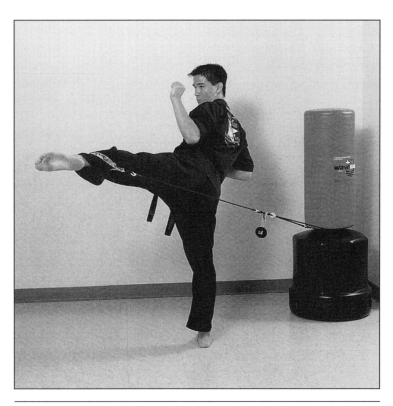

Figure 21.10 Karate round kick (end position).

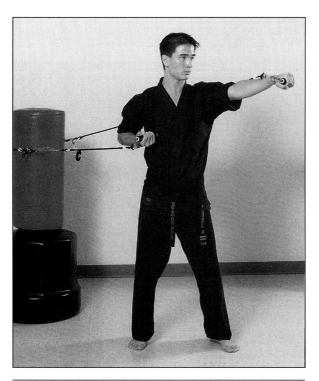

Figure 21.11 Karate jab with left hand.

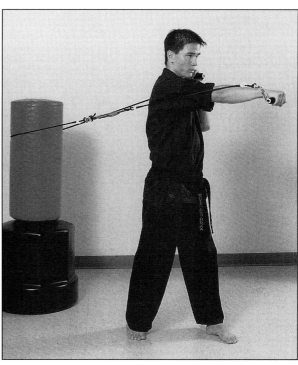

Figure 21.12 Karate rear hand punch with right hand.

Eccentric Muscle Training

I also recommend using the Thera-Band to perform slow, controlled, eccentric deceleration movements to create the eccentric strengthening response to prepare the muscles for performance, minimize delayed-onset muscle soreness, and prevent injuries (Chu and Plummer 1984; Chu 1996; Davies and Ellenbecker 1992). Using the eccentric training as a different stimulus to the muscle should help improve the end ROM performance, which is so important when the athlete is repeating a kick or performing combinations with the same leg. Figures 21.13 and 21.14 demonstrate one method of eccentric training for the karate front kick. The muscle-tendon unit needs to be able to eccentrically decelerate the kicking leg, and then the athlete must use the plyometric stretch-shortening cycle concept to facilitate the power for the follow-up kick. This technique can be applied with both short arc and full ROM exercises.

"Overspeed" Training With Elastic Resistance

Elastic resistance also is used for overspeed training to increase the speed of a kick or a punch, as

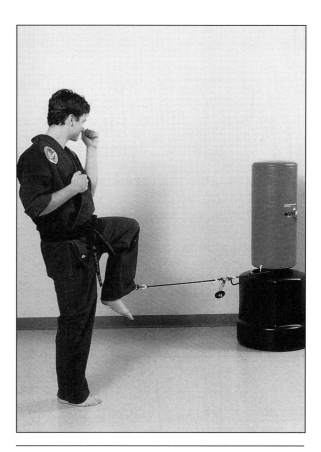

Figure 21.13 Eccentric front leg front kick (chamber position).

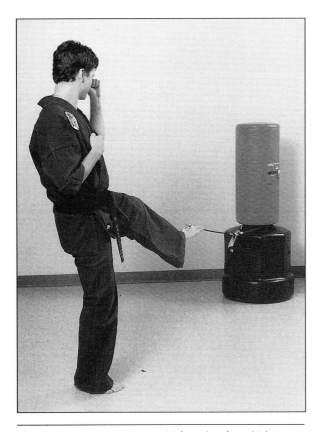

Figure 21.14 Karate (eccentric) front leg, front kick.

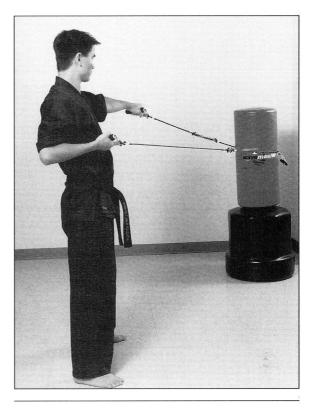

Figure 21.15 Over speed training for hand speed: karate front hand jab.

illustrated in figures 21.15 and 21.16. There are many anecdotal stories of athletes using overspeed training with a variety of activities for improving performance, such as sprinting and improving 40-yd dash times. However, there is minimal research in this area. The concept is related to kinesthetic training, where the body part is forced to go even faster than the red-line speed that the martial artists thinks he or she is capable of achieving. Overperforming with the speed may cause a disinhibition in the nervous system and actually improve the speed of performance. This technique is performed by placing the hands or feet into a position of stretch on the elastic band and then letting the elastic band go. The elastic resistance pulls the limb with exaggerated acceleration through the ROM. The goal is to improve the speed of the technique. This technique is demonstrated in figures 21.17 and 21.18, where the elastic resistance tubing is "pulling" the kick faster than it is normally performed. It is important to minimize the number of repetitions used with this type of overspeed training because of the potential for microtraumatic overuse injuries.

These training techniques are applicable for martial artists of many ages. Even older or mature martial

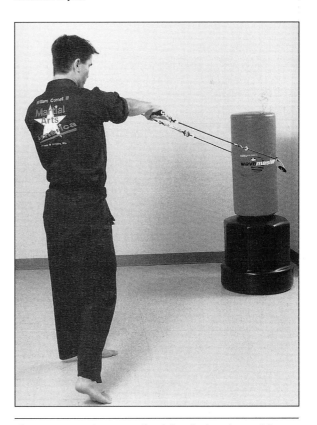

Figure 21.16 Over speed training for hand speed: karate rear hand punch.

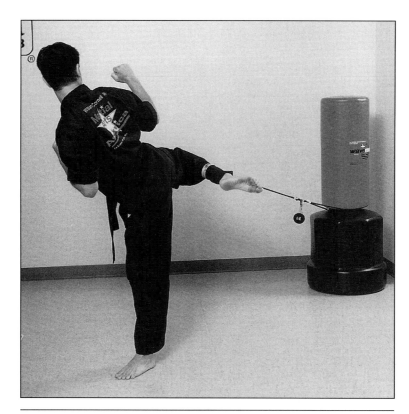

Figure 21.17 Over speed training for karate round kick (chamber position).

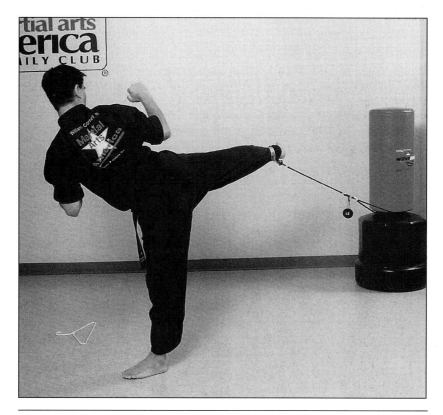

Figure 21.18 Over speed training for karate round kick.

artists can generate a lot of height, speed, and power in the kicks by using these training methods.

When many of these techniques are applied in a practical manner, they can be deadly, as described by Oler et al. (1991). Figures 21.19 through 21.21 demonstrate a technique that has been documented to kill an opponent. Although the figures demonstrate three distinct steps in executing the spinning hook kick, it actually occurs in milliseconds.

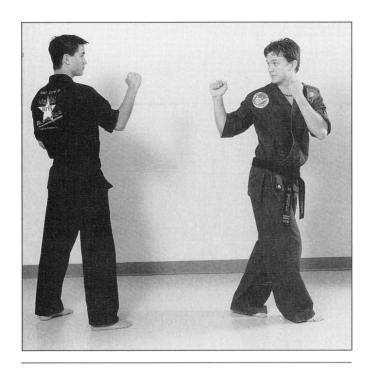

Figure 21.19 Karate spinning hook kick.

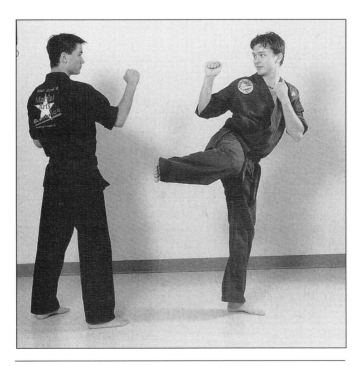

Figure 21.20 Karate spinning hook kick (chamber position).

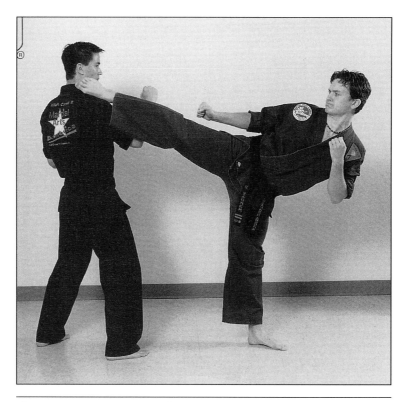

Figure 21.21   Karate spinning hook kick (end position).

Conclusion

This chapter provided a brief introduction to the exciting world of martial arts. I briefly described a historical perspective and a variety of concepts regarding strength and conditioning with particular emphasis on martial arts training. I described various techniques that are used to increase strength and power for martial arts training and conditioning to enhance performance. Elastic resistance training can be integrated in training programs to enhance a variety of performance variables for martial arts.

References

Baechle, T.R., ed. 1994. *Essentials of Strength Training and Conditioning*. Champaign, IL: Human Kinetics.

Birrer, R.B. 1996. "Trauma Epidemiology in the Martial Arts. The Results of an Eighteen-Year International Survey." *American Journal of Sports Medicine* 24: S72-9.

Bompa, T.O. 1993. *Periodization of Strength: The New Wave in Strength Training*. Toronto: Veritas.

Bompa, T.O. 1995. *Power Training for Sport*. New York: Mosaic Press.

Brown, C. 1998. *The Law and Martial Arts*. Santa Clarita, CA: Ohara.

Brown, D.D., W.G. Mucci, R.K. Hetzler, and R.G. Knowlton. 1989. "Cardiovascular and Ventilatory Responses During Formalized T'ai Chi Chuan Exercises." *Research Quarterly* 60: 246-50.

Callister, R., R.J. Callister, R.S. Staron, S.J. Fleck, P. Tesch, and G.A. Dudley. 1991. "Physiological Characteristics of Elite Judo Athletes." *International Journal of Sports Medicine* 12: 196-203.

Cavanagh, P.R., and J. Landa. 1976. "A Biomechanical Analysis of the Karate Chop." *Research Quarterly* 47: 610-8.

Chu, D.A. 1996. *Explosive Power and Strength*. Champaign, IL: Human Kinetics.

Chu, D.A., and L. Plummer. 1984. "The Language of Plyometrics." *National Strength and Conditioning Association Journal* 6: 30-5.

Cook, A.S., and M. Woollacott. 1995. *Motor Control: Theory and Practical Applications*. Baltimore: Williams & Wilkins.

Costello, F., and E.J. Kreis. 1993. *Sports Agility*. Nashville, TN: Taylor Sports.

Davies, G.J. 1992. *A Compendium of Isokinetics in Clinical Usage*. Onalaska, WI: S & S.

Davies, G.J. 1996. "Playing Through the Pain." *Biomechanics* 2: 37-40.

Davies, G.J. In press. "Mechanisms of Injuries That Create Common Injuries in Martial Arts." *Sports Medicine Update*.

Davies, G.J., C. Durall, and D.C. Fater. 2001. "Biomechanical Approach to Sports Rehabilitation: Martial Arts." In *Sport Injury Rehabilitation*, ed. E. Shamus. New York: McGraw-Hill.

Davies, G.J., and T.S. Ellenbecker. 1992. "Eccentric Isokinetics." *Orthopedic Physical Therapy Clinics of North America* 1: 297-336.

Davies, G.J., K. Wilk, and T.S. Ellenbecker. 1997. "Assessment of Strength." Pp. 225-56 in *Orthopedic and Sports Physical Therapy*, ed. T.R. Malone, T.G. McPoil, and A.J. Nitz. St. Louis: Mosby.

Dintiman, G.B., and R.D. Ward. 1988. *Sport Speed.* Champaign, IL: Leisure.

Feld, M.S., R.W. McNair, and S.R. Wilk. 1979. "The Physics of Karate." *Scientific American* 240: 150-8.

Fleck, S.J., and W.J. Kraemer. 1996. *The Ultimate Training System: Periodization Breakthrough.* New York: Advanced Research Press.

Fleck, S.J., and W.J. Kraemer. 1997. *Designing Resistance Training Programs.* 2nd ed. Champaign, IL: Human Kinetics.

Francescato, M.P., T. Talon, and P.R. diPrampero. 1995. "Energy Cost and Energy Sources in Karate." *European Journal of Applied Physiology* 71: 355-61.

Hirano, K., and M. Seto. 1973. "Dangers of Karate." *Journal of the American Medical Association* 226: 1118-9.

Imamura, H., Y. Yoshimura, S. Nishimura, A.T. Nakazawa, C. Nishimura, and T. Shirota. 1999. "Oxygen Uptake, Heart Rate and Blood Lactate Responses During and Following Karate Training." *Medicine and Science in Sports and Exercise* 31: 342-7.

Imamura, H., Y. Yoshimura, and K. Uchida, A. Tanaka, S. Nishimura, and A.T. Nakazawa. 1996. "Heart Rate Response and Perceived Exertion During Twenty Consecutive Karate Sparring Matches." *Australian Journal of Science and Medicine in Sport* 28: 114-5.

Imamura, H., Y. Yoshimura, K. Uchida, A. Tanaka, S. Nishimura, and A.T. Nakazawa. 1997. "Heart Rate, Blood Lactate Responses and Ratings of Perceived Exertion to 1,000 Punches and 1,000 Kicks in Collegiate Karate Practitioners." *Applied Human Science* 16: 9-13.

Jaffe, L., and J. Minkoff. 1988. "Martial Arts: A Perspective on Their Evolution, Injuries and Training Formats." *Orthopaedic Review* 17: 208-21.

Kim, S.H. 2000. *Martial Arts After 40.* Hartford, CT: Turtle Press.

Koiwai, E.K. 1981. "Fatalities Associated With Judo." *The Physician and Sportsmedicine.* 9: 61-6.

Koiwai, E.K. 1987. "Deaths Allegedly Caused by the Use of Choke Holds (Shimewaza)." *Journal of Forensic Science* 32: 419-32.

Lai, J.S., C. Lan, M.K. Wong, and S.H. Tseng. 1995. "Two-Year Trends in Cardiorespiratory Function Among Older Tai Chi Chuan Practitioners and Sedentary Subjects." *Journal of the American Geriatrics Society* 43: 1222-7.

Lan, C., J.S. Lai, S.Y. Chen, and M.K. Wong. 1998. "12 Month Tai Chi Training in the Elderly: Its Effect on Health Fitness." *Medicine and Science in Sports and Exercise* 30: 345-51.

Lan, C., J.S. Lai, M.K. Wong, and M. Yu. 1996. "Cardiorespiratory Function, Flexibility, and Body Composition Among Geriatric Tai Chi Chuan Practitioners." *Archives of Physical Medicine and Rehabilitation* 77: 612-6.

Lannuzel, A., T. Moulin, D. Amsallem, J. Galmiche, and L. Rumbach. 1994. "Vertebral-Artery Dissection Following a Judo Session: A Case Report." *Neuropediatrics* 25: 106-8.

Matsumoto, T., S. Nakagawa, S. Nishida, and R. Hirota. 1997. "Bone Density and Bone Metabolic Markers in Active Collegiate Athletes: Findings in Long Distance Runners, Judoists, and Swimmers." *International Journal of Sports Medicine* 18: 408-12.

Norris, C. 1975. *Winning Tournament Karate.* Santa Clarita, CA: Ohara.

Oler, M., W. Tomson, H. Pepe, Yoon D, Branoff R, Branch, J. 1991. "Morbidity and Mortality in the Martial Arts: A Warning." *Journal of Trauma* 21: 251-3.

Owens, R.G., and E.J. Ghadiali. 1991. "Judo as a Possible Cause of Anoxic Brain Damage: A Case Report." *Journal of Sports Medicine and Physical Fitness* 31: 627-8.

Pieter, F., and W. Pieter. 1995. "Speed and Force of Selected Tae Kwon Do Techniques." *Biology of Sport* 12: 257-66.

Ratamess, N.A. 1998. "Weight Training for Jiu Jitsu." *Strength and Conditioning Journal* 20: 8-15.

Reay, D.T., and J.W. Eisle. 1982. "Death From Law Enforcement Neck Holds." *American Journal of Forensic Medicine and Pathology* 3: 253-8.

Russel, S.M., and A. Lewis. 1975. "Karate Myoglobinuria." *New England Journal of Medicine* 293: 941.

Sanders, M.S., and J. Antonio. 1999. "Strength and Conditioning for Submission Fighting." *Strength and Conditioning Journal* 21: 42-5.

Schmidt, R.J. 1975. "Fatal Chest Trauma in Karate Trainers." *Medicine and Science in Sports* 7: 59-61.

Schneider, D., and R. Leung. 1991. "Metabolic and Cardiorespiratory Responses to the Performance of Wing Chun and Tai Chi Chuan Exercises." *International Journal of Sports Medicine* 12: 319-23.

Shaw, D.W., and D.T. Deutsch. 1982. "Heart Rate and Oxygen Uptake Response to Performance of Karate Kata." *Journal of Sports Medicine and Physical Fitness* 22: 461-8.

Shumway-Cook, A., and M. Woollacott. 1995. *Motor Control.* Philadelphia: Williams and Wilkins.

Staley, C.I. 1996. *Special Topics in Martial Arts Conditioning.* Santa Barbara, CA: Myo-Dynamics.

Staley, C.I. 1999. *The Science of Martial Arts Training.* Burbank, CA: Multi-Media Books.

Stricevic, M., T. Okazaki, A.J. Tanner, N. Mazzarella, and R. Merola. 1980. "Cardiovascular Responses to the Karate Kata." *The Physician and Sportsmedicine* 8: 57-67.

Takahashi, R. 1992. "Plyometrics: Power Training for Judo: Plyometric Training With Medicine Balls." *National Strength and Conditioning Association Journal* 14: 66-71.

Vos, J.A., and R.A. Brinkhorst. 1966. "Velocity and Force of Some Karate Arm Movements." *Nature* 211: 89-90.

Walker, J. 1975. "Karate Strikes." *American Journal of Physics* 43: 845-9.

Wolf, S.L., C. Coogler, and W. Tingsen. 1997. "Exploring the Basis for Tai Chi Chuan as a Therapeutic Exercise Approach." *Archives of Physical Medicine and Rehabilitation* 8: 886-92.

Young, D.R., L.J. Appel, S. Jee, and E.R. Miller. 1999. "The Effects of Aerobic Exercises and Tai Chi on Blood Pressure in Older People: Results of a Randomized Trial." *Journal of the American Geriatrics Society* 47: 277-86.

Zatsiorsky, V.M. 1995. *Science and Practice of Strength Training*. Champaign, IL: Human Kinetics.

Zehr, E.P., S.G. Sale, and J.J. Dowling. 1997. "Ballistic Movement Performance in Karate Athletes." *Medicine and Science in Sports and Exercise* 29: 1366-73.

Zigun, J.R., and S.M. Schneider. 1988. "'Effort' Thrombosis (Paget-Schroetter's Syndrome) Secondary to Martial Arts Training." *American Journal of Sports Medicine* 16: 189-90.

CHAPTER 22

Sport-Specific Training for Skiing

• • • • •

Burt Johnson, ATC
Howard Head Sports Medicine Centers

Jeff Carlson, PT
Howard Head Sports Medicine Centers

Skiing is an extremely demanding sport that requires coordination and strength of the lower body and trunk. It is no wonder that ski injuries are so prevalent among recreational and professional racers. The Steadman-Hawkins Sports Medicine Foundation, which has conducted survey research over the past decade, has reported that approximately 32 to 48% of all ski injuries are related to the knee. Most commonly seen are medial collateral ligament (MCL) injuries followed by the anterior cruciate ligament and the meniscus (Briggs and Steadman 1998). Thus, our strength and rehabilitation protocols focus on the musculature surrounding the knee joint.

To maximize turning ability and maintain sufficient speed through a turn, a skier must maintain balance by controlling the center of gravity relative to the base of support. The skier accomplishes this by using various muscles of the lower body and trunk and by limb positioning. Torry, Decker, and Steadman (in press) described four phases of turning: preparation, turn initiation, fall line, and turn completion. Throughout these phases, the quadri-

ceps, hamstrings, gastrocsoleus complex, hip adductors, gluteals, and low back and abdominal muscles are responsible for timing and loading of the ski. Eccentric contractions of these muscles have been shown to exhibit the most control during the turning phases. These muscles do not simultaneously cocontract during a ski turn, but rather each portion of each muscle has its own specific sequence of firing (Hintermeister et al. 1995; Hintermeister, Lange, and O'Connor 1993). For example, it has been found that the vastus medialis and the vastus lateralis produce greater electromyographic activity on the downhill leg than the uphill leg (Hintermeister et al. 1993). Thus, rehabilitation and strengthening techniques focus on eccentric contractions of the vastii muscle groups, because this most closely simulates the muscle's actions during an active ski turn (Hintermeister et al. 1998; Silverskiold et al. 1988). Also, the gluteus maximus shows a unilateral dominance on the downhill leg. The adductors are active at high levels throughout the phases of a ski turn, suggesting that they stabilize the knee and hip joint during skiing (Hintermeister,

Lange, and O'Connor 1993), so they require adequate attention when training.

Ski-Specific Elastic Resistance Exercises

Through the research of the Steadman-Hawkins Sports Medicine Foundation and Topper Sports Medicine, a series of ski-specific elastic resistance exercises have been developed to emphasize ski-specific motions for conditioning.

Double-Knee Bends

While the athlete stands with feet facing forward and about shoulder-width apart, the elastic cord is placed under the athlete's feet so that with no resistance the handles come just above the knee. The handles then are pulled up to the waist and held there for the duration of the exercise. To begin the motion, the person slowly lowers his or her body to the ground, stopping at about 60° of knee flexion, and then returns to the starting position. At the

top of the movement it is very important not to "lock" the knees. The best results are obtained when the quadriceps are under continuous tension, and 3 sets of 50 repetitions are recommended during each session. This exercise focuses primarily on strengthening the quadriceps (figure 22.01).

Single-Knee Bends

This exercise is similar to the double-knee bend, also focusing on the quadriceps. The uninvolved lower extremity is held in the air, or the person can balance with a toe on the ground. To get the proper form it helps to hold something, enabling the athlete to drop his or her weight back instead of keeping the knees over the toes (figure 22.02).

Balance Squats

This exercise increases proprioception, which can help prevent injury and improve performance. This exercise requires balance and strength, because it is deeper and more difficult than single-knee bends. This exercise is performed approximately 1 to 2 months before the patient returns to skiing. The

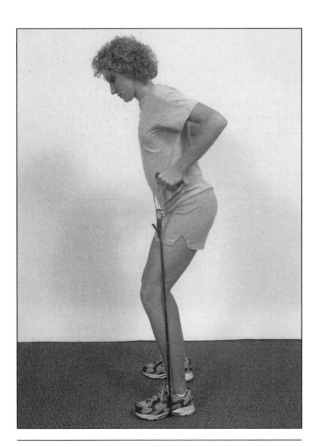

Figure 22.01   Double knee bends.

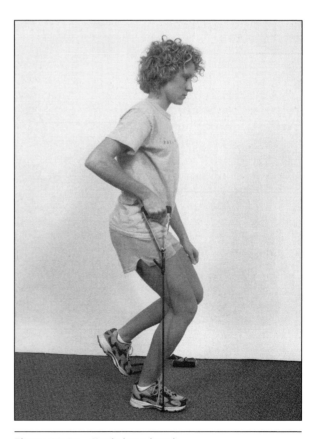

Figure 22.02   Single knee bends.

motion is done without resistance first, and then tension is added to the elastic cord. To start, the person stands erect with the uninvolved leg extended behind the body, balancing on a chair. The motion is a single-leg squat from roughly 30 to 80° of knee flexion, which primarily strengthens the quadriceps and gluteals (figure 22.03; Hintermeister et al. 1998).

Tuck Squats

This exercise has been shown to train similar muscle groups as the downhill tuck position in skiing (Torry, Decker, and Steadman 2000). This exercise, which is aimed at training the quadriceps and gluteal muscles in a deep squat position, is an excellent way to train the muscles anaerobically. Electromyography was used to show muscle-firing patterns during the exercise. These electromyographic results show the increase in muscle activity as time increased in a 2.5-min trial. The athlete can perform this exercise by using one or two elastic cords on both extremities. The athlete sits on a low chair, leans forward, and places the cords under each foot. The elastic cords are loaded under the metatarsal heads.

Standing up from the chair increases resistance as the cords are stretched. The athlete should try to perform this exercise in the range of 90 to 100° of knee flexion, but if this range is uncomfortable, the athlete can try the 70 to 80° range (figure 22.04).

Hamstring Drags

The athlete begins by sitting on the edge of a chair with an elastic cord secured in a door or to a wall. The opposite end of the elastic cord is attached to the ankle of the exercise leg. The athlete slides the chair back until there is resistance on the cord with the leg fully extended. The exercise is done by pointing the toes into the ground and slowly flexing the knee to 90°. (See chapter 5, p. 80.) The toe should remain pointed to strengthen the hamstrings and gastrocsoleus together. At the end of the motion, the athlete lifts the toe off the ground and slowly extends the knee to the starting position. This exercise targets and isolates the distal portion of the hamstrings. This area of the muscle tendon junction is responsible for stabilizing the knee through cocontraction in skiing (Hintermeister et al. 1998).

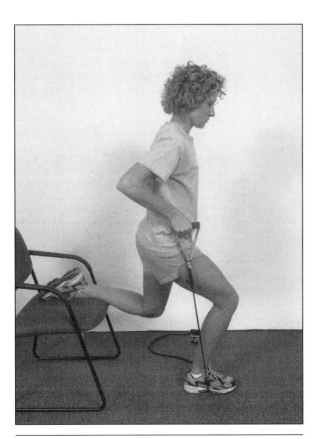

Figure 22.03　Balance squats.

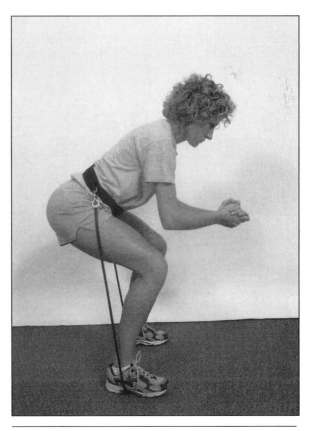

Figure 22.04　Tuck squats.

Hip Exercises

Strengthening the hip musculature is extremely important for control of the lower body. The athlete should focus on hip extension, abduction, and flexion using the elastic cord. (See chapter 5, figures 5.03-5.17, pp. 71-77.)

Forward/Backward Jogging

Forward/backward jogging is used to develop plyometric muscle control. With the elastic cord attached to the door, put the waist belt through the handles and attach to the athlete's waist. Facing away from the door, the athlete steps away until he or she feels tension on the cord, then steps away approximately 6 in. more. The athlete should slowly lower and raise the body, using alternating legs (figure 22.05). Each knee should be bent approximately 30°. The athlete should start slowly and maintain control, while developing strength by increasing the depth and speed of the bends. The athlete should perform the same exercise

facing the door where the cord is attached (figure 22.06; Hintermeister et al. 1998).

Side-to-Side Lateral Agility

Side-to-side lateral agility allows the individual to simulate the giant slalom turn with resistance. The components of the lateral agility exercise allow the individual to increase muscle endurance, strength, power, and control in muscles that are active during the ski turn. This exercise requires a high level of proprioception, which will aid in transitioning between ski turns. The athlete should face the involved hip toward the attachment with the waist belt and handles secured around the body. The athlete steps out until he or she feels tension on the cord and then moves 3 to 4 in. further out from the attachment. The athlete should bend the knees to approximately 30 to 40°. Place a piece of tape near the outer edge of the foot closest to the door. This foot should hit the marker after each repetition. To start, the athlete takes a step away from the door, maintaining the bend in

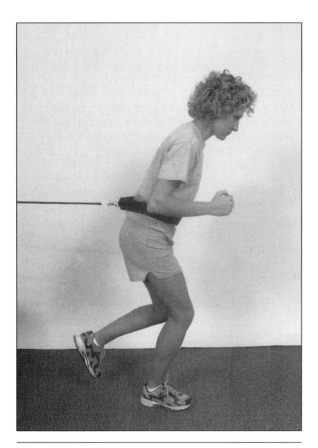

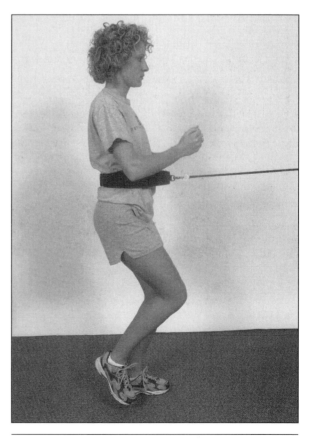

Figure 22.05 Forward jogging.

Figure 22.06 Backward jogging.

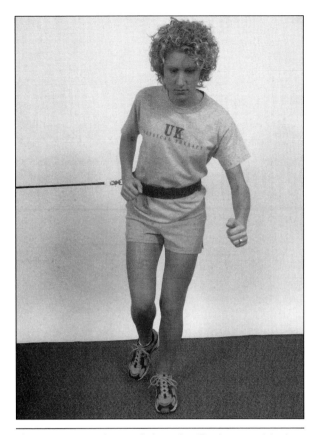

Figure 22.07 Side-to-side lateral agility (start position).

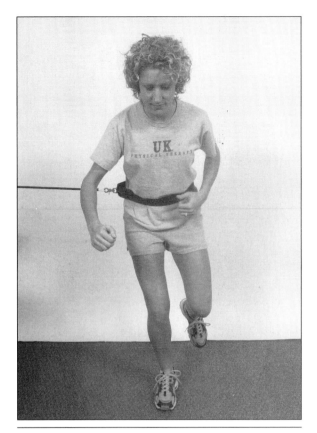

Figure 22.08 Side-to-side lateral agility (end position).

the knee (figure 22.07). The athlete slowly returns to the marker and flexes slowly with the inside leg (figure 22.08). Now the athlete should try pushing off, not just stepping. The goal is to jump laterally approximately 1 m, landing on the outside leg. The athlete holds this position and then returns to the inside leg, absorbing body weight slowly during landing. This exercise is done in sets of 2 to 3, with 40 repetitions.

The exercise should be performed in a slow and controlled manner to emphasize proper form and technique. This allows for a greater muscle contraction, which increases muscle control.

Conclusion

This chapter has outlined basic knee strengthening exercises that can be useful for preseason conditioning of the recreational skier as well as rehabilitation of the injured knee, with appropriate modifications, for return to skiing after a significant knee injury. The use of elastic resistance is an important part in the overall conditioning and training program for skiers.

References

Briggs, K.B., and J.R. Steadman. 1998. *Pre-Placement Screening Program for the Ski Resort Industry.* Vail, CO: Steadman-Hawkins Foundation.

Hintermeister, R.A., M.J. Bey, G.W. Lange, J.R. Steadman, and C.J. Dillman. 1998. "Quantification of Elastic Resistance Knee Rehabilitation Exercises." *Journal of Orthopaedic and Sports Physical Therapy* 28: 40-50.

Hintermeister, R.A., G.W. Lange, and D.D. O'Connor. 1993. "Muscle Activity of the Inside Leg and Outside Leg in Slalom and Giant Slalom Skiing." Pp. 142-9 in *Science and Skiing,* ed. E. Muller, H. Schwameder, E. Kornexel, and C. Raschner. New York: Chapman & Hall.

Hintermeister, R.A., D.D. O'Connor, C.J. Dillman, C.L. Suplizio, G.W. Lange, and J.R Steadman. 1995. "Muscle Activity in Slalom and Giant Slalom Skiing." *Medicine and Science in Sports and Exercise* 27: 315-22.

Silfverskiold, J.P., J.R. Steadman, R.W. Higgins, T. Hagerman, and J.A. Atkins. 1988. "Rehabilitation of the Anterior Cruciate Ligament in the Athlete." *Sports Medicine* 6: 308-19.

Torry, M.R., M.J. Decker, and J.R. Steadman. 2000. "EMG Activity in the Tuck Position During Simulated Downhill Skiing." Unpublished data, Steadman-Hawkins Foundation.

Torry, M.R., M.J. Decker, and J.R. Steadman. In press. "Alpine Skiing." In *Physical Therapy for Sports Medicine,* ed. E. Shamus. New York: McGraw-Hill.

PART V

SPECIAL POPULATIONS

The final section of this book presents several more recent applications of elastic resistance exercise. Research has shown the benefits of regular exercise and strength training for older adults, people with disabilities, and persons with chronic disease. The following chapters describe the scientific rationale and specific clinical application of elastic resistance exercise in these special populations.

CHAPTER 23

Elastic Resistance Training for Older Adults

• • • • •

Robert Topp, PhD, RN

School of Nursing, Medical College of Georgia

In the United States, the older adult population is expanding faster than any other age group, which is increasing the mean age of the U.S. population. This pattern of advancing age within the population is also occurring within most other developed countries. By the year 2020, approximately 20% of Americans will be age 65 or older. It is projected that by the year 2050, there will be 15 to 30 million individuals in the United States over the age of 85, with women significantly outnumbering men and outliving men by an average of 7 to 8 years (O'Brien and Vertinsky 1991). However, later life is often accompanied by chronic illness, which reduces the quality of life and decreases the individual's ability to perform activities of daily living (ADLs; Fiatarone and Evans 1990; Fisher, Pendergast, and Calkins 1991). Roughly 80% of all older adults exhibit at least one chronic health condition, and a substantial proportion of this group exhibit multiple comorbid conditions. Morbidity associated with the aging process has led many developed countries to consider aging their most important health issue (Lexell 1995).

This chapter explores the impact that resistance training can have on older adults. The process of aging, which commonly includes a cycle of declin-ing activity levels, declining functional capacity, and increasing chronic disease, can be interrupted with resistance training. After I review the impact of resistance training on the health and functioning of older adults, I present three components of designing an elastic resistance training program for older adults: conducting the pretraining evaluation, formulating the exercise prescription, and maintaining and enhancing compliance.

The Effect of Resistance Training on Aging

Muscles are the most prevalent type of tissue in the body. Roughly 45% of the human body weight is muscle, and if the 450 skeletal muscles of the body contracted simultaneously 25 tons of force could be generated (Siegel 1986). Muscle tissue is responsible not only for transporting objects, including the body itself, within the environment but also for moving substances that are being transported within the body. Total muscle mass based on urinary creatinine excretion declines by approximately 50% between the ages of 20 and 90 years (Tzankoff and

Norris 1978). This decline in muscle mass that appears to accompany aging is more marked in Type 2 muscle fibers (fast twitch), which decrease from an average of 60% among young sedentary men to less than 30% among sedentary 80-year-old men (Larsson 1983). Peak muscle strength commonly is realized before age 30 years (Larsson, Grimby, and Karlsson 1979). Peak strength has been observed to decline by 15% per decade among sedentary individuals after age 50 (Harries and Bassey 1990; Murray et al. 1985).

Muscle strength is an important predictor of independence, and decreases in muscle mass accompanied by decreases in strength have been implicated as factors in the loss of independence among older adults (Bassey et al. 1992; Fiatarone and Evans 1990). In addition, loss of muscle mass combined with decreasing bone mass has been associated with an increased incidence of debilitating injuries resulting from falls (Fisher, Pendergast, and Calkins 1991). In persons 65 years and over, falls are the leading cause of accidental death (Nelson et al. 1994; O'Brien and Vertinsky 1991). The progressive decline in muscle mass in later life is a major public health problem, which costs an estimated $10 billion in acute care for fall-related fractures and another $7 billion in health care costs that can be attributed to the inability to perform ADLs (Tseng et al. 1995).

Declining functional ability, including the ability to carry out ADLs, has been associated with declines in health and increased dependency among older adults. Functional ability has been inversely correlated with the need for assisted living and with short-term morbidity among older adults. Guralnik et al. (1994) reported that strength, postural control, and the functional abilities of rising from a chair and gait speed were independent predictors of short-term mortality and nursing home admissions among a sample of 5,000 community-dwelling older adults. Williams and Hornberger (1984) observed that poor ability to ambulate and poor manual dexterity in institutionalized elders were significant predictors of transfer to a skilled nursing facility. These findings support the results of Speare, Avery, and Lawton (1991), who reported significant correlations between declines in the ability to perform ADLs and an increased likelihood of declines in residential mobility and more dependent living arrangements among older adults. Thus, declines in functional ability in later life seem to be associated with an increased need for assisted living and with short-term morbidity.

Muscle weakness, which commonly accompanies the aging process, is an important link in the cycle that includes declines in functional ability and an increased risk for chronic disease in later life. Functional ability in later life is defined as the ability to complete ADLs or activities required for independent living (Lueckenotte 1996). As figure 23.01 indicates, inactivity in later life contributes to skeletal muscle atrophy. Skeletal muscle atrophy or loss of muscle mass in turn leads to declines in muscle strength. It is theorized that declines in muscle strength among older adults contribute to declines in functional ability, which diminish the individual's confidence to perform functional tasks. These declines in functional ability and confidence contribute to additional declines in activity and contribute to the development and progression of a number of common chronic diseases. The development and progression of chronic disease among older adults then contribute to additional declines in activity and the cycle begins anew. This cycle continues until the older individual becomes unable to perform critical functional activities necessary to maintain functional independence and thus becomes dependent on others to complete activities required for independent living.

This cycle, which includes muscle weakness leading to a loss of functional ability and chronic disease, can be arrested and possibly reversed through regular exercise. Exercise is defined as planned, structured, and repetitive physical activity that involves muscle contraction and that is done to improve or maintain one or more components of physical fitness (Pate et al. 1995). Resistance training is a form of exercise in which the resistance against which a muscle generates force is progressively increased over time, resulting in an increased muscle strength and/or endurance (Mazzeo et al. 1998). Previous researchers have concluded that resistance training by older adults can improve strength approximately 10 to 30%. This training response to resistance training is similar to that observed among younger adults (Buchner et al. 1993). A large number of investigators have reported that resistance training improves muscle strength (Fiatarone and Evans 1990; Frontera et al. 1988; Morgan et al. 1995; Topp et al. 1993) even among frail older adults (Fiatarone et al. 1994). Muscle strength has been reported to be an important predictor of older adults' ability to perform specific functional tasks (Dayhoff et al. 1998; Topp et al. 1998, 2000; Woolley et al. 1999). Resistance training designed to improve muscle strength also has been shown to improve the ability to perform selected functional tasks (Cress et al. 1999) such as rising from a chair (McMurdo and Rennie 1993; Noble et

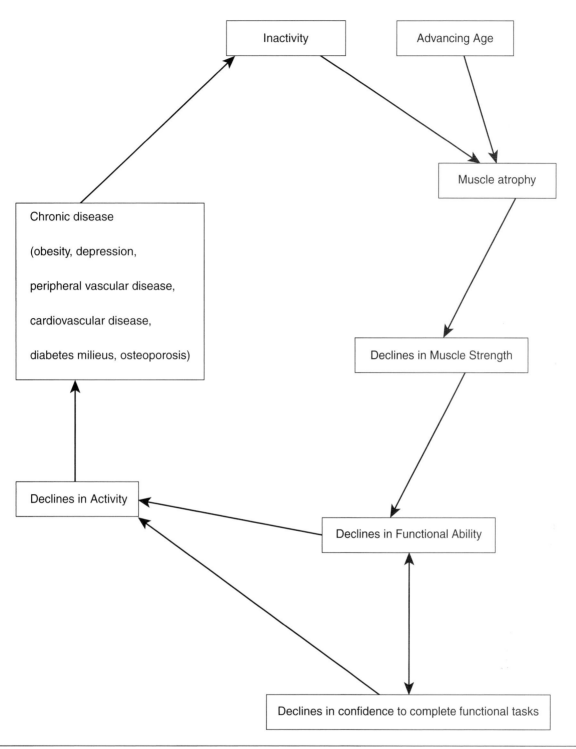

Figure 23.01   Model of inactivity and disease among older adults.

al. 1994) as well as to improve walking speed (Fiatarone and Evans 1990; Topp et al. 1996) and self-reported functional ability (Borchelt and Steinhagen-Thiessen 1992; Hyatt et al. 1990). Resistance training also appears to attenuate or reverse bone loss (osteoporosis; Layne and Nelson, 1992), decrease the risk for falls among older adults, and improve mobility (Buchner et al. 1996; Lamb, Morse, and Evans 1995). Thus, resistance training by older adults appears to have the potential to break the cycle of inactivity, muscle weakness, loss of functional ability, and chronic disease.

In the introduction to the symposium entitled "Resistance Training for Health and Disease" for the ACSM, Pollock and Evans (1999) briefly compared the outcome similarities and differences between aerobic and resistance training. These authors concluded that both pure aerobic and pure resistance training positively affect functional ability, skeletal integrity, and cardiovascular fitness indexes. However, resistance training appears to result in superior gains in muscle strength, basal metabolism, and possibly functional ability over aerobic training. Conversely, these authors concluded that aerobic training appears to be superior to resistance training in eliciting gains in body composition and measures of maximum aerobic capacity. Hurley and Hagberg (1998) reached a similar conclusion, that cardiovascular fitness is optimally enhanced through aerobic training whereas muscle mass, functional ability, and muscle strength are best improved through resistance training. Consistent with this conclusion is the finding of Booth, Weeden, and Tseng (1994), who asserted that muscle strength is a more important predictor of mobility and the ability to perform ADLs in older adults than aerobic capacity. Results of the Fitness Arthritis and Seniors Trial (FAST) among subjects with osteoarthritis of the knee concluded that participation in either resistance or aerobic training modestly reduced disability and pain (Ettinger et al. 1997) and improved postural sway or balance (Messier et al. 2000). On closer inspection of the data, the subjects in the strength training group improved their muscle strength more than the aerobic and control groups, whereas the subjects in the aerobic group improved their measures of aerobic fitness more than the strength and control groups. Finally, the data indicate that both the aerobic and resistance training groups demonstrated significantly better measures of postural sway than the control group. The conclusions of Pollock and Evans (1999) along with those of Booth, Weeden, and Tseng (1994), that resistance training appears to improve the ability

to perform functional tasks to a greater extent than aerobic training, seem logical, because it appears that the functional tasks encountered by older adults primarily involve muscle strength and a minimal amount of aerobic capacity. Thus, it appears that resistance training has a greater potential than aerobic training to maintain and enhance older adults' ability to perform functional tasks.

A number of empirical studies have examined the impact of resistance training with elastic resistance on the strength of older adults. Jette et al. (1999) reported that after 3 and 6 months of resistance training with elastic bands of varying resistance, lower extremity strength improved 6 to 12%, tandem gait improved 20%, and subjects reported a 15 to 18% decrease in disability. These investigators used a partially supervised in-home training program and achieved an 89% compliance rate among the older adult sample over the 6-month project. These findings are consistent with a previous study that also used elastic resistance training among elders with functional limitations (Krebs, Jette, and Assmann 1998). These authors reported that the intervention resulted in moderate gains in strength along with improvements in gait characteristics. Damush and Damush (1999) also reported that an 8-week resistance training program that used elastic bands as the mode of resistance resulted in 14 to 26% improvements in strength among community-dwelling older women. In a similar study, significant improvements in isokinetic strength and training volumes were observed among older adults (mean age = 71.7 years) after 12 weeks of resistance training with elastic bands (Mikesky et al. 1994). These findings that even short-term resistance training can increase muscle strength are consistent with the findings of Jette, Harris, and Sleeper (1996), who reported that 12 to 15 weeks of resistance training with elastic bands significantly increased skeletal muscle strength. Skelton et al. (1995) reported limited improvements in strength as a result of 12 weeks of elastic resistance training and no change in their measures of functional ability among a sample of women 75 years and older. Brill et al. (1995) also reported a minimal impact of 11 weeks of elastic resistance training on their sample of elder nursing home residents with dementia. Both of these studies that reported nonsignificant results after elastic resistance training may have measured their older participants before measurable changes occurred in the outcome variables as a result of the elastic resistance training interventions. Thus, these studies appear to demonstrate that older adults can achieve similar gains in strength by using elastic resistance compared with more traditional modes of resistance training if the training is longer than 14 to 16 weeks (McCartney et al. 1996; Meuleman et al. 2000).

Advantages of Elastic Resistance Exercise for Older Adults

Elastic resistance training offers three advantages to older adults over more conventional modes of resistance training. First, elastic resistance appears to be a safe mode of generating resistance to increase strength among older adults, including older adults with severe physical and cognitive limitations. Previous investigators who have used elastic resistance have reported no major injuries and only minor musculoskeletal discomfort similar to that reported in resistance programs that use free weights or strength training machines. Second, elastic bands cost less than more traditional modes of resistance training. Cost of the exercise equipment may be an important consideration to older adults, who may be limited by a fixed income. Finally, elastic bands appear to be as effective as traditional modes of resistance training in eliciting strength gains among older adults.

Older adults may be more likely to maintain a resistance training program that uses elastic bands rather than free weights or strength training machines. A higher rate of compliance with an elastic resistance training program may be attributed to the portability of the training devices. Home-based strength training with elastic bands allows older individuals to train privately at their convenience and thus may facilitate compliance with the training program. Resistance training machines and free weights are difficult to transport or store in one's home and are costly and difficult to incorporate into a home-based training program. Community-dwelling older adults can easily maintain their resistance training schedule by transporting the elastic bands while traveling. Finally, elastic resistance is appealing to older adults, who may have limited functional ability attributable to chronic health problems, because obstacles such as facility access, transportation, and psychological barriers are minimized (Dishman, Sallis, and Orenstein 1985).

Thus, maintaining functional ability in later life is essential to successful aging (Rowe and Kahn 1997). Functional ability, or the ability to complete functional tasks required for independent living, depends on muscle strength in later life. Regular resistance training by older adults has been shown to not only increase their muscular strength but also favorably impact their performance of functional tasks. Because a majority of functional tasks encountered in later life depend on muscle strength rather than aerobic capacity, it appears logical that older adults should emphasize resistance training versus aerobic training to maintain and enhance their abilities to perform functional tasks. Resistance training with elastic bands has a number of advantages for older adults over more traditional modes of resistance training. Elastic bands appear to be just as effective in enhancing muscle strength as other modes of resistance training while being less expensive and possibly more easily integrated into the older adult's lifestyle. The next section describes the components of an elastic resistance training program designed specifically for older adults.

Designing a Resistance Training Program for Older Adults

A resistance training program for older adults consists of three components. The pretraining evaluation determines the presence of potential risks involved with beginning a resistance training program. This evaluation also provides the basis for establishing the resistance training prescription. The next component of the program is designing the resistance training prescription, which is based on the same training principles as resistance programs designed for younger adults (McArdle, Katch, and Katch 1991). The final component of a resistance training program for older adults includes techniques for maintaining or enhancing compliance with the resistance training program.

Pretraining Evaluation

A pretraining evaluation is completed to ensure the participant's safety as well as to collect data to formulate the resistance training prescription. The ACSM recommends a physician-supervised stress test for anyone more than 50 years old who wants to begin a vigorous training program (ACSM 2000). A number of factors may confound achieving a true maximal exercise performance among older adults including exercise-induced cardiovascular abnormalities, joint disease, deconditioning, muscle weakness, fear of overexertion, commonly prescribed medications, and lack of experience with exercise at or near maximum capacity (Åstrand 1960, 1968; Martinez-Caro et al. 1984). Evans (1999) recommended that if an older adult wishes to begin a walking program or participate in resistance training, a maximum exercise test is probably not necessary. However, Maria Fiatarone, MD (in Evans 1999) recommended that older adults be screened by a series of questions before beginning a resistance training program (see below). An older adult who responds yes to any of these questions should not begin a resistance training program before undergoing a history and physical and receiving clearance from a physician to begin the program. Other significant contraindications to beginning a resistance training program include recent myocardial infarction, aortic stenosis, dissecting aortic aneurysm, uncompensated congestive heart failure, unstable angina, recent myocarditis, acute pulmonary embolism, uncontrolled hypertension, or ventricular or other serious cardiac arrhythmia (ACSM 2000; Evans 1999)

Resistance training screening questions

If the individual responds "yes" to any of the following questions he or she will need physician clearance prior to beginning a resistance training exercise program:

1. Do I get chest pains while at rest and/or during exertion?
2. If the answer to question #1 is "yes", is it true that I have not had a physician diagnose these pains yet?
3. Have I ever had a heart attack?
4. If the answer to question #3 is "yes", was my heart attack within the last year?
5. Do I have high blood pressure?
6. If you do not know the answer to question #5, answer this: Was my blood pressure reading more than 150/100?
7. Am I short of breath after extremely mild exertion and sometimes even at rest or at night in bed?
8. Do I have any ulcerated wounds or cuts on my feet that do not seem to heal?
9. Have I lost 10 pounds or more in the past 6 months without trying and to my surprise?
10. Do I get pain in my buttocks or the back of my legs—my thighs and calves—when I walk?

11. While at rest, do I frequently experience fast irregular heartbeats or, at the other extreme, very slow beats? (Although a low HR can be a sign of an efficient and well-conditioned heart, a very low rate can also indicate a nearly complete heart block.)
12. Am I currently being treated for any heart or circulatory condition, such as vascular disease, stroke, angina, hypertension, congestive heart failure, poor circulation in the legs, valvular heart disease, blood clots, or pulmonary disease?
13. As an adult, have I ever had a fracture of the hip, spine, or wrist?
14. Did I fall more than twice in the past year (no matter what the reason)?
15. Do I have diabetes?

The pretraining component also should include an assessment of the older adult's ability to engage in resistance training. This assessment not only will provide the basis for prescribing the resistance training but also will lend insight into components of the program that will help the older individual realize his or her fitness goals. This assessment consists of determining the individual's fitness goals, identifying previous participation in fitness programs, determining activity level, establishing perceived benefits and barriers to engaging in exercise, determining level of motivation to begin and maintain the program, and defining personal preferences when engaging in exercise. Fitness goals include five components. The first component is that the fitness goals should be significant to the individual older adult. Second, the fitness goal should be objectively measurable or quantifiable. The third component is that the goal should be realistically attainable by the individual. Fourth, the goal should directly relate to the participant. For example, a person may wish to engage in exercise training to improve his or her appearance to others. In this example, the outcome of the training is unrelated to the person engaging in the training and thus is difficult or even impossible to attain. The fifth component of a fitness goal is a timeline that indicates when the goal is expected to be attained. A simple pneumonic to remember these five components of a fitness goal is SMART (significant, measurable, attainable, related to the target, time dependent). Some examples of well-stated fitness goals for older adults are as follows:

• After 10 weeks of resistance training, I will be able to climb a flight of 20 stairs in less than 15 s.

- After 8 weeks of resistance training, I will be able to lift myself out of a bathtub without assistance.

These are examples of poorly stated fitness goals:

- I will walk better after the resistance training program.
- After the first session, I will be stronger.

The initial assessment should include identifying the older adult's previous participation in fitness programs. This assessment should include determining older adults' present and past activity levels, establishing their perceived benefits and barriers to engaging in exercise, determining their level of motivation to begin and maintain the program, and defining their personal preferences when engaging in exercise. Identifying past and present fitness participation and activity levels may indicate modes of training with which the individual may or may not be likely to comply. For example, an older adult who has led an active lifestyle that has included participating in competitive team sports

may be more compliant with resistance training programs that are moderate to high intensity and that incorporate group or team activities. A large number of health behavior theories have indicated that perceived barriers and benefits to engaging in a fitness program are important predictors of adopting and maintaining the fitness program (Bandura 1997; see figure 23.02). The older adult's perceived benefits of and barriers to engaging in a resistance training program should be clarified and enlightened with the current findings and prevailing practice in the area. If the older individual has unrealistic expectations, he or she will be disappointed when these perceived benefits are not attained. Similarly, an older adult who has unrealistic perceptions of the barriers to participating in a resistance program may never begin such a program or may perceive any setback as proof that the barriers to engaging in the program are, in fact, insurmountable.

Once the fitness goals and perceived benefits and barriers have been identified, they can be incorporated into a resistance training prescription for the older adult. Because older adults' muscles adapt to

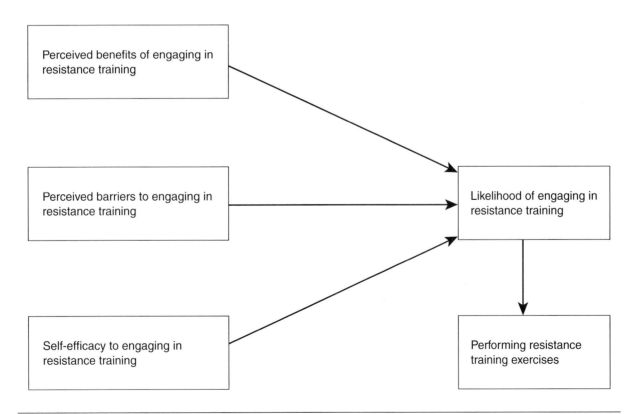

Figure 23.02   Model of factors influencing engagement in resistance training.

Data from A. Bandura, 1997. *Self-Efficacy: The Exercise of Control.* New York: Freeman Press.

resistance training in a similar fashion as younger adults' muscles (Foster-Burns 1999), the five principles of resistance training are the same for older adults as for younger adults. The principles that should be considered when prescribing resistance training to older adults include the overload principle, training progression, reversibility, specificity, and individual differences (McArdle, Katch, and Katch 1991).

A resistance training program should stress the muscles beyond what is encountered during regular daily activity. This principle of overloading the muscle beyond what the muscle is accustomed to will result in adaptations by both the muscle and the nerves supplying the muscle, resulting in greater muscular strength (Fleck and Kraemer 1987). Because muscles and nerves adapt to overloading after a couple of weeks of training, the stress imposed by the resistance training program must be increased continually to ensure that gains in muscle strength continue. This principle of training progression indicates that as muscles adapt to increasing levels of stress in the form of resistance training, the resistance must be progressively increased to continue to increase muscle strength. Conversely, if the older adult stops training, his or her muscles will adapt to the reduced level of stress by declining in strength. Muscle strength will continue to decline to a level necessary to adapt to the reduced level of stress. The loss of strength resulting from cessation of resistance training is an example of the reversibility principle.

Not only does resistance training need to be progressive, but it also must be specific to the older individual's fitness goals. The specificity principle indicates that resistance training should emphasize the specific muscle groups involved in the individual's fitness goals. For example, if the individual's fitness goal involves climbing stairs, resistance training should primarily emphasize training the muscles of the legs. In addition, the more closely the resistance training exercise mimics the actual activity stated in the fitness goal, the greater the progression toward the goal. For the fitness goal of stair climbing, single-leg squats from 0 to 45° of knee flexion would likely result in superior gains in stair climbing than knee extensions with resistance from 0 to 120° while seated. The final principle of resistance training is the principle of individual differences. This principle indicates that adaptations to resistance training will vary between individuals based on their initial level of strength. Thus, it is critical to attempt to match the stress induced by the resistance training program with the older adult's initial level of strength and ability to complete the prescribed resistance pro-

gram. Older adults who have led an inactive lifestyle devoid of exercise should be advised to begin a resistance training program with little resistance, because almost any activity will impose an overload capable of increasing strength. These five principles should be incorporated into the resistance training prescription for older adults.

Formulating an Elastic Resistance Exercise Prescription for the Older Adult

Once the resistance training goals are determined, a specific prescription of resistance with the elastic training device (ETD) can be developed. Four factors of a resistance training program can vary between individuals based on their fitness goals. These components include mode of training, muscle groups involved in the exercise, training volume (sets × repetitions × resistance), and frequency of training (Feigenbaum and Pollack 1999; Fleck and Kraemer 1997). The mode of the training is the mechanism by which resistance is applied to the muscle. Mode of resistance training can be isotonic (static degree of resistance across a range of motion), isokinetic (static speed of muscle lengthening across a range of motion), isometric (static muscle length across a duration of time), or variable resistance (variable resistance across a range of motion). Elastic resistance exercise is best defined as variable resistance because the resistance increases as the ETD is stretched. Thus, the mode of training with an ETD is variable resistance.

A number of resistance training exercises that use ETD have been developed for older adults, emphasizing all of the major muscle groups (Topp, Mikesky, and Bawl 1994). Figures 23.03 through 23.31 present specific exercises for the older adult using elastic resistance. The specific exercises incorporated into the resistance program are dictated by the individual's fitness goals. After the clinician reviews the individual's fitness goals, the muscle groups involved in the goal can be identified. Once these muscle groups are identified, specific resistance training exercises can be selected to increase the strength of the muscles involved in the activity. For example, if the individual's fitness goal involves getting out of a chair without assistance, the muscles involved with this activity should be emphasized in training. The muscles involved in this activity include the quadriceps, gluteals, and hamstrings (and triceps if the individual uses the arms to assist in rising from the chair). If we invoke the principle

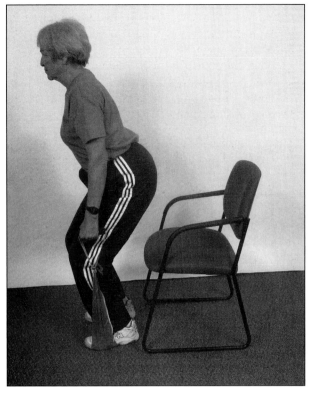

Figure 23.03 Chair squat (start position).

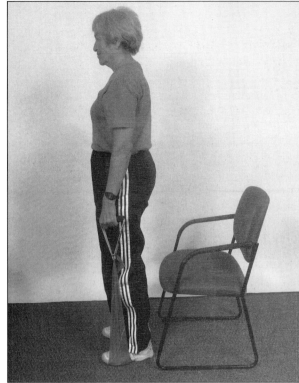

Figure 23.04 Chair squat (end position).

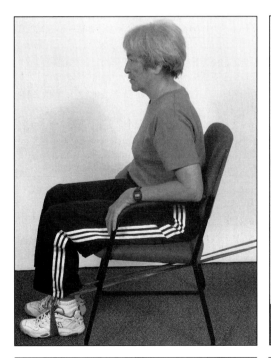

Figure 23.05 Leg extension (start position).

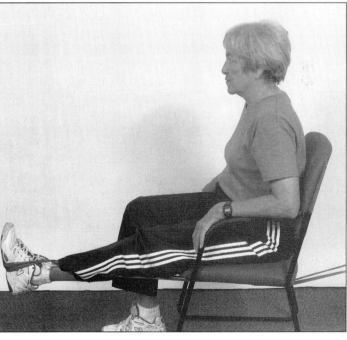

Figure 23.06 Leg extension (end position).

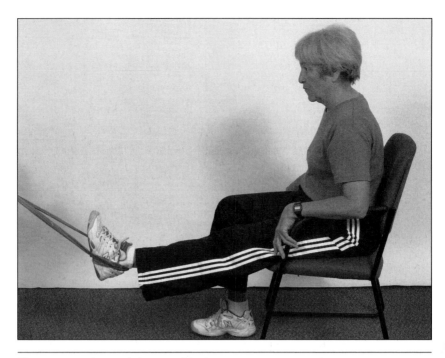

Figure 23.07 Leg curls (start position).

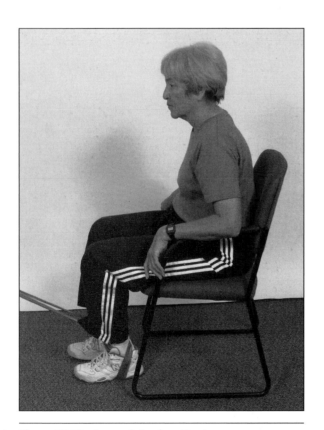

Figure 23.08 Leg curls (end position).

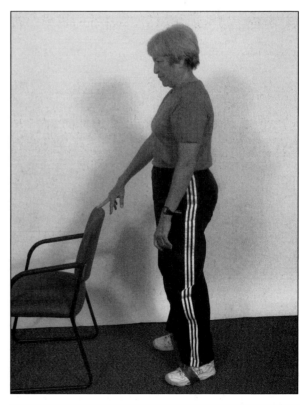

Figure 23.09 Hip flexion (start position).

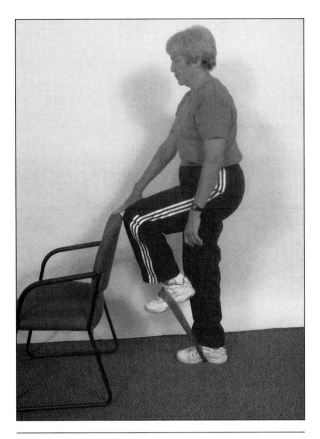

Figure 23.10   Hip flexion (end position).

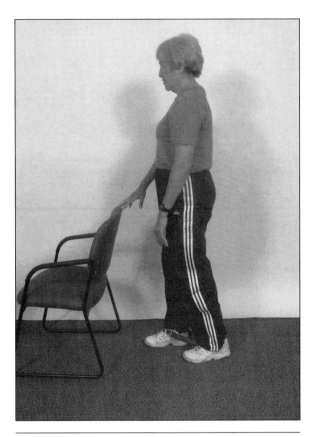

Figure 23.11   Hip extension (start position).

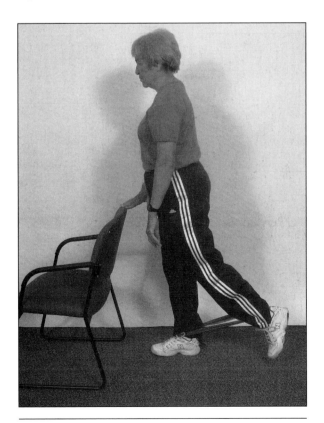

Figure 23.12   Hip extension (end position).

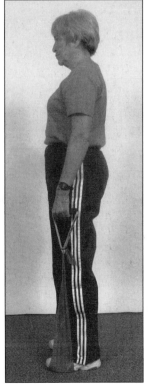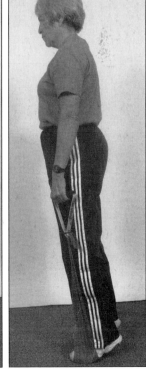

Figure 23.13a and b   Calf raise (start position) (a); calf raise (end position) (b).

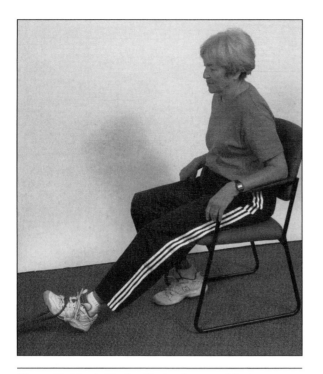

Figure 23.14 Ankle dorsiflexion (start position).

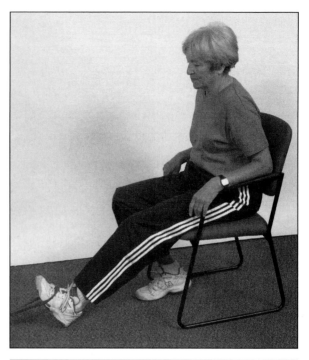

Figure 23.15 Ankle dorsiflexion (end position).

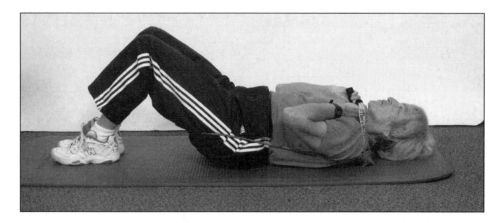

Figure 23.16 Abdominal curls (start position).

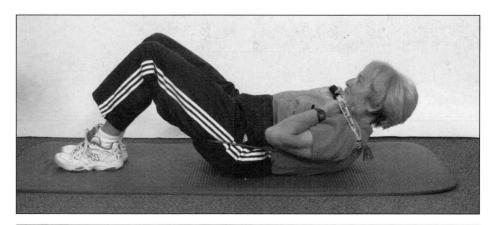

Figure 23.17 Abdominal curls (end position).

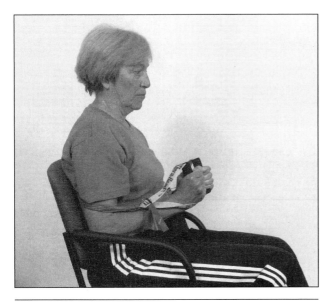

Figure 23.18 Chest press (start position).

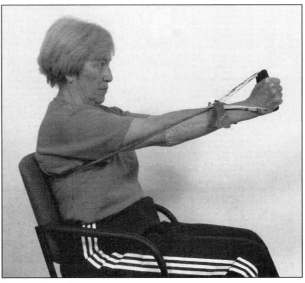

Figure 23.19 Chest press (end position).

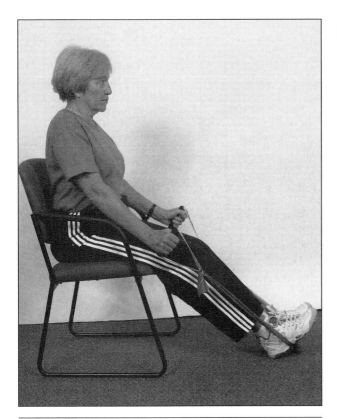

Figure 23.20 Seated rows (start position).

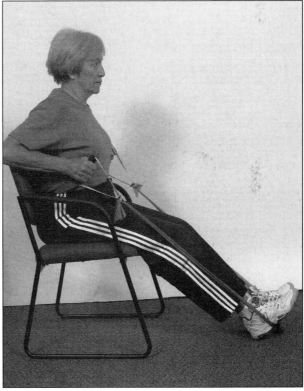

Figure 23.21 Seated rows (end position).

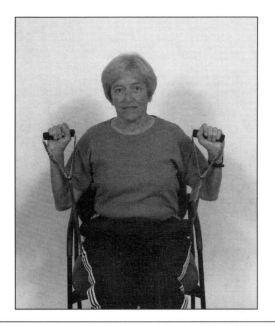

Figure 23.22 Overhead or military press (start position).

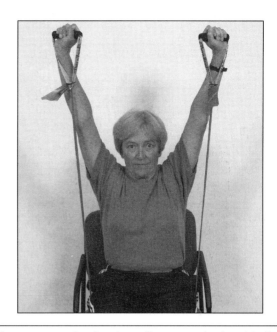

Figure 23.23 Overhead or military press (end position).

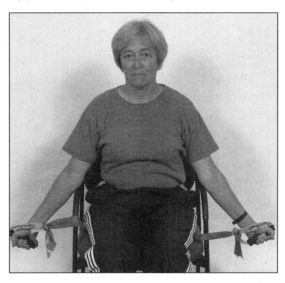

Figure 23.24 Lateral shoulder raises (start position).

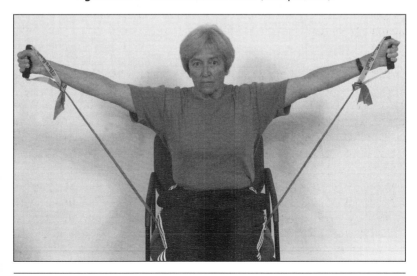

Figure 23.25 Lateral shoulder raises (end position).

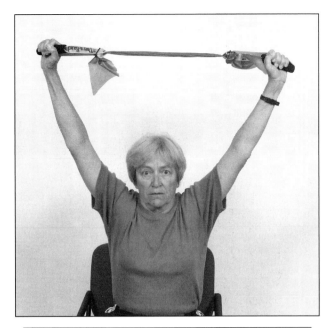

Figure 23.26 Overhead pull-downs (start position).

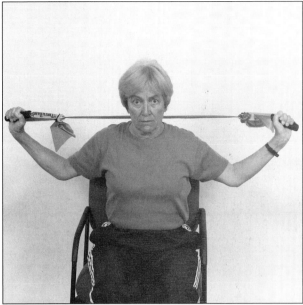

Figure 23.27 Overhead pull-downs (end position).

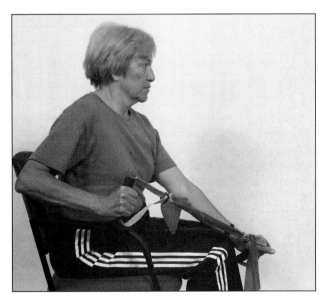

Figure 23.28 Triceps extension (start position).

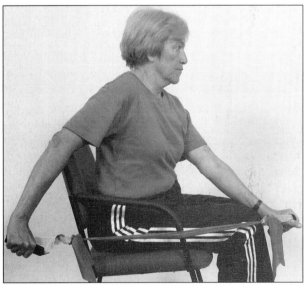

Figure 23.29 Triceps extension (end position).

of specificity, the resistance exercise best suited for advancing the individual toward the goal would be squats down to and up from a chair (figure 23.03). The principle of progression may be applied by encouraging the individual to complete the training with increasingly greater resistance by using heavier ETDs. Simply stated, the resistance exercises included in the individual's resistance training prescription should mimic as closely as possible the activities included in the individual's fitness goals.

Determining the training resistance volume considers repetitions, sets, and resistance. Tables have

been developed to quantify training volume in pounds when Thera-Band elastic bands are used (see tables in the appendix, page 339). These tables operationalize training volume, expressed in pounds, as the product of the number of repetitions multiplied by the number of sets of the exercise multiplied by the resistance provided by the degree of stretch of the elastic band (Thera-Band). Thus, stretching a red Thera-Band 10 repetitions to 100% of elongation (e.g., from 12 in. to 24 in.) will result in a training resistance volume of 39 lb. If the number of elongations of the red elastic bands to 100%

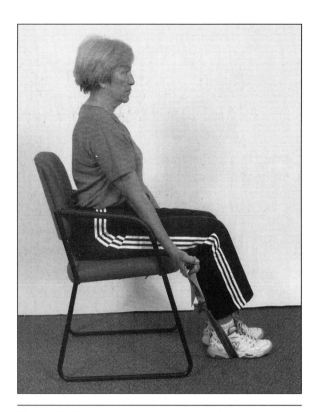

Figure 23.30   Biceps curls (start position).

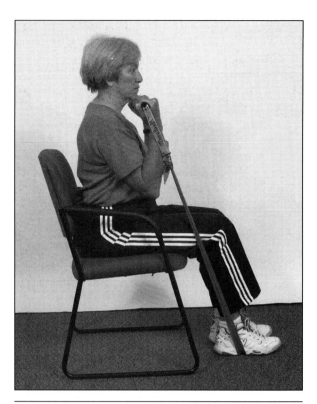

Figure 23.31   Biceps curls (end position).

is increased to 20 repetitions, the training resistance volume increases in a linear fashion to 78 lb. With these tables, increases in resistance, repetitions, and sets can be specifically quantified as changes in training resistance volume.

Initial training volume can be determined easily and again should be based on the individual's fitness goals. The number of repetitions, performed with proper form before fatigue is an important consideration when the clinician establishes initial training volume. If the activities described in the fitness goals involve brief bursts of muscle exertion, or muscle strength, then fewer repetitions should be prescribed. The greatest gains in muscle strength have been observed from resistances that yield fatigue after 4 to 10 repetitions before exhaustion (Carpenter et al. 1991; McDonagh and Davies 1984). If the fitness goal activities involve numerous muscle contractions over a period of time, or muscle endurance, the resistance should be reduced to allow 20 to 25 contractions before failure to complete the exercise attributable to fatigue. The most important factor for developing muscular strength is the resistance of the training, whereas total resistance training volume (sets × resistance × repetitions) is more important for the development of muscle endurance (Fleck and Kraemer 1997; Messier and Dill 1985; Silvester et al. 1984; Starkey et al. 1996). It is recommended that moderate-intensity resistance

training, which is commonly recommended for older adults, consist of a resistance that produces fatigue after 8 to 12 repetitions. If the individual has limited experience with resistance training and reports a sedentary lifestyle, the initial 2 weeks of the resistance training prescription should emphasize proper training form and adherence to the number of repetitions instead of performing repetitions during training to fatigue. Commonly, inactive individuals who begin resistance training develop delayed muscle soreness 24 to 48 hr after training. Older adults have reported anecdotally that this delayed muscle soreness begins to appear during the first week of resistance training, peaks after 2 to 3 weeks of training, and declines after 6 weeks of consistent resistance training. The clinician can minimize this delayed muscle soreness by encouraging proper form and by not training the participant to fatigue during the initial 2 weeks of resistance training.

The optimal number of sets to develop muscular strength remains controversial. An early study by Berger (1962) indicated that multiple sets were superior to a single set in eliciting strength gains among college-age males. Although statistically significant, the difference in increases in strength between the groups in this study was small (3%). A majority of more recent studies conducted with middle-aged adults have found improvements in strength to be independent of the number of sets performed (Carpinelli and Otto 1998; Starkey et al. 1996). With the exception of Berger's study, the literature indicates that a single set of resistance training is sufficient to result in strength gains (Graves, Pollock, and Forester 1990). To date no study has examined the efficacy of a single set versus multiple sets of resistance training with ETDs, although considering the similarities in strength gains observed between ETD and other types of resistance training, we can assume that a single set with an ETD would result in similar strength gains as multiple sets. Thus, it is recommended that to increase muscular strength, older adults should complete a single set of 8 to 12 repetitions. If the goal of training is to increase muscular endurance, up to 3 sets of 20 to 25 repetitions of a resistance training exercise are recommended.

The third component of a resistance training prescription is the frequency of training. The period between strength training sessions must be sufficient to allow the muscle to rest and avoid overtraining. Conversely, a protracted period of rest between training sessions will result in detraining. Thus, a rest period of 48 hr between training periods has been recommended (Fleck and Kraemer, 1997), which corresponds with a frequency of strength training of 3 days per week (Feigenbaum and Pollock 1999). This frequency of training is generally recommended, although specific muscle groups respond differently to varying frequencies of training (DeMichele et al. 1997; Shephard 1987). On the basis of the inconclusive studies, there appears to be no single best frequency of resistance training for every skeletal muscle group. Thus, it is up to the clinician developing the resistance training prescription to consider the individual's time availability and fitness goals when recommending the frequency of resistance training. Minimally, resistance training should be performed at least 2 days per week. Initially, a 2-day/week frequency of resistance training is recommended. This initial frequency will allow a greater time for recuperation, decrease the risk of injuries from overtraining, and thus possibly enhance adherence to the resistance training prescription. Feigenbaum and Pollock (1999) extensively reviewed the literature and reported that 2-day/week resistance training programs resulted in 80 to 90% of the strength benefits when compared with resistance training programs that involved more frequent training. Once the individual has consistently performed the resistance training program, he or she may choose to increase the frequency of training to 3 days/week to achieve maximum gains.

The final component of a resistance training program is the rate of progression of training intensity. The rate of progression is always specific to the individual's fitness goals, motivation, and ability to perform the resistance exercises to fatigue. Generally, if the older individual is able to perform the prescribed number of sets and repetitions to fatigue consistently for 2 weeks, the resistance should be increased such that the training volume for a single set of resistance training increases by 5 to 10%. For example, an older adult has been prescribed to perform a single set of 6 to 10 repetitions of biceps curls 3 times per week while elongating the red Thera-Band 100% of the initial length. After 3 weeks of consistent training, the participant is able to perform 1 set of 10 repetitions of this exercise while reporting minor to moderate fatigue. The training volume for this exercise according to table A.02 in the appendix is 39 lb. Because the repetitions are preset in the individual's training prescription and the elongation percentage based on the anatomical characteristics of the individual will not change, the participant should be advised to change the resistance offered by the elastic band. To achieve a 5 to 10% increase in training volume (approximately 2-4 lb), the individual should be advised to perform 6 repetitions of the same exercise, elongating the blue Thera-Band to 100%. This progression skips over the next level of Thera-Band (green), which would provide a training volume of only 30 lb after 6 repetitions. Using the blue band will increase the training volume 5 to 10%, to 42.6 lb. Thus, progression would continue in this fashion until the individual achieved his or her fitness goals. Once these fitness goals are achieved, the individual can maintain the resistance training program to maintain strength and functioning.

Maintaining Compliance With Strength Training

As Bandura's theory of health behavior indicates, the likelihood of complying with a health behavior can be attributed directly to the perceived benefits of and barriers to performing the behavior and the individual's self-efficacy to engage in the behavior (Bandura 1997). Self-efficacy is the individual's belief that he or she can perform a particular behavior. The approach to facilitating compliance with resistance training can be multifactorial. Applying this theory to encourage resistance training by older adults may result in a variety of diverse, individualized possible interventions. Previous studies have found that convenient, easily accessible facilities with adjacent parking (Dishman, Sallis, and

Orenstein 1985) that are available at convenient times (Dishman and Ikes 1981) and can be adapted to weather changes significantly improve adherence with a program of regular exercise. Availability of facilities to train, including parking, is a strong determinant of self-efficacy among older adults to engage in a resistance training program. Previous research has found that behavioral techniques of personal goal setting, self-monitoring, and behavioral contracts enhance the benefits and decrease the barriers to participating in regular exercise programs (Martin et al. 1984). Social reinforcement or social support also is a strong cue to action in a program of regular exercise. Before beginning a program of resistance training, older adults might be requested to sign a behavioral contract that outlines exactly their personal fitness goals and how the resistance training will advance them toward achieving their goals. Group identification is also a strong benefit to older adults engaging in resistance training. Inexpensive incentives that identify the older adult as part of a resistance training group have been shown to enhance compliance with resistance training. Finally, recognition of achieving even small advancements toward the fitness goal enhances perceived benefits and decreases the perceived barriers to continuing with the resistance training program. Recognizing progression toward fitness goals also has a profound effect on enhancing self-efficacy.

Conclusion

The number and percentage of older adults in developed countries is expanding at a rate never before seen in human history. By the year 2020, only four working adults will support the health and retirement benefits of each individual over age 65. These later years are frequently accompanied by inactivity and declines in strength and functional ability, which commonly contribute to chronic disease and a cycle of inactivity. Thus, many developed countries have identified aging as their most important health issue. Muscular strength has been shown to be an essential factor for successful aging and maintaining functional ability among older adults. It is postulated that strength may even be more critical than aerobic capacity to maintaining functional ability in later life. Numerous studies have indicated that regular resistance training among older adults improves strength and functional ability. A variety of modes of generating resistance for these programs of resistance training have been used, including elastic training devices.

A resistance training program designed for older adults is based on the same training principles as a program designed for younger adults. A resistance training program designed for older adults should include pretraining evaluation, resistance training prescription, and techniques for maintaining or enhancing compliance.

References

American College of Sports Medicine. 2000. *Guidelines for Exercise Testing and Prescription*. 5th ed. Baltimore: Williams & Wilkins.

Åstrand, P.O. 1960. "Aerobic Work Capacity in Men and Women With Special Reference to Age." *Acta Physiologica Scandinavica* 49: 1-12.

Åstrand, P.O. 1968. "Physical Performance as a Function of Age." *Journal of the American Medical Association* 205(11): 729-33.

Bandura, A. 1997. *Self-Efficacy: The Exercise of Control*. New York: Freeman Press.

Bassey, E.J., M.A. Fiatarone, E.F. O'Neill, M. Kelly, W.J. Evans, and L.A. Lipsitz. 1992. "Leg Extensor Power and Functional Performance in Very Old Men and Women." *Clinical Science* 82(3): 321-7.

Berger, R.A. 1962. "Effect of Varied Weight Training Programs on Strength." *Research Quarterly* 33: 168-81.

Booth, F.W., S.H. Weeden, and B.S. Tseng. 1994. "Effect of Aging on Human Skeletal Muscle and Motor Function." *Medicine and Science in Sports and Exercise* 26(5): 556-60.

Borchelt, M.F., and E. Steinhagen-Thiessen. 1992. "Physical Performance and Sensory Functions as Determinants of Independence in Activities of Daily Living in the Old and the Very Old." *Academic Science* 673: 350-61.

Brill, P.A., A.M. Drimmer, L.A. Morgan, and N.F. Gordon. 1995. "The Feasibility of Conducting Strength and Flexibility Programs for Elderly Nursing Home Residents With Dementia." *The Gerontologist* 35(2): 263-6.

Buchner, D.M., M.E. Cress, P.C. Esselman, A.J. Margherita, B.J. de Lateur, A.J. Campbell, and E.H. Wagner. 1996. "Factors Associated With Changes in Gait Speed in Older Adults." *Journal of Gerontology: Biological and Medical Science* 51(6): M297-302.

Buchner, D.M., M.E. Cress, E.H. Wagner, B.J. de Lateur, R. Price, and I.B. Abrass. 1993. "The Seattle FICSIT/Move It Study: The Effect of Exercise on Gait and Balance in Older Adults." *Journal of the American Geriatrics Society* 41(3): 321-5.

Carpenter, D.M., J.E. Graves, M.L. Pollock, S.H. Leggett, D. Foster, B. Holmes, and M.N. Fulton. 1991. "Effect of 12 and 20 Weeks of Resistance Training on Lumbar Extension Torque Production." *Physical Therapy* 71(8): 580-8

Carpinelli, R.N. and R.M. Otto. 1998. "Strength Training. Single Versus Multiple Sets." *Sports Medicine* 26(2): 73-84.

Cress, M.E., D.M. Buchner, K.A. Questad, P.C. Esselman, B.J. de Lateur, and R.S. Schwartz. 1999. "Exercise: Effects on Physical Functional Performance in Independent Older Adults." *Journal of Gerontology, Biological and Medical Science* 54(5): M242-8.

Damush, T.M. and J.G. Damush, Jr. 1999. "The Effects of Strength Training on Strength and Health-Related Quality of Life in Older Adult Women." *The Gerontologist* 39(6): 312-8.

Dayhoff, N.E., J. Suhrheinrich, J. Wigglesworth, R. Topp, and S. Moore. 1998. "Balance and Muscle Strength as Predictors of Frailty Among Older Adults." *Journal of Gerontology of Nursing* 24(7): 18-27.

DeMichele, P.L., M.L. Pollock, J.E. Graves, D.N. Foster, D. Carpenter, L. Garzarella, W. Brechue, and M. Fulton. 1997. "Isometric Torso Rotation Strength: Effect of Training Frequency on Its Development." *Archives of Physical Medicine and Rehabilitation* 78(1): 64-9.

Dishman, R.K., and W. Ickes. 1981. "Self-Motivation and Adherence to Therapeutic Exercise." *Journal of Behavioral Medicine* 4(4): 421-38.

Dishman, R.K., J.F. Sallis, and D.R. Orenstein. 1985. "The Determinants of Physical Activity and Exercise." *Public Health Reports* 100(2): 158-71.

Ettinger, W.H., Jr., R. Burns, S.P. Messier, W. Applegate, W.J. Rejeski, T. Morgan. S. Shumaker, M.J. Berry, M. O'Toole, J. Monu, and T. Craven. 1997. "A Randomized Trial Comparing Aerobic Exercise and Resistance Exercise With a Health Education Program in Older Adults With Knee Osteoarthritis. The Fitness and Seniors Trial (FAST)." *Journal of the American Medical Association* 277: 25-31.

Evans, W.J. 1999. "Exercise Training Guidelines for the Elderly." *Medicine and Science in Sports and Exercise* 31: 12-7.

Feigenbaum, M.S., and M.L. Pollock. 1999. "Prescription of Resistance Training for Health and Disease." *Medicine and Science in Sports and Exercise* 31(1): 38-45.

Fiatarone, M.A., and W.J. Evans. 1990. "Exercise in the Oldest Old." *Topics of Geriatric Rehabilitation* 5: 63-77.

Fiatarone, M.A., E.F. O'Neill, N.D. Ryan, K.M. Clements, G.R. Solares, M.E. Nelson, S.B. Roberts, J.J. Kehayias, L.A. Lipsitz, and W.J. Evans. 1994. "Exercise Training and Nutritional Supplementation for Physical Frailty in Very Elderly People." *New England Journal of Medicine* 330(25): 1769-75.

Fisher, N.M., D.T. Pendergast, and E. Calkins. 1991. "Muscle Rehabilitation in Impaired Elderly Nursing Home Residents." *Archives of Physical Medicine and Rehabilitation* 72(3): 181-5.

Fleck, S.J., and W.J. Kraemer. 1987. *Designing Resistance Training Programs*. Champaign, IL: Human Kinetics.

Fleck, S.J., and W.J. Kraemer. 1997. *Designing Resistance Training Programs*. 2nd ed. Champaign, IL: Human Kinetics.

Foster-Burns, S.B. 1999. "Sarcopenia and Decreased Muscle Strength in the Elderly Woman: Resistance Training as a Safe and Effective Intervention." *Journal of Women and Aging* 11(4): 75-85.

Frontera, W.R., C.N. Meredith, K.P. O'Reilly, H.G. Knuttgen, and W.J. Evans. 1988. "Strength Conditioning in Older Men: Skeletal Muscle Hypertrophy and Improved Function." *Journal of Applied Physiology* 64: 1038-44.

Graves, J.E., M.L. Pollock, and D.N. Forester. 1990. "Effect of Training Frequency and Specificity on Isometric Lumbar Extension Strength." *Spine* 15(3): 504-9.

Guralnik, J.M., E.M. Simonsick, L. Ferrucci, R.J. Glynn, L.F. Berkman, D.G. Blazer, P.A. Scherr, and R.B. Wallace. 1994. "A Short Physical Performance Battery Assessing Lower Extremity Function: Association With Self-Reported Disability and Prediction of Mortality and Nursing Home Admission." *Journal of Gerontology* 49: M85-94.

Harries, U.J., and E.J. Bassey. 1990. "Torque-Velocity Relationships for the Knee Extensors in Women in their 3rd and 7th Decades." *European Journal of Applied Physiology and Occupational Physiology* 60(3): 187-90.

Hurley, B.F., and J.M. Hagberg. 1998. "Optimizing Health in Older Persons: Aerobic or Strength Training?" *Exercise and Sport Sciences Reviews* 26: 61-89.

Hyatt, R.H., M.N. Whitlaw, A. Bhat, S. Scott, and J.D. Maxwell. 1990. "Association of Muscle Strength With Functional Status of Elderly People." *Age and Aging* 19: 330-6.

Jette, A.M., B.A. Harris, and L. Sleeper. 1996. "A Home-Based Exercise Program for Nondisabled Adults." *Journal of the American Geriatrics Society* 44: 644-6.

Jette, A.M., M. Lachman, M.M. Giorgetti, S.F. Assmann, B.A. Harris; C. Levenson, M. Wernick, and D. Krebs. 1999. "Exercise—It's Never Too Late: The Strong-For-Life Program." *American Journal of Public Health* 89: 66-72.

Krebs, D.E., A.M. Jette, and S.F. Assmann. 1998. "Moderate Exercise Improves Gait Stability in Disabled Elders." *Archives of Physical Medicine and Rehabilitation* 79: 1489-95.

Lamb, S.E., R.E. Morse, and J.G. Evans. 1995. "Mobility after Proximal Femoral Fracture: The Relevance of Leg Extensor Power, Postural Sway and Other Factors." *Age and Ageing* 24(4): 308-14.

Larsson, L. 1983. "Histochemical Characteristics of Human Skeletal Muscle During Aging." *Acta Physiologica Scandinavica* 117: 469-71.

Larsson, L.G., G. Grimby, and J. Karlsson. 1979. "Muscle Strength and Speed of Movement in Relation to Age and Muscle Morphology." *Journal of Applied Physiology* 46: 451-6.

Layne, J.E., and M.E. Nelson. 1992. "The Effects of Progressive Resistance Training on Bone Density: A Review." *Medicine and Science in Sports and Exercise* 1: 25-30.

Lexell, J. 1995. "Human Aging, Muscle Mass, and Fiber Type Composition." *Journals of Gerontology. Series A, Biological Sciences and Medical Sciences* 50: 11-16.

Lueckenotte, A.C. 1996. *Gerontological Nursing*. St. Louis: Mosby.

Martin, J.E., P.M. Dubbert, A.D. Katell, J.K. Thompson, J.R. Raczynski, M. Lake, P.O. Smith, J.S. Webster, T. Sikora, and R.E. Cohen. 1984. "Behavioral Control of Exercise in Sedentary Adults: Studies 1 Through 6." *Consulting Clinical Psychology* 52(5): 795-811.

Martinez-Caro, D., E. Alegria, D. Lorente, J. Azpilicueta, J. Calabuig, and R. Ancin. 1984. "Diagnostic Value of Stress Testing in the Elderly." *European Heart Journal* 11(5) (Suppl. E): 63-7.

Mazzeo, R.S., P. Cavanagh, W.J. Evans, M. Fiatarone, H. Hagberg, E. McAuley, and J. Startzell. 1998. "ACSM Position Stand on Exercise and Physical Activity for Older Adults." *Medicine and Science in Sports and Exercise* 30(6): 992-1008.

McArdle, W.D., F.I. Katch, and V.L. Katch. 1991. *Exercise Physiology: Energy Nutrition and Human Performance*. 3rd ed. Philadelphia: Lea & Febiger.

McCartney, N., A.L. Hicks, J. Martin, and C.E. Webber. 1996. "A Longitudinal Trial of Weight Training in the Elderly: Continued Improvements in Year 2." *Journal of Gerontology, Biological Science* 51A(B4): 25-33.

McDonagh, M.J., and C.T. Davies. 1984. "Adaptive Response of Mammalian Skeletal Muscle to Exercise With High Loads." *European Journal of Applied Physiology and Occupational Physiology* 52(2): 139-55.

McMurdo, M.E., and L. Rennie. 1993. "A Controlled Trial of Exercise by Residents of Old People's Homes." *Age and Ageing* 22: 11-5.

Messier, S.P., and M.E. Dill. 1985. "Alterations in Strength and Maximal Oxygen Uptake Consequent to Nautilus Circuit Weight Training." *Research Quarterly in Exercise and Sport* 56: 345-51.

Messier, S.P., T.D. Royer, T.E. Craven, M.L. O'Toole, R. Burns, and W.H. Ettinger, Jr. 2000. "Long-Term Exercise and its Effect on Balance in Older, Osteoarthritic Adults: Results From the Fitness, Arthritis, and Seniors Trial (FAST)." *Journal of the American Geriatrics Society* 48(2): 131-8.

Meuleman, J.R., W.F. Brechue, P.S. Kubilis, and D.T. Lowenthal. 2000. "Exercise Training in the Debilitated Aged: Strength and Functional Outcomes." *Archives of Physical Medicine and Rehabilitation* 81(3): 312-8.

Mikesky, A., R. Topp, J. Wigglesworth, J. Harsha, and J. Edwards. 1994. "Efficacy of a Home-Based Resistance Training Program for Older Adults Using Elastic Tubing." *European Journal of Applied Physiology* 69(10): 316-20.

Morgan, A.L., J.D. Ellison, M.P. Chandler, and W.J. Chodzko-Zajko. 1995. "The Supplemental Benefits of Strength Training for Aerobically Active Postmenopausal Women." *Journal of Aging and Physical Activity* 3: 332-9.

Murray, M.P., E.H. Duthie, Jr., S.R. Gambert, S.B. Sepic, and L.A. Mollinger. 1985. "Age-Related Differences in Knee Muscle Strength in Normal Women." *Journal of Gerontology* 40(3): 275-80.

Nelson, M.E., M.A. Fiatarone, C.M. Morganti, I. Trice, R.A. Greenberg, and W.J. Evans. 1994. "Effects of High-Intensity Strength Training on Multiple Risk Factors for Osteoporotic Fractures. A Randomized Controlled Trial." *Journal of the American Medical Association* 272(24): 1909-14.

Noble, L.J., R. Salcido, M.K. Walker, J. Atchinson, and R. Marshall. 1994. "Improving Functional Mobility Through Exercise." *Rehabilitation Nursing Research* 2: 23-9.

O'Brien, S.J., and P.A. Vertinsky. 1991. "Unfit Survivors: Exercise as a Resource for Aging Women." *The Gerontologist* 31(3): 347-57.

Pate, R.R., M. Pratt, S.N. Blair, W.L. Haskell, C.A. Macera, C. Bouchard, D. Buchner, W. Ettinger, G.W. Heath, and A.C. King. 1995. "Physical Activity and Public Health. A Recommendation From the Centers for Disease Control and Prevention and the American College of Sports Medicine." *Journal of the American Medical Association* 273(5): 402-7.

Pollock, M.L., and W.J. Evans. 1999. "Resistance Training for Health and Disease: Introduction." *Medicine and Science in Sports and Exercise* 31(1): 10-1.

Rowe, J.W., and R.L. Kahn. 1997. "Successful Aging." *The Gerontologist* 37(4): 433-40.

Shephard, R.J. 1987. *Physical Activity and Aging*. 2nd ed. Rockville, MD: Aspen.

Siegel, I.M. 1986. *Muscle and Its Diseases*. Chicago: Year Book Medical.

Silvester, L.J., J. Stiggins, C. McGown, and G.R. Bryce. 1984. "The Effect of Variable Resistance and Free Weight Training Programs on Strength and Vertical Jump." *Journal of the National Strength and Conditioning Association* 5(3): 33.

Skelton, D.A., A. Young, C.A. Greig, and K.E. Malbut. 1995. "Effects of Resistance Training on Strength, Power, and Selected Functional Abilities of Women Aged 75 and Older." *Journal of the American Geriatrics Society* 43: 1081-7.

Speare, A., Jr., R. Avery, and L. Lawton. 1991. "Disability, Residential Mobility, and Changes in Living Arrangements." *Journal of Gerontology* 46(3): 133-42.

Starkey, D.B., M.L. Pollock, Y. Ishida, M.A. Welsch, W.F. Brechue, J.E. Graves, and M.S. Feigenbaum. 1996. "Effect of Resistance Training Volume on Strength and Muscle Thickness." *Medicine and Science in Sports and Exercise* 28: 1311-20.

Topp, R., A. Mikesky, and K. Bawl. 1994. "Developing a Strength Training Program for Older Adults: Planning, Programming, and Potential Outcomes." *Rehabilitation Nursing* 19(5): 266-73, 97.

Topp, R., A. Mikesky, N. Dayhoff, and W. Holt. 1996. "Effect of Resistance Training on Strength, Postural Stability, and Gait Speed of Older Adults." *Clinical Nursing Research* 5(4): 407-27.

Topp, R., A. Mikesky, K. Thompson, and A. Myere. 1998. "Determinants of Four Functional Tasks Among Older Adults: An Exploratory Regression Analysis." *Journal of Orthopaedic and Sports Physical Therapy* 27(2): 144-53.

Topp, R., A. Mikesky, J. Wigglesworth, and J. Edwards. 1993. "The Effect of a 12-Week Dynamic Strength Training Program on Gait Velocity and Balance of Older Adults." *The Gerontologist* 33(4): 501-6.

Topp, R., S. Woolley, S. Khuder, J. Hornyak, and A. Bruss. 2000. "Predictors of Four Functional Tasks in Patients With Osteoarthritis of the Knee." *Orthopaedic Nursing* 19(5): 49-58.

Tseng, B.S., D.R. Marsh, M.T. Hamilton, and F.W. Booth. 1995. "Strength and Aerobic Training Attenuate Muscle Wasting and Improve Resistance to the Development of Disability With Aging." *Journals of Gerontology. Series A, Biological Sciences and Medical* 50: 113-9.

Tzankoff, S.P., and A.H. Norris. 1978. "Longitudinal Changes in Basal Metabolism in Man." *Journal of Applied Physiology* 45(4): 536-9.

Williams, M.E., and J.C. Hornberger. 1984. "A Quantitative Method of Identifying Older Persons at Risk for Increasing Long Term Care Services." *Journal of Chronic Diseases* 37(9-10): 705-11.

Woolley, S., R. Topp, S. Khuder, B. Kahaleh, and J. Commager. 1999. "Function: Which Factors Predict Ability in OA Patients?" *Biomechanics* 17(1): 77-84.

CHAPTER 24

Rehabilitation of Persons With Physical Disabilities

● ● ● ● ●

Mark A. Anderson, PhD, PT, ATC
University of Oklahoma Health Sciences Center

Kathleen Curtis, PhD, PT
California State University at Fresno

James Laskin, PhD, PT
University of Montana at Missoula

The use of elastic resistance in rehabilitation can be expanded beyond those patients with typical musculoskeletal dysfunction to patients with specific rehabilitation needs, depending on their disability. This chapter focuses on the use of elastic resistance in the functional training of persons with disabilities, specifically persons with spinal cord injury, lower extremity amputation, and cerebral palsy. We present disability-specific pathomechanics and pathophysiology along with examples of specific rehabilitation techniques with elastic resistance to meet the needs of patients with these disabilities. One word of caution should be noted. Many patients with physical disabilities have a latex allergy that can result in anaphylaxis if the patient accidentally comes in contact with latex. These patients should use nonlatex elastic tubing or bands.

Spinal Cord Injury

An estimated 235,000 individuals with spinal cord injury (SCI) live in the United States. Most individuals with SCI are male and are injured in early adulthood (Maddox 1990). Early, effective treatment of individuals with SCI has increased the life expectancy in this population (Gellman, Sie, and Waters 1988; Pentland and Twomey 1991, 1994; Sie et al. 1992). With individuals using a wheelchair 40 to 50 years, there is an increase in the prevalence of degenerative conditions associated with the aging and overuse of the upper extremities.

Upper limb pain is much more prevalent in wheelchair users than in non–wheelchair users (Nichols, Norman, and Ennis 1979; Pentland and Twomey 1991, 1994). The prevalence of shoulder pain in individuals with SCI has been reported between 30 and 100% in the literature (Bayley, Cochran, and Sledge 1987; Campbell and Koris 1996; Curtis et al. 1995a, 1995b; Gellman, Sie, and Waters 1988; MacKay-Lyons 1994; Nichols, Norman, and Ennis 1979; Pentland and Twomey 1991, 1994; Sie et al. 1992; Silfverskiold and Waters 1991).

Over half (53%) of all persons with SCI have involvement at the cervical level, resulting in tetraplegia (Maddox 1990). Shoulder pain has been documented to be a serious and persistent problem for individuals with tetraplegia (Campbell and Koris 1996; Curtis et al. 1999a, 1999b; MacKay-Lyons 1994; Scott and Donovan 1981; Sie et al. 1992; Silfverskiold and Waters 1991; Waring and Maynard 1991). Recent studies have documented that wheelchair users with tetraplegia report both a higher intensity and higher prevalence of pain during functional activities than do wheelchair users with paraplegia (Curtis et al. 1999a, 1999b).

The high prevalence of chronic shoulder pain seems to be related to increased physical demands and overuse, in that wheelchair users rely exclusively on their upper extremities for their mobility and transfers (Nichols, Norman, and Ennis 1979; Pentland and Twomey 1991, 1994), which eventually results in degenerative structural or physiological joint changes (Bayley, Cochran, and Sledge 1987). This may explain why a majority of long-term wheelchair users experience chronic shoulder problems (Gellman, Sie, and Waters 1988; Nichols, Norman, and Ennis 1979; Pentland and Twomey 1991, 1994; Silfverskiold and Waters 1991). However, shoulder pain cannot be attributed totally to degenerative joint changes in the wheelchair user. Shoulder pain may develop during the acute rehabilitation period and persist chronically (Scott and Donovan 1981).

Upper extremity strength and proper function are essential components of independent living for wheelchair users. Although shoulder pain may not initially limit the ability to perform activities independently, it may have functional costs such as fatigue, loss of endurance, decreased speed or efficiency of movement, low tolerance for prolonged work or leisure activity, decreased cardiorespiratory endurance, chronic postural deviations, and elimination of positioning or activities that are painful (Curtis et al. 1995a, 1995b).

Muscle tightness of the anterior shoulder, combined with weakness of the posterior shoulder musculature, seems to contribute to development of shoulder pain in wheelchair users (Burnham et al. 1993; Millikan, Morse, and Hedrick 1991; Powers et al. 1994). This may be attributed, in part, to the repetitive nature of the stroke pattern involved in wheelchair propulsion (Millikan, Morse, and Hedrick 1991). This may lead to protraction and elevation of the scapula with relative internal rotation of the humerus. Pain often results as the soft tissues of the rotator cuff become impinged in the narrowed subacromial space during humeral elevation (Apple, Cody, and Allen 1996; Burnham, Curtis, and Reid 1995; Powers et al. 1994).

Paralysis and spasticity in the individual with tetraplegia may further complicate muscle imbalance around the shoulder (Silfverskiold and Waters 1991). As a result of this imbalance, active or passive exercise may lead to abnormal glenohumeral motion, subluxation, and chronic stresses leading to synovial and capsular inflammation or rotator cuff or bicipital tendinitis. Inflammation that causes pain may increase spasticity, creating a vicious cycle (Silfverskiold and Waters 1991). A functional balance is needed in the shoulder girdle musculature to maintain proper joint function and prevent impingement of the soft tissue structures about the shoulder.

The shoulder joint relies on ligamentous and muscular components for stability (Apple, Cody, and Allen 1996). The rotator cuff muscles control upward migration of the humeral head created by the pull of the deltoid muscles during humeral elevation. In addition, these muscles control the upward thrust from axial loading of the arm during wheelchair propulsion and upper extremity weight-bearing activities (Burnham, Curtis, and Reid 1995). Encroachment of the subacromial space with resultant impingement of the subacromial bursa and rotator cuff tendons results from repetitive shoulder motions, namely abduction and internal rotation (Apple, Cody, and Allen 1996).

Maintaining muscular balance through a progressive strengthening program has been reported to reduce pain, restore shoulder function, and prevent recurrent injury in the non-wheelchair-dependent individual (Curtis et al. 1999b; Davis and Shephard 1990). Several studies suggest the importance of an intervention aimed at preventing shoulder pain and dysfunction for the individual who uses a wheelchair (Barber and Gall 1991; Ferrara et al. 1992; Millikan, Morse, and Hedrick 1991; Pentland and Twomey 1991; Sie et al. 1992).

Several authors have proposed interventions to prevent the onset of shoulder pain or to treat chronic shoulder pain (Burnham, Curtis, and Reid. 1995; Burnham et al. 1993; Millikan, Morse, and Hedrick 1991). These interventions include increasing the flexibility of the anterior musculature, including the pectoralis and biceps muscles, and increasing the muscle strength of the weaker muscles in the posterior shoulder complex that are responsible for shoulder external rotation, shoulder adduction, and scapular retraction.

Curtis et al. (1999b) examined the effect of a 6-month program of shoulder strengthening with elastic resistance and stretching exercises on shoulder pain experienced during functional activities in wheelchair users randomly assigned to a treatment and control group. All subjects completed a self-report questionnaire and the Wheelchair Users Shoulder Pain Index (Curtis et al. 1995a, 1995b) initially and at bimonthly intervals during the 6-month intervention. Subjects in the treatment group decreased their shoulder pain scores by an average of 39.9%, compared with decreases of only 2.5% in the control group (Curtis et al. 1999b). This pilot study demonstrates a general decrease in reported shoulder pain, especially in subjects with paraplegia, during the performance of exercises to increase shoulder strength and flexibility. A simple exercise program that uses flexibility and strengthening exercises is described next.

Exercise Program for Persons With Spinal Cord Injury

To maintain or improve flexibility, the following exercises should be repeated twice a day every day. Each stretch should be held at the end position for 20 to 30 s for best results. A dowel or broomstick may be used to stretch the pectoral or anterior chest musculature. Stretching both heads (sternal and clavicular) of the pectoralis major is recommended. When stretching the sternal head, the patient elevates the right arm as far as possible, using the left hand to facilitate the stretch. When stretching the clavicular head, the patient brings the right arm out to the side as far as possible using the left hand to facilitate the stretch. If a dowel is not available, the patient can perform this stretch inside of a doorway using the same arm positions.

To stretch the shoulder external rotators, the individual grasps the dowel and places it behind the head, slowly lowering the dowel to rest behind the shoulders. The individual then moves the hands into a comfortable position in which he or she can hold or maintain the stretch for 20 to 30 s. Both of these stretches should be repeated with each arm.

Shoulder strengthening exercises should be done one arm at a time. Before starting each exercise, the person should stretch and adjust the length of the band to take up the slack. During the exercise, the patient should pull the band to create resistance. Individuals may feel fatigued while performing these exercises but they should not feel a sharp pain. Each exercise should be repeated a minimum of 10 repetitions, gradually increasing to 3 sets of 10 to 15 repetitions. The patient should perform exercises 3 to 5 times per week for maximum benefit.

To strengthen the scapular retractors, the individual should hold either end of the elastic band in each hand with arms elevated to chest level (figure 24.01). The individual should slowly pull one arm back in a rowing motion and return to the starting position. The exercise should be repeated with other arm.

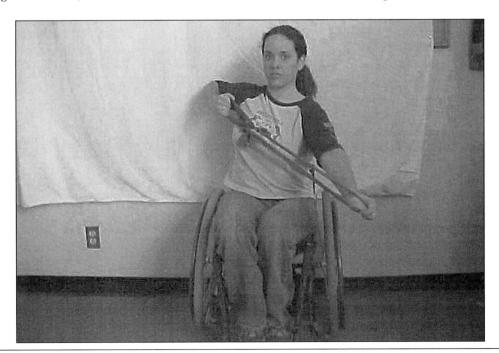

Figure 24.01 Spinal cord injury: scapular retraction.

The individual can strengthen the shoulder external rotators by keeping the elbows bent to a 90° angle, with the arms at the sides. The patient holds the band in one hand, pulling the other hand out to the side, moving only the arm below the elbow. The elbow should remain at the side and bend to 90° throughout the motion (figure 24.02). The arm is then slowly returned to the starting position. The exercise is repeated with the opposite arm.

The patient also can perform exercises to strengthen the shoulder adductors (figure 24.03). The individual should tie a large knot in one end of a long elastic band and place the knot in a doorway, securing the band by closing the door. The knot should be placed higher than shoulder level. The wheelchair should be positioned at a 90° angle to the door with the arm at shoulder height and the elbow straight. The person holds the band with the

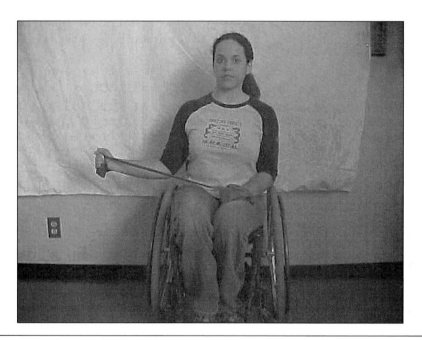

Figure 24.02 Spinal cord injury: shoulder external rotation.

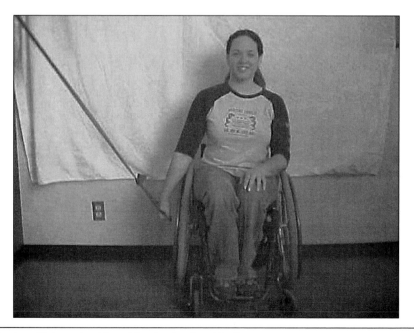

Figure 24.03 Spinal cord injury: shoulder adduction (end position).

hand that is closest to the door and pulls the arm down toward the side while keeping the elbow straight and thumb pointed down. The person then slowly returns the arm to the starting position and repeats the exercise with the opposite arm.

A simple stretching and strengthening program can help to counteract the stresses of daily wheelchair use. This program takes 10 to 15 min to perform and has been shown to reduce shoulder pain in wheelchair users.

Lower Extremity Amputation

Exercise of the residual limb is a critical part to the rehabilitation of the patient with lower extremity amputation (Kegel et al. 1981). Begun in the preprosthetic phase, exercise improves circulation, increases muscle power, maintains flexibility, decreases sensitivity, and helps to develop the individual's proprioceptive sense in the recently amputated limb (Eisert and Tester 1954). During this early rehabilitation, exercises should focus on maintaining or increasing flexibility as well as strengthening specific muscles or muscle groups that will be used during prosthetic training. In addition, these exercises should emphasize coordinated movement between the residual limb and the rest of the body, to prepare the individual for the kinds of movements he or she will use while walking on the prosthesis (Eisert and Tester 1954; May 1988). Although many of the exercises will be the same, it is important to recognize the specific rehabilitation needs of the individual who has an above-knee (AK) or transfemoral amputation from the specific needs of the individual with a below-knee (BK) or transtibial amputation.

It has been shown that the higher the level of amputation, the more muscles are involved and the more changes will appear in the remaining muscles (Jaegers, Arendzen, and de Jongh 1995). Jaegers, Arendzen, and de Jongh (1995) demonstrated that in people with AK or transfemoral amputations, the hip flexors, particularly the iliopsoas and vastus musculature, showed increased atrophy with increasing level of amputation. The same was true of the hip adductors. Although the hip extensor, the gluteus maximus, showed some atrophy, the hamstring muscles all showed severe atrophy. The amount of hip abductor (gluteus medius and minimus) atrophy depended on the level of amputation, and the tensor fascia latae atrophied severely in all individuals after AK amputation (Jaegers, Arendzen, and de Jongh 1995). Partridge, Kreuter, and Belding (1997) recommended selective

strengthening of the hip flexors, extensors, abductors, and adductors as part of their program for regaining optimal function for individuals after AK amputation.

For those with a BK or transtibial amputation, the attachments of the quadriceps and hamstrings are typically intact, as are the proximal muscles of the hip and pelvis. However, for satisfactory prosthetic ambulation, good strength is needed in the knee extensors and flexors as well as the hip extensors and abductors (Lusardi and Owens 2000; May 1988; Partridge, Kreuter, and Belding 1997; Powers et al. 1996). There is also an increased risk of hip and knee flexion contractures. Contracture development may be related to prolonged sitting, a pain-related protective flexion withdrawal response, lower extremity muscle imbalances secondary to the loss of distal muscle attachments, or the loss of sensory input generated by weight bearing on the sole of the foot (Lusardi and Owens 2000).

Exercise Program for Persons With Lower Extremity Amputation

The goals of a strengthening program after lower extremity amputation are remediation of specific muscle weakness identified during the evaluation and maximization of overall strength and muscular endurance that will lead to a safe, efficient prosthetic gait (Lusardi and Owens 2000). This means that active and resistance exercises for the trunk, uninvolved lower extremity, and upper extremities should be initiated immediately after surgery (May 1988). The focus should be on functional activities that emphasize coordination between the extremities and the trunk rather than on individual muscles or muscle groups. The therapist should gradually progress the individual from bed and mat exercises to upright exercises that facilitate the development of proper gait technique.

Initial gait training of people with recent lower extremity amputation traditionally begins with exercises designed to equalize weight bearing while they are standing. These exercises, such as weight shifting, alternate knee bending, and repetitive stance and swing drills, are part of a sequential rehabilitation approach designed to simulate components of the total movement pattern of walking (Thompson 2000).

In people with AK amputations, the contribution of pelvic motion is critical in the development of efficient gait and proper prosthetic function

(Saunders, Inman, and Eberhart 1953). Improper control of the pelvis leads to many common prosthetic gait deviations. During the swing phase, the individual must advance the prosthetic limb by rotating the pelvis on the side of the amputation forward. Failure to accomplish this maneuver robs the prosthetic socket segment of the velocity that is necessary to produce prosthetic knee flexion. Therefore, people must learn to use a combination of prosthetic hip flexion and forward pelvic rotation on the amputated side to advance the prosthesis (Eisert and Tester 1954; Thompson 2000). This skill may be practiced on the parallel bars in the clinic or at home with support of chairs or counters by having the individual practice repeated and rapid stepping with the prosthetic limb, emphasizing forward rotation of the pelvis as the prosthetic limb advances. As the individual's strength and balance improve, resistance can be added to this exercise through the use of elastic bands, aligned to provide resistance to forward pelvic rotation during swing phase (figure 24.04).

Hip extensor strength is critical in the development of early stance phase stability. Patients use their hip extensors along with prosthetic characteristics to counteract the tendency toward hip flexion that is produced by ground reaction force. By forcefully extending the hip against the posterior wall of the prosthesis at heel strike, the person moves the prosthetic knee joint into terminal extension. Hip extension against resistance may be accomplished

in a side-lying position. However, to make the exercise more specific to how the hip extensors function during gait, supine is the position of choice for performing the classic bridging exercise. The person lies supine with a firm object under the distal residual limb. The person then extends the hip on the residual limb by pushing the thigh posteriorly against the support and lifting the pelvis off the surface (figure 24.05). Elastic resistance can be applied over the proximal thigh or pelvis on the residual limb side to increase the difficulty of this exercise (Eisert and Tester 1954).

Individuals also can perform the bridging exercise with the intact limb. While holding the bridge with the intact limb, the individual then lowers and raises the pelvis on the amputated side (Thompson 2000). This strengthens the hip and pelvis musculature and assists with forward pelvic rotation on the amputated side. As with bridging on the amputated side, elastic resistance can be applied to increase the difficulty of this exercise (figure 24.06).

An imbalance of the hip abductor and adductor moments at the residual limb hip joint and prosthetic socket interface may result in lateral trunk lean toward the prosthetic side during the midstance phase of gait. This is indicative of either inadequate stabilization of the residual limb within the socket or functional weakness of the hip abductors, especially the gluteus medius and tensor fasciae latae. If socket fit is optimal, the therapist must focus on developing the individual's ability to force-

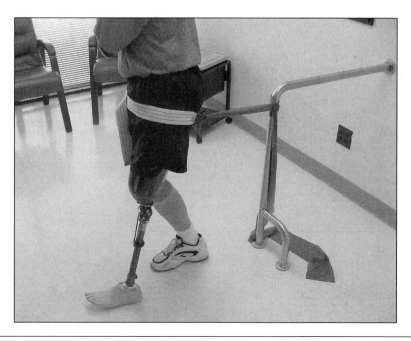

Figure 24.04 Amputee: anterior pelvic rotation.

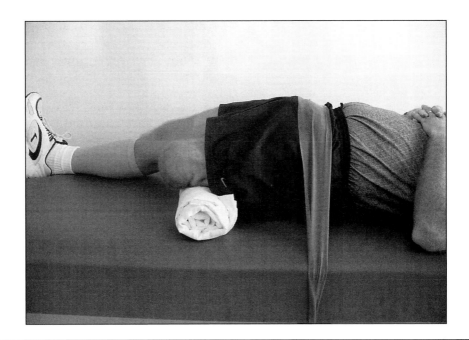

Figure 24.05   Amputee: bridging, supine residual limb (end position).

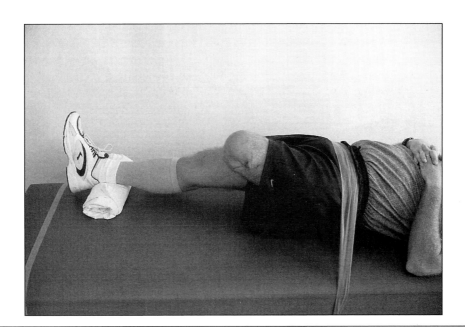

Figure 24.06   Amputee: bridging, supine intact limb (end position).

fully activate the hip abductors within the socket to minimize or eliminate the lateral lean (Thompson 2000). Bridging exercises can be performed in the side-lying position on the amputated side. The intact limb is flexed at the hip and knee and placed on a small stool or other firm object. A small towel roll is placed under the distal lateral residual limb. The person then pushes against the towel roll to elevate the pelvis off the surface. Care should be taken to prevent the patient from substituting with stronger hip muscles by rolling the pelvis backward or forward (Eisert and Tester 1954). As strengthening improves, elastic resistance may be placed over the lateral pelvis on the intact side (figure 24.07).

After an AK amputation, a large portion of the hip adductors and their distal attachments are lost, resulting in an imbalance between the hip adductors and abductors. This increases the chance that the gluteus maximus will shorten over time without its adductor antagonists. To minimize this, it is important to strengthen the residual hip adductor musculature (Thompson 2000). The patient may be positioned side-lying on the intact side, with the intact limb flexed at the hip and knee. The residual limb remains extended and supported on a firm surface such as a padded low stool. The person then pushes the medial thigh of the residual limb downward into the stool, attempting to lift the pelvis slightly from the surface. An elastic band can be placed over the pelvis to increase the resistance to lateral pelvic elevation (figure 24.08).

To achieve clearance of the prosthetic limb during swing phase, the person with an AK amputation must initiate flexion in the prosthetic knee during

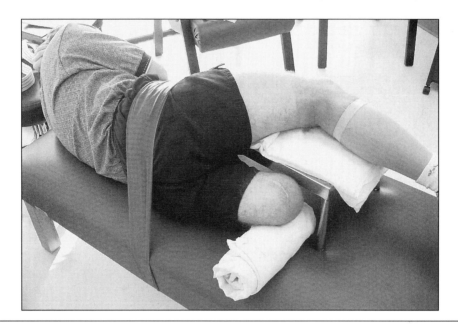

Figure 24.07   Amputee: bridging, sidelying.

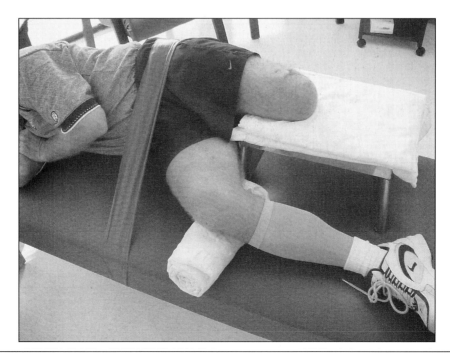

Figure 24.08   Amputee: bridging, sidelying on intact side.

preswing. If this flexion is inadequate, the person may drag the toe as swing phase is initiated. In normal gait, flexion is initiated by a combination of momentum, hip flexor activity, and weight shift to unload the extremity. The hip flexors contract to lift the thigh at the initiation of the swing phase, which is critical to developing propulsive energy to the gait cycle (Inman, Ralston, and Todd 1981). People with AK prostheses must initiate a rapid but brief concentric contraction of the hip flexors to accelerate the prosthetic socket to achieve this propulsive energy and, through reaction forces at the prosthetic knee, to produce knee flexion. This action, along with forward pelvic rotation, allows the knee to flex during the swing phase (Thompson 2000). To strengthen the hip flexors, elastic resistance may be applied to the proximal thigh of the residual limb and aligned to provide resistance to hip flexion during swing phase (figure 24.09).

For individuals with BK amputations, exercises to strengthen the knee extensors and flexors, such as muscle sets and short arc exercises, can be initiated early in the rehabilitation program. However, progressive resistance exercise should be delayed until there is evidence of adequate healing at the surgical site (Lusardi and Owens 2000). Once adequate healing has taken place, resistance to knee extension and or flexion can be initiated, either through manual resistance by the therapist or with elastic resistance. With the individual in a sitting position, elastic bands can be placed around the tibial residual limb and aligned to provide resistance

to knee extension (figure 24.10). With the person in a prone position, the elastic band can be positioned to resist knee flexion (figure 24.11). The hip and pelvis exercises described for people with an AK amputation are just as important those with a BK amputation. General strengthening of the trunk and upper extremities is also an essential component of an effective prosthetic rehabilitation program (Lusardi and Owens 2000).

Cerebral Palsy

The reported incidence of cerebral palsy (CP) in the United States of America is 1.5 to 2.5 cases per 1,000 live births (Mutch et al. 1992). The medical model defines CP as a constellation of nonprogressive conditions or syndromes of the brain that occur during the early stages of development. Although the lesion or anomaly is considered static, the presentation of symptoms is not (Mutch et al. 1992). Cerebral palsy may result from a number of prenatal (e.g., congenital brain malformations or maternal substance abuse), perinatal (e.g., delivery-related anoxia or direct brain trauma), or postnatal events (e.g., meningitis, traumatic head injuries, or near drowning; DeLuca 1996). Typically, postnatal onset CP is defined as events occurring before age 2 (DeLuca 1996). The International Paralympic Committee and the Cerebral Palsy–International Sport and Recreation Association also use the term *cerebral palsy* to describe athletes with physical disabilities who fit

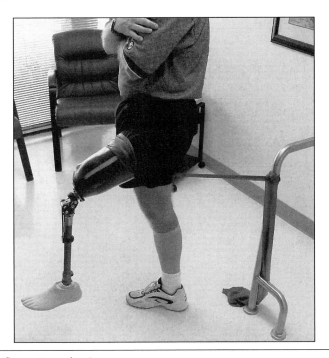

Figure 24.09 Amputee: hip flexor strengthening.

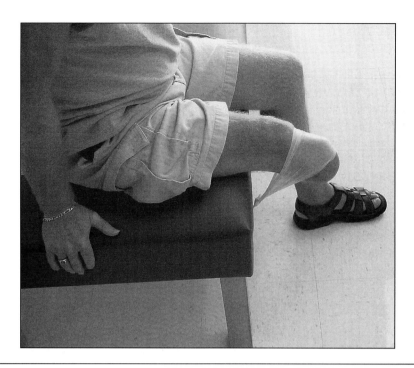

Figure 24.10 Amputee: knee extension strengthening.

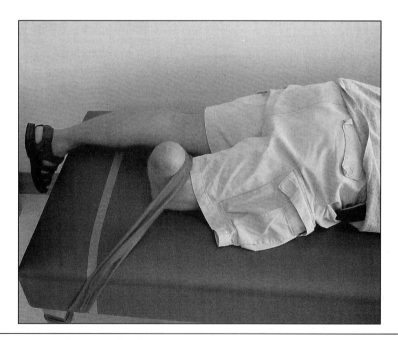

Figure 24.11 Amputee: knee flexion strengthening.

the medical definition as well as any other individual with a nonprogressive brain injury such as tumor, cerebral vascular accident, and traumatic brain injury after age 2 (DePauw and Gavron 1995).

A number of classification systems are used to define and describe the presentation of an individual with CP. Classification based on the observed movement disorder is typically most clinically relevant (Davis and Shephard 1990). Table 24.01 presents the movement disorders commonly observed with the classifications of spastic CP, dyskinetic CP, and mixed CP. Spasticity is defined as an increase in the resting muscle tone that interferes with normal movement. The intensity and speed of the intended movement can mediate the degree of abnormal muscle tone, as can the individual's arousal

Table 24.01 Cerebral Palsy (CP) Classification System by Movement Disorder

CP classification	Movement disorder
Spastic CP (subcategories: diplegia, hemiplegia, monoplegia, paraplegia, quadriplegia, and triplegia)	Spasticity: present in ~65% of those with CP; diplegia most common subcategory; typically greater lower extremity involvement than upper extremity; involves flexors, adductors, and internal rotators greater than their antagonists; hypotonia at birth progressing to spasticity after infancy; hypotonicity often remains in the trunk; increased deep tendon reflexes, clonus; abnormal postural reflexes.
Dyskinetic CP	Ataxia: uncoordinated, voluntary movements; wide-based gait with genu-recurvatum; mild intention tremors; in the infant, generalized hypotonia; normal deep tendon reflexes.
	Apraxia: mild form of ataxia that results in an inability to perform coordinated voluntary gross and fine motor skills.
	Athetosis: slow, writhing motions of the extremities; present in ~25% of those with CP; impairment of postural reflexes; nonrhythmic involuntary movement; signs of athetosis increase with anxiety, absent during sleep; commonly present with the communication disorders of dysarthria (disrupted speech) and dysphagia (disrupted swallowing).
	Chorea: state of excessisve, spontaneous, irregularly timed, nonrepetitive and abrupt movements; present in ~25% of those with CP.
	Dystonia: sustained muscle contractions that result in twisting and repetitive movement or abnormal posture; present in 15-25% of those with CP; persists throughout life, joint contractures or deformities not typically present because of continuous dystonic movements.
Mixed CP	Present in ~20% fo those with CP; both spastic and dyskinetic components.

Adapted from A.L. Albright, 1996. "Spasticity and Movement Disorders in Cerebral Palsy." *Journal of Child Neurology,* 11 (Suppl.),S1-4 and D.W. Davis, 1997, "Review of Cerebral Palsy. Part II: Identification and Intervention." *Neonatal Network,* 16(4), 19-25.

level, environmental factors, and noxious stimuli. Typically, spastic CP results in abnormally high muscle tone in one or more limbs. However, the trunk often demonstrates hypotonicity or decreased muscle tone. This combination of increased tone in the extremities and decreased tone in the trunk leads to dysfunctional movement patterns in adults and alters the development of normal movement patterns in children (Olney and Wright 2000). Individuals who present with dyskinetic CP demonstrate one or more of the following movement disorders: apraxia, ataxia, athetosis, chorea, and dystonia (Davis and Shephard 1990).

Clinicians must be aware of the client's current pharmacological regime and previous surgical interventions before initiating an elastic resistance program. The pharmacological component attempts to normalize muscle tone and minimize the disruptive influences of dyskinetic movement disorders (Pranzatelli 1996). Surgical interventions such as bone/joint stabilization, soft tissue releases, and tendon transfers are used to enhance function. These surgeries are deemed necessary as a result of the deformities caused by the abnormal muscle tone so commonly observed with CP (Renshaw et al. 1996; Van Heest, House, and Cariello 1999).

When assessing an individual with CP prior to the exercise prescription, the clinician should be aware of the following potential concerns. Abnormal muscle tone has already been addressed, but its affect on movement quality cannot be overlooked. Coordination and control of gross motor movements may be impaired in the involved limbs because of the motor dysfunctions listed in Table 24.01. The

impaired coordination and motor control also may
be a result of abnormal motor development during
childhood or incomplete recovery during rehabilitation from a traumatic event. Many individuals with
CP demonstrate the presence of primitive reflexes.
The appearance and disappearance of primitive reflexes are critical components of early motor development. The continued existence of a primitive reflex can seriously alter normal movement patterns
and limit functional activities. The symmetrical tonic
neck reflex is an example of a primitive reflex that
normally appears during the 4th to 6th month and
is integrated by the 8th to 12th month. This reflex
facilitates the upper extremity flexion when the neck
is extended and upper extremity extension when the
neck is flexed (O'Sullivan and Schmitz 2001).

Associated reactions are another form of normal
reactions to activity that can facilitate movement
when under control but can seriously impair movements in persons with CP (O'Sullivan and Schmitz
2001). An example of an associated reaction in the
nondisabled population is that when a person performs a maximal open-chain knee extension exercise, we typically see the ankle plantar flex. Although this is a normal response to a maximal effort
in the nondisabled person, ankle plantar flexion that
occurs with each knee extension effort would make
ambulation difficult.

Contractures or permanent limitations in joint
range of motion can occur in individuals with CP
secondary to alterations in muscle tone and posture (O'Sullivan and Schmitz 2001). Individuals
with spasticity of the lower extremities (e.g., spastic diplegia) typically develop hip adductor and
plantar flexion contractures attributable to the
chronic effects of those muscle groups' increased
tone (Tecklin 1999). For those who are full-time
wheelchair users, their long-term sitting postures
may limit hip and knee extension. In addition to
the motor impairments that contribute to the difficulty with exercise prescription for clients with CP,
fully 25% of these individuals present with communication disorders, 40 to 50% with visual distur-
bances, and 25% with hearing impairments. In addition, cognitive status may be affected in as many
as 75% of persons with CP (Olney and Wright 2000).

Exercise Program for Persons With Cerebral Palsy

Persons with CP benefit greatly from a well-
constructed, individualized warm-up. Typically,

the warm-up would begin with a period of large
muscle group cardiovascular exercise (Ferrara
and Laskin 1997). The specific mode, intensity,
and duration will depend on the client's functional capabilities and current fitness level
(ACSM 1998). However, slow to moderate velocity, low intensity, and reciprocal-type activities
will provide the most benefits in terms of dimin-
ishing spasticity (Ferrara and Laskin 1997).
Stretching should follow the principles of target-
ing large muscle groups; the person should use
long-duration, slow, controlled movements, remain in a stable position, and use only a gentle
stretching force (Olney and Wright 2000; Rimmer
1994). Focused relaxation is key to facilitating a
successful stretching program in individuals with
CP. As with any other client, the warm-up protocol also can be used for the postexercise cool-down.

The choice of exercises is based on the functional
abilities of the client and the clinician's determina-
tion of the exercise program required; the specific
exercises are well documented in other sections of
this text. However, elastic resistance provides some
unique exercise opportunities, especially for the
seriously involved client. Figure 24.12 shows an individual with severe spastic quadriplegia using his
only truly functional limb to perform a rowing activity. In this case, resistance is minimal and the client performs 5 min of continuous exercise, using
the activity to enhance muscular endurance and
significantly increase his heart rate. This individual
was unable to use any of the traditional forms of
arm or leg ergometry, so creative use of elastic resistance provided the clinician with unlimited exercise possibilities. Figure 24.13 shows an individual with spastic diplegia performing a reciprocal
elbow flexion exercise. For this individual, the clinician could address either cardiovascular endurance or muscular strengthening. Figure 24.14 shows
this same individual performing a similar activity
for reciprocal knee flexion. In both figures 24.13 and
24.14, the reciprocal nature of the activity helps reduce spasticity and enhance the quality of the
movement.

Figure 24.15 illustrates the person with spastic
quadriplegia using elastic resistance to strengthen
his shoulder girdle and elbow flexors in a diagonal
pattern going from an extended, elevated position
to a flexed, across-the-body position. This activity
is an attempt to reproduce one of the typical diagonal patterns used in proprioceptive neuromuscular
facilitation. A rule to use for all clients with CP, especially those presenting with spasticity, ataxia, and
athetosis, is to emphasize the eccentric component

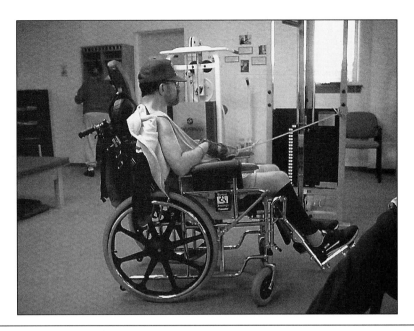

Figure 24.12   Cerebral Palsy: rowing.

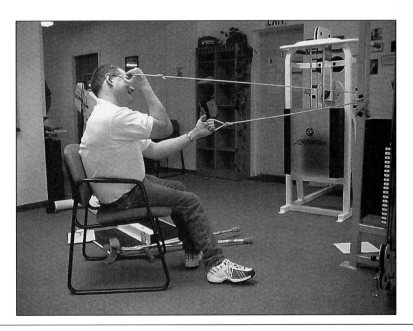

Figure 24.13   Cerebral Palsy: reciprocal elbow flexion.

of the movement. Figure 24.16 demonstrates the use of elastic resistance for an individual with minimal lower extremity strength. In this case, the individual cannot produce any observable movement of his lower extremities; however, on palpation of the hamstring tendons, a moderately strong contraction occurs. Eccentric control is particularly difficult for these clients, and in terms of function, eccentric control is critical.

Figure 24.17 demonstrates the use elastic resistance to strengthen the functional activity of "sit to stand." The tubing provides resistance when the person moves from a sitting position into standing. Besides strengthening the hip, knee, and back extensors, providing additional resistance to an activity often helps decrease athetosis and ataxia, which will enhance the quality of the movement. Figure 24.18 shows a client with

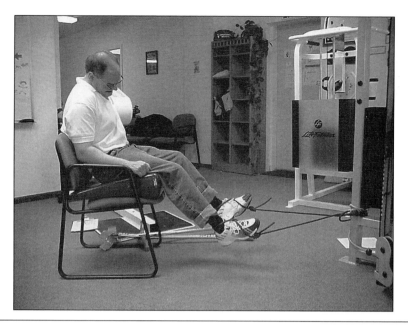

Figure 24.14   Cerebral Palsy: reciprocal knee flexion.

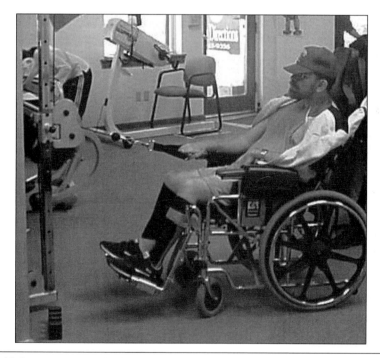

Figure 24.15   Cerebral Palsy: upper extremity D-2 extension pattern.

spastic quadriplegia performing a rowing activity with his severely affected right arm. In this case, he has no functional grip in the right hand. The clinician has overcome this limitation by using an assistive exercise device.

When using elastic resistance, the clinician should be aware that individuals with CP are susceptible to diminished quality of the intended activity because of fatigue. Although exercise has been shown to mediate spasticity, athetosis, and ataxia, fatigue may increase these symptoms (Ferrara and Laskin 1997; Olney and Wright 2000). The clinician should be vigilant and terminate the activity when the quality of the movement dimin-

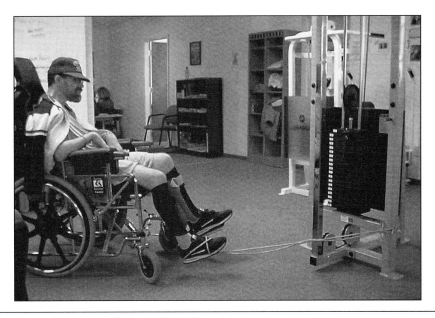

Figure 24.16 Cerebral Palsy: isometric facilitated knee flexion.

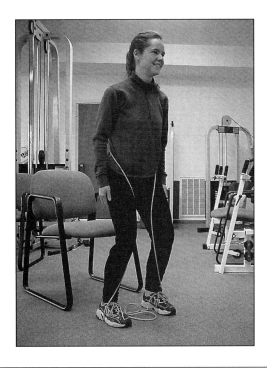

Figure 24.17 Cerebral Palsy: sit to stand.

2000). Clinicians also must respect the existing limitations in range of motion. Forcing movements beyond the client's available range will only cause pain and increase abnormal motor responses. Because of potential cognitive deficits, learning disabilities, communication difficulties, or vision/hearing impairments, individuals with CP may be slow in learning new skilled movements (Ferrara and Laskin 1997). Finally the clinician must ensure that each exercise chosen is functional, goal oriented, and age/ability appropriate.

Because of the diverse nature of CP and the unique way in which each individual is affected, elastic resistance is a logical choice for an exercise modality. Elastic resistance exercise provides a safe, inexpensive, and effective way to prescribe exercise to individuals with CP. Regardless of the functional ability of the individual, the clinician will be able to devise an exercise program using elastic resistance.

ishes. The loss of quality could be the client's inability to continue perform the activity through the full available range of motion, an increase in spasticity or tremor, increased asthenic movements, or the increased presence of primitive reflexes or associated reactions (Olney and Wright

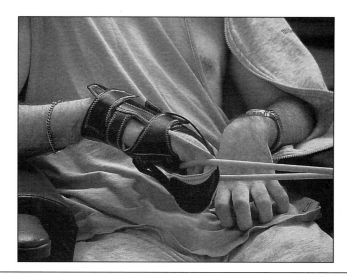

Figure 24.18   Cerebral Palsy: adapted hand grip.

Conclusion

The rehabilitation of persons with physical disabilities presents the therapist with a unique set of challenges. The clinician must modify traditional exercise programs, in terms of both the exercise prescription and the logistics of how the patient performs the exercise. Exercise modalities that are easily modifiable to fit the specific needs of the patient are of great benefit to the busy clinician. The use of elastic resistance, which is limited only by the therapist's imagination, fits this requirement.

References

Albright, A.L. 1996. "Spasticity and Movement Disorders in Cerebral Palsy." *Journal of Child Neurology* 11 (Suppl. 1): S1-4.

American College of Sports Medicine. 1998. *ACSM's Resource Manual for Guidelines for Exercise Testing and Prescription.* 3rd ed. Philadelphia: Lippincott, Williams & Wilkins.

Apple, D.F., R. Cody, and A. Allen. 1996. "Overuse Syndrome of the Upper Limb in People With Spinal Cord Injury." In *Physical Fitness: A Guide for Individuals With Spinal Cord Injury,* ed. D.F. Apple. Washington, DC: Department of Veterans Affairs, Rehabilitation Research and Development Service Scientific, and Technical Publications Section.

Barber, B., and G.G. Gall. 1991. "Osteonecrosis: An Overuse Injury of the Shoulder in Paraplegia: Case Report." *Paraplegia* 29: 423-6.

Bayley, J.C., P.C. Cochran, and C.B. Sledge. 1987. "The Weight Bearing Shoulder: The Impingement Syndrome in Paraplegics." *Journal of Bone and Joint Surgery* 69(5): 676-8.

Burnham, R.S., K.A. Curtis, and D.C. Reid. 1995. "Shoulder Problems in the Wheelchair Athlete." In *Athletic Injuries of the Shoulder,* ed. F.A. Petrone. New York: McGraw-Hill.

Burnham, R.S., L. May, E. Nelson, R. Steadward, and D.C. Reid. 1993. "Shoulder Pain in Wheelchair Athletes: The Role of Muscle Imbalance." *American Journal of Sports Medicine* 21(2): 238-42.

Campbell, C.C., and M.J. Koris. 1996. "Etiologies of Shoulder Pain in Cervical Spinal Cord Injury." *Clinical Orthopaedics and Related Research* 322: 140-5.

Curtis, K.A., G. Drysdale, R. West, R. Vitolo, M. Kolber, and D. Lanza. 1999a. "Comparison of the Prevalence and Intensity of Shoulder Pain in Individuals With Tetraplegia and Paraplegia." *Archives of Physical Medicine and Rehabilitation* 80(4): 453-7.

Curtis, K.A., K.E. Roach, E.B. Applegate, T. Amar, C.S. Benbow, T.D. Genecco, and J. Gualano. 1995a. "Development of the Wheelchair User's Shoulder Pain Index (WUSPI)." *Paraplegia* 33: 290-3.

Curtis, K.A., K.E. Roach, E.B. Applegate, T. Amar, C.S. Benbow, T.D. Genecco, and J. Gualano 1995b. "Reliability and Validity of the Wheelchair User's Shoulder Pain Index (WUSPI)." *Paraplegia* 33: 595-601.

Curtis, K.A., T.M. Tyner, L. Zachary, G. Lentell, D. Brink, T. Didyk, J. Hall, M. Hooper, J. Klos, S. Lesina, and B. Pacillas. 1999b. "Effect of a Standard Exercise Protocol on Shoulder Pain in Long-Term Wheelchair Users." *Spinal Cord* 37: 421-9.

Davis, D.W. 1997. "Review of Cerebral Palsy, Part II: Identification and Intervention." *Neonatal Network* 16(4): 19-25.

Davis, G.M., and R.J. Shephard. 1990. "Strength Training for Wheelchair Users." *British Journal of Sports Medicine* 24(1): 25-30.

DeLuca, P.A. 1996. "The Musculoskeletal Management of Children With Cerebral Palsy." *Pediatric Clinics in North America* 43(5): 1135-50.

DePauw, K.P., and S.J. Gavron. 1995. *Disability and Sport.* Champaign, IL: Human Kinetics.

Eisert, O., and O.W. Tester. 1954. "Dynamic Exercises for Lower Extremity Amputees." *Archives of Physical Medicine and Rehabilitation* 35(11): 695-704.

Ferrara, M.S., W.E. Buckley, B.C. McCann, T.J. Limbird, J.W. Powell, and R. Robl. 1992. "The Injury Experience of the Competitive Athlete With a Disability: Prevention Implications." *Medicine and Science in Sports and Exercise* 24(2): 184-8.

Ferrara, M., and J. Laskin. 1997. "Cerebral Palsy." In *ACSM's Exercise Management for Persons With Chronic Diseases and Disabilities.* Champaign, IL: Human Kinetics.

Gellman, H., I. Sie, and R.L. Waters. 1988. "Late Complications of the Weight-Bearing Extremity in the Paraplegic Patient." *Clinical Orthopaedics and Related Research* 233: 132-5.

Inman, V.T., H.J. Ralston, and F. Todd. 1981. *Human Walking.* Baltimore: Williams & Wilkins.

Jaegers, S.M.H.J., J.H. Arendzen, and H.J. de Jongh. 1995. "Changes in Hip Muscles After Above-Knee Amputation." *Clinical Orthopedics and Related Research* 319: 276-84.

Kegel, B., E.M. Burgess, T.W. Starr, and W.K. Daly. 1981. "Effects of Isometric Training on Residual Limb Volume, Strength, and Gait of Below-Knee Amputees." *Physical Therapy* 61(10): 1419-26.

Lusardi, M.M., and L.L.F. Owens. 2000. "Postoperative and Preprosthetic Care." In *Orthotics and Prosthetics in Rehabilitation*, ed. M.M. Lusardi and C.C. Nielsen. Boston: Butterworth-Heinemann.

MacKay-Lyons, M. 1994. "Shoulder Pain in Patients With Acute Quadriplegia: A Retrospective Study." *Physiotherapy Canada* 46(4): 255-8.

Maddox, S. 1990. "Spinal Cord Injury: The Statistical Picture." Pp. 38 in *The Spinal Network.* Boulder, CO: The Spinal Network.

May, B.J. 1988. "Preprosthetic Management for Lower Extremity Amputations." In *Physical Rehabilitation: Assessment and Treatment*, ed. S.B. O'Sullivan and T.J. Schmitz. 2nd ed. Philadelphia: Davis.

Millikan, T., M. Morse, and B. Hedrick. 1991. "Prevention of Shoulder Injuries." *Sports 'n Spokes* 17(2): 35-8.

Mutch, L., E. Alberman, B. Hagberg, B. Kodama, and M.V. Perat. 1992. "Cerebral Palsy Epidemiology: Where Are We Now and Where Are We Going?" *Developmental Medicine and Child Neurology* 34: 574-51.

Nichols, P.J.R., P.A. Norman, and J.R. Ennis. 1979. "Wheelchair User's Shoulder? Shoulder Pain in Patients With Spinal Cord Lesions." *Scandinavian Journal of Rehabilitation Medicine* 11: 29-32.

Olney, S.J., and M.J. Wright. 2000. "Cerebral Palsy." In *Physical Therapy for Children*, ed. S.K. Campbell, D.W. Vander Linden, and R.J. Palisano. 2nd ed. Philadelphia: Saunders.

O'Sullivan, S.B., and T.J. Schmitz. 2001. *Physical Rehabilitation: Assessment and Treatment.* 4th ed. Philadelphia: Davis.

Partridge, W., P. Kreuter, and S. Belding. 1997. *Exercises for the Lower Extremity Amputee: A Program for Regaining Optimal Function.* Redmond, WA: Medic.

Pentland, W.E., and L.T. Twomey. 1991. "The Weight-Bearing Upper Extremity in Women With Long Term Paraplegia." *Paraplegia* 29: 521-30.

Pentland, W.E., and L.T. Twomey. 1994. "Upper Limb Function in Persons With Long Term Paraplegia and Implications for Independence: Part I and II." *Paraplegia* 32: 211-24.

Powers, C.M., L.A. Boyd, C.A. Fontaine, and J. Perry. 1996. "The Influence of Lower-Extremity Muscle Force on Gait Characteristics in Individuals With Below-Knee Amputations Secondary to Vascular Disease." *Physical Therapy* 76(4): 369-77.

Powers, C.M., C.J. Newsam, J.K. Gronley, C.A. Fontaine, and J. Perry. 1994. "Isometric Shoulder Torque in Subjects With Spinal Cord Injury." *Archives of Physical Medicine and Rehabilitation* 75: 761-5.

Pranzatelli, M.R. 1996. "Oral Pharmacotherapy for the Movement Disorders of Cerebral Palsy." *Journal of Child Neurology* 11 (Suppl 1): S13-22.

Renshaw, T.S., N.E. Green, P.P. Griffin, and L. Root. 1996. "Cerebral Palsy: Orthopaedic Management." *Instructional Course Lectures* 45: 475-90.

Rimmer, J.H. 1994. *Fitness and Rehabilitation Programs for Special Populations.* Madison, WI: Brown & Benchmark.

Saunders, J.B., V.T. Inman, and H.D. Eberhart. 1953. "The Major Determinants in Normal and Pathological Gait." *Journal of Bone and Joint Surgery* 35: 543-58.

Scott, J.A., and W.H. Donovan. 1981. "The Prevention of Shoulder Pain and Contracture in the Acute Tetraplegia Patient." *Paraplegia* 19: 313-9.

Sie, I.H., R.L. Waters, R.H. Adkins, and H. Gellman. 1992. "Upper Extremity Pain in the Post-Rehabilitation Spinal Cord Injured Patient." *Archives of Physical Medicine and Rehabilitation* 73(1): 44-8.

Silfverskiold, J., and R.L. Waters. 1991. "Shoulder Pain and Functional Disability in Spinal Cord Injury Patients." *Clinical Orthopaedics and Related Research* 272(11): 141-5.

Tecklin, J.S. 1999. *Pediatric Physical Therapy.* 3rd ed. Philadelphia: Lippincott, Williams & Wilkins.

Thompson, D.M. 2000. "Rehabilitation for Persons With Transfemoral Amputation." In *Orthotics and Prosthetics in Rehabilitation*, ed. M.M. Lusardi and C.C. Nielsen. Boston: Butterworth-Heinemann.

Van Heest, A.E., J.H. House, and C. Cariello. 1999. "Upper Extremity Surgical Treatment of Cerebral Palsy." *Journal of Hand Surgery* 24A: 323-30.

Waring, W.P., and F.M. Maynard. 1991. "Shoulder Pain in Acute Traumatic Quadriplegia." *Paraplegia* 29: 37-42.

CHAPTER 25

Elastic Resistance Exercise for Chronic Disease

● ● ● ● ●

Phillip Page, MS, PT, ATC, CSCS
Benchmark Physical Therapy, Baton Rouge, LA
The Hygenic Corporation

Melvin Manning, MD
Texas Sports Medicine Group, Dallas, Texas

The human body is genetically programmed for physical activity. Without physical activity, the body loses its ability to function properly, thus hindering normal physiological maintenance. This leads to numerous physical ailments linked to inactivity, such as obesity, diabetes, osteoporosis, and cardiovascular disease. Although physical activity prevents many chronic diseases, it is also considered an effective treatment to manage or reverse these conditions.

Exercise is one of the most important and beneficial treatments in many chronic diseases. This was known as far back as Hippocrates, who treated many illnesses with exercise rather than medication. Because of our fast-paced lives and need of a "quick fix," our society has focused more on rest and medication-based management for many diseases. Although medication is the treatment of choice in many illnesses, it is important for health-care practitioners to include exercise in their prescription. This is difficult, unfortunately, because of the lack of research and education on specific exercise programs for chronic disease. The purpose of this chapter is to draw on available literature to discuss the use of elastic resistance exercise in the management of chronic disease.

The Epidemic of Inactivity and Disease

Worldwide, society is experiencing an epidemic of inactivity in addition to an increase in the population and life expectancy (figure 25.01). Although the number of diseased individuals is somewhat small, as the population increases, the numbers of persons at risk and those with disease increase proportionally (Brown, personal communication).

Consequently, an epidemic of chronic disease has developed. More than 90 million Americans live with chronic illnesses, and these diseases account for 70% of all deaths in the United States (Centers for Disease Control and Prevention[CDC] 2001). Twenty-five percent of adults in the United States are sedentary, and nearly one third of the population does not achieve the recommended amount of physical activity (CDC 2001). This has led the U.S. government to issue a proclamation to improve health and promote physical activity by 2010 (United States Department of Health and Human Services 2001).

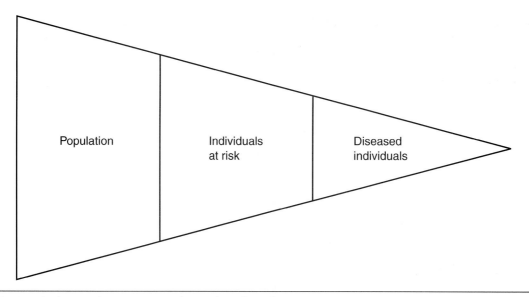

Figure 25.01 As the population increases, the number of at-risk and diseased individuals increases proportionally.

Benefits of Physical Activity in Chronic Disease

The role of physical activity in chronic disease is threefold: prevention, management, and reversal of disease. In a review of the literature on physical activity and fitness, Blair (1993) demonstrated strong evidence that physical activity decreases mortality, coronary artery disease, hypertension, obesity, diabetes (type 2), osteoporosis, and colon cancer. Physical activity is also an integral part in the management of arthritis, Parkinson's disease, and multiple sclerosis. Therefore, physical activity should be a regular part of every individual's lifestyle.

Increasing physical activity can simply involve using stairs instead of elevators or can entail a comprehensive exercise program including cardiovascular and resistance training. Resistance exercise has been shown to have positive effects on several systems of the body. In addition to improving muscular strength and bone mineral density, resistance exercise has been shown to reverse atrophy, improve insulin sensitivity, increase basal metabolic rate, decrease blood pressure, and improve blood lipids (Hurley et al. 1988).

Exercise Prescription in Chronic Disease

Obviously, exercise is an essential component in the prevention and management of chronic disease. It is often thought that exercise would be a very potent and effective medication if it could be put into a bottle. Although it is beneficial, it can also be dangerous if not prescribed properly; therefore, it should be dosed and prescribed just as medication. There is a well-documented dose-response to exercise in most individuals (Franklin 2000). The ACSM (Durstine 1997) has recommended a specific exercise prescription for most individuals without chronic disease. Table 25.01 provides these recommendations based on three different modes of exercise: cardiorespiratory fitness, muscular fitness, and musculoskeletal flexibility.

Because the dose-response for exercise varies among individuals, the ACSM recommends specific and individualized exercise prescription for cardiac and pulmonary disease patients, children, the elderly, pregnant women, and individuals with chronic disease (Franklin 2000). Medication and comorbidity for these populations also alter the exercise dose-response. In many cases, close medical supervision is required during exercise; therefore, this type of exercise prescription has been termed *medical exercise*. This type of management requires an integrated team approach to patient care including the patient, physician, therapist, and exercise specialist. Communication between members of the team is essential. This coordinated team approach facilitates a "continuum of care" from therapy to fitness (figure 25.02). The goal in managing chronic disease is to effectively treat the disease with therapy in its acute stages and ultimately promote a healthy lifestyle by using medical exercise to prevent further exacerbation of the condition.

Table 25.01 ACSM Guidelines for Exercise Prescription in a Well Population

Exercise mode	Recommendations
Cardiorespiratory fitness	Exercise large muscle groups with rhythmic and aerobic movement
	3-5 days per week
	55/65-95% maximum heart rate
	20-60 min (continuous or intermittent)
Muscular fitness	8-10 exercises for major muscle groups (table 25.02)
	2-3 days per week
	1 set of 8-12 repetitions to fatigue for each exercise
	1 set of 10-15 repetitions to fatigue for older adults chronic disease
Musculoskeletal flexibility	Use static or proprioceptive neuromuscular facilitation (PNF) stretching for all major muscle groups
	2-3 days per week
	3-4 repetitions per stretch
	Hold position of mild discomfort for 10-30 s (with or without preliminary 6-s PNF contraction

Data from B.A. Franklin, ed. 2000, *ACSM's Guidelines for Exercise Testing and Prescription*. 6th ed. Philadelphia: Lippincott, Williams and Wilkins.

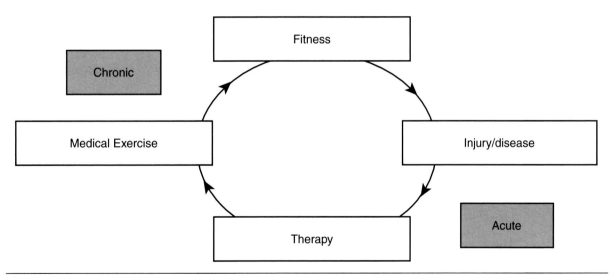

Figure 25.02 The continuum of care from therapy to fitness.
Reprinted, by permission from The Hygenic Corporation.

Individualized Medical Exercise Prescription

The first and most important step in developing an individualized medical exercise prescription is to have physician clearance for physical activity. Next, a thorough evaluation should be performed to determine response to exercise, specific problems that can be addressed through exercise, and the need for supervision during exercise. Because a detailed explanation of the methods of exercise testing and evaluation is beyond the scope of this chapter, we recommend *ACSM's Guidelines for Exercise Testing and Prescription* (Franklin 2000). It is extremely important to be aware of the contraindications associated with exercise for each medical condition.

The next step in the process is to develop a detailed problem list and realistic goals with appropriate interventions based on the individual. Other factors to consider in the prescription include comorbidity, medications, and compliance level. Implementing the appropriate intervention can be termed *exercise dosing*. Finally, reassessment of problems and modification of goals should be performed periodically (2-4 weeks) to ensure program efficacy and patient compliance.

Medical Exercise Dosing

As stated previously, much work has been done on appropriate cardiovascular and muscular fitness exercise dosing in healthy populations including appropriate mode, intensity, frequency, and dura-

tion. A well-rounded exercise prescription includes cardiovascular, strengthening, flexibility, and balance activities. Obviously, cardiovascular fitness is the most important component of any exercise prescription and remains the focus of most research on exercise in chronic disease. Unfortunately, little research has been done on the dose-response relationship of resistance exercise in chronic disease. Therefore, biological plausibility, experience, and clinical judgment must be used in prescribing resistance exercise in these special populations.

Resistance Exercise Dosing

Typically, exercise programs for persons with chronic disease are directed toward maintenance and are performed as part of a home program. Although cardiovascular exercise requires no special equipment, resistance training usually requires some form of external resistance. Compound movements involving multiple joint motion are both beneficial and efficient (Fleck and Kraemer 1997; table 25.02).

Table 25.02 Exercises for Major Muscle Groups

Region	Exercise	Muscles involved
Upper body	Chest press	Pectoralis major Triceps
	Seated row	Rhomboids Trapezius Biceps
	Pull-down	Latissimus dorsi Trapezius Biceps
	Overhead press	Deltoid Trapezius Rotator cuff
Lower body	Squat/leg press	Quadriceps Gluteus maximus
	Knee extension	Quadriceps
	Knee flexion	Hamstrings
	Calf raise	Gastrocsoleus
Trunk	Abdominal curl	Rectus abdominis Obliques
	Lumbar extension	Multifidus Paraspinals

The benefits of elastic resistance (convenience, versatility, safety, progression, and compliance) have been discussed extensively in this book. Elastic resistance produces results similar to those provided by other forms of resistance training. Elastic resistance exercise is also ideal for individuals with chronic disease because it allows them to perform their resistance training at home or on the road, thus improving compliance.

In dosing resistance exercise, the clinician must consider several parameters: mode (free weights, selectorized machines, pulley systems, or elastic resistance), volume (sets and repetitions), frequency (times per week), duration (length of training), and intensity. Intensity, rather than volume, is the most important factor in improving strength (Feigenbaum and Pollock 1999; McDonagh and Davies 1994).

The intensity traditionally is based on a percentage of the maximum weight lifted during one repetition of a particular exercise (1 repetition maximum, or RM). However, in diseased populations, it may be difficult and unsafe to determine 1 RM baselines. Others (Fleck and Kraemer 1997) recommend using a "multiple RM" approach to intensity dosing. In this method, the intensity is based on the amount of weight one can lift a certain number of repetitions to fatigue. For example, a 10 RM resistance is a resistance that can be moved only 10 times. Finally, the Borg (1998) rating of perceived exertion (RPE) scale can be used to estimate resistance exercise intensity. For example, a moderate level of resistance training corresponds to an RPE level of 13 (somewhat hard) (Borg 1998). Although the Borg RPE scale has been shown valid and reliable for cardiovascular exercise (Borg 1998), little research has proven the Borg RPE scale valid or reliable in estimating resistance training intensity. However, the Borg scale has been used effectively to determine the intensity of resistance training in several training studies that used elastic resistance (Aniansson et al. 1984; Christopherson et al. 1998; Damush and Damush 1999; Heislein, Harris, and Jette 1994).

Resistance Exercise Dosing in Chronic Disease

In this section, several chronic diseases are discussed briefly, including the rationale for resistance exercise and suggested dosage. It is imperative to have physician clearance before beginning any exercise program in these populations. In general, resistance exercise for chronic disease involves higher repetitions (10 or 15-20) at a low to moderate resistance

The Borg RPE Scale for Perceived Exertion

While exercising we want you to rate your perception of exertion, i.e., how heavy and strenuous the exercise feels to you. The perception of exertion depends mainly on the strain and fatigue in your muscles and on your feeling of breathlessness or aches in the chest.

Look at this rating scale; we want you to use this scale from 6 to 20, where 6 means "no exertion at all" and 20 means "maximal exertion."

6 No exertion at all
7
   Extremely light
8
9 Very light
10
11 Light
12
13 Somewhat hard
14
15 Hard (heavy)
16
17 Very hard
18
19 Extremely hard
20 Maximal exertion

Borg RPE scale
© Gunnar Borg, 1970, 1985, 1994, 1998
Reprinted, by permission, from G. Borg, 1998, *Borg's Perceived Exertion and Pain Scales*, Champaign, IL: Human Kinetics, 47.

(7-13 RPE) for at least 2 days per week (Feigenbaum and Pollock 1999). One set of 8 to 10 different exercises that train major muscle groups should be performed. Table 25.02 provides specific exercise programming for major muscle groups. In addition, resistance training should always be combined with aerobic exercise training in people with chronic disease. These specific diseases can be divided into five basic categories (Durstine 1997): cardiovascular and pulmonary diseases, metabolic diseases, immunological/hematological diseases, orthopedic diseases, and neuromuscular diseases.

Cardiovascular and Pulmonary Diseases

Several factors influence cardiovascular responses to resistance training (McCartney 1998); therefore, resistance exercise dosing should be specific and individualized. Recently, several agencies including the Agency for Health Care Policy and Research (Wenger 1995), the American Association of Cardiovascular and Pulmonary Rehabilitation (1995), the American Heart Association (Fletcher et al. 1995), and ACSM (Franklin 2000) have recommended strength training to improve skeletal muscle strength and endurance in clinically stable coronary patients. High-intensity resistance exercise demonstrates more favorable blood flow to the heart compared with isometric or treadmill exercise (Featherstone, Holly, and Amsterdam 1993; McCartney 1998), thus making it ideal for use in cardiovascular disease.

A common response to resistance exercise is the pressor response. During this acute physiological response, heart rate and blood pressure increase in response to high-intensity muscle contractions, particularly isometric contractions. Resistance training decreases this pressor response and may decrease the cardiac demands of general activities of daily life (Pollock et al. 2000). Resistance training also reduces cardiac risk factors (Hurley et al. 1988). Finally, resistance training may improve accessory breathing muscle strength and increase blood flow to working muscles, thus improving circulation throughout the body.

Coronary Artery Disease

Coronary artery disease is characterized by atherosclerosis (plaque lining the vessel walls) of the coronary vessels and is a major risk factor for myocardial infarction. Resistance training decreases cardiac events either directly (through cardiovascular effects) or indirectly (by modifying risk factors; Goldberg 1989). Exercise training improves coronary artery blood flow (perfusion) in patients with coronary artery disease (Hambrecht et al. 2000). In general, a strengthening program for people with coronary artery disease is based on traditional prescription for individuals without disease, although the program must not induce myocardial symptoms. The recommended intensity of exercise is based on the degree of risk. Hurley et al. (1988) found that resistance training lowered coronary risk factors without changing cardiovascular endurance or body composition. In particular, subjects demonstrated improved lipid profiles, improved insulin sensitivity, and decreased blood pressure. Faigenbaum et al. (1990) also noted that aerobically trained patients with coronary artery disease could perform moderate to heavy resistance exercise without complications.

Congestive Heart Failure

Congestive heart failure is a decrease in the heart's ability to deliver oxygen to the rest of the body, usually because of a decrease in cardiac output. Muscle weakness is common in these patients, thus making them excellent candidates for resistance training (McCartney 1998). Unfortunately, much research remains to be performed on resistance training in this population. Recently, Maiorana et al. (2000) reported improvements in functional capacity and muscular strength after circuit weight training in patients with congestive heart failure. Barnard et al. (2000) also studied the addition of a high-intensity (60-80% 1 RM) strengthening program to aerobic training in stable patients with congestive heart failure. The authors noted an average increase in strength by 26% with no abnormal responses.

Hypertension

Individuals with blood pressures greater than 140/90 generally are considered to be hypertensive. Most research demonstrates a trend toward decreased blood pressures with resistance training, although these findings are not as definitive as findings that aerobic training reduces blood pressure (Kelley and Kelley 2000). Therefore, resistance training is not recommended as the primary form of exercise training but is recommended as a component of a well-rounded fitness program.

Orthostatic Hypotension

Orthostatic hypotension is a sudden decrease in blood pressure as a result of changing position quickly, such as rising from a chair, causing dizziness and light-headedness. Orthostatic hypotension is particularly common among older adults and may be a risk factor in falls among the elderly (Tinetti et al. 1994). Little research has been done on the effects of resistance training in orthostatic hypotension. Brilla and colleagues (1998) demonstrated that strength training at 80% of 1 RM significantly improved response to positional changes in older adults with orthostatic hypotension, without changing resting blood pressure. More recently, Zion, DeMeersman, and Bloomfield (2001) reported that a home-based elastic resistance training program was safe and viable to promote activity in older adults with orthostatic hypotension.

Myocardial Infarction

Myocardial infarction is a coronary event resulting from ischemia of cardiac tissue, leading to death of heart tissue. Patients recovering from myocardial infarction (particularly postoperative patients) usually undergo cardiac rehabilitation under close medical supervision. Mild to moderate resistance training can be performed safely as early as 2 to 3 weeks postmyocardial infarction in Phases 2 to 4 in low- to moderate-risk patients (Franklin 1997). Adams et al. (1999) reported that Phase 2 cardiac rehabilitation patients can improve their strength significantly by combining high-intensity (60-80% 1 RM) strength and aerobic training. Ghilarducci, Holly, and Amsterdam (1989) also showed that resistance training at high as 80% 1 RM is safe in stable patients after myocardial infarction. Those undergoing coronary artery bypass surgery should not begin resistance training until 3 months after surgery to allow for adequate soft tissue healing (Pollock et al. 2000).

Elastic resistance exercise has been suggested (Franklin 2000; Pollock et al. 2000; Verrill et al. 1992) for cardiac patients because of its ability to provide low-level resistance training. Christopherson et al. (1998) demonstrated significant improvements in strength when subjects used elastic bands, without adverse hemodynamic or electrocardiogram problems. In general, resistance exercise dosing during cardiac rehabilitation should incorporate 8 to 10 exercises using 1 to 3 sets of 10 to 15 repetitions at 40 to 50% of 1 RM (RPE 11-14); the subject should avoid the Valsalva maneuver (Franklin 1997; Pollock et al. 2000). Resistance training should be performed 2 to 3 days per week for 4 to 6 months. The large muscle groups of the upper and lower body should be exercised (table 25.02). Brubaker et al. (2000) suggested that a home-based maintenance program for cardiac rehabilitation could be offered as an alternative to center-based programs.

Metabolic Diseases

Resistance training affects metabolic diseases by increasing muscle mass, one of the most metabolic tissues in the body. Resistance training also stimulates hormone activity that may affect these diseases.

Obesity

Obesity is excess body fat that significantly impairs health, and this disease is reaching epidemic proportions worldwide. Obesity is classified by a body mass index greater than 30. Many chronic diseases can be linked to obesity, such as cardiovascular disease, hypertension, diabetes, osteoarthritis, and cancer (Grundy et al. 1999). Although diet is important in reducing body fat, exercise is possibly the most important component of any obesity management program. In fact, a recent study determined that exercise alone is effective in reducing obesity and related comorbidities (Ross, Freeman, and Janssen

2000). Decreasing caloric intake without exercise decreases lean body mass. Aerobic exercise is the most effective mode of training to burn calories to reduce body fat; however, resistance training increases lean body mass (muscle mass) in addition to burning calories during the activity. The increase in muscle mass increases the basal metabolic rate at rest, thus increasing caloric expenditure after exercise. Therefore, resistance training is an essential component of any obesity management program. The general principles of resistance training in apparently healthy adults should be followed, as outlined in table 25.01.

Diabetes Mellitus

Type 2 diabetes mellitus is also called adult-onset or non-insulin-dependent diabetes. It is characterized as a decrease in the body's ability to metabolize blood sugar with insulin, leading to hyperglycemia. Complications include peripheral neuropathy, kidney disease, and eye diseases. Type 2 diabetes is usually associated with obesity and generally can be managed through diet and exercise.

Aerobic exercise has been the main focus of exercise training for diabetes mellitus, but resistance training has been shown safe and effective as an adjunct to aerobic exercise (Ettinger and Afable 1994). When muscle mass and strength are increased, glycogen stores increase and insulin improves in its ability to control blood glucose (Durak, Jovanovic-Peterson, and Peterson 1990; Eriksson et al. 1997; Ishii et al. 1998; Miller, Sherman, and Ivy 1994). Ishii and colleagues (1998) demonstrated that a moderate resistance exercise program in patients with diabetes mellitus improved insulin sensitivity without altering maximal oxygen uptake. The ACSM position stand on exercise and type 2 diabetes (ACSM 2000) also suggested including resistance training at least 2 days per week, whereby the individual performs 8 to 10 exercises with the major muscle groups for 1 set of 10 to 15 repetitions to near fatigue.

Finally, it is important for individuals with diabetes mellitus to monitor their blood glucose during exercise and to follow the general precautions of exercise for persons with diabetes (ACSM 2000), particularly those with associated retinopathy, neuropathy, or coronary artery disease.

Immunological/Hematological Diseases

Patients with immunological disease usually suffer local and systemic damage, leading to body "wasting" and deconditioning. Additionally, the treatment for these diseases can be damaging to the body. In these diseases, resistance training helps maintain or increase physical strength lost during treatment.

Cancer

Cancer comprises many different diseases, each of which is characterized by abnormal cell proliferation. Cancer treatment continues to evolve; however, treatment may be as debilitating as the cancer itself, usually causing side effects and excessive fatigue. Until recently, exercise has not been considered appropriate in the management of cancer patients. Aerobic exercise has been shown to improve physical performance of patients recovering from high-dose chemotherapy (Dimeo et al. 1997). Exercise training not only helps the person regain or maintain strength and function during remission, but exercise training may actually be preventive in some cancers, particularly colorectal (Thune and Lund 1996) and breast cancer (Thune et al. 1997).

Unfortunately, there is little evidence for the specific resistance exercise dosing in cancer patients. Few studies have specifically evaluated resistance training in cancer patients (Durak and Lily 1998). For resistance training, the guidelines established for healthy adults may be used (table 25.01) with individual modifications for lower intensity. Deconditioned patients or those experiencing serious side effects may need to modify their duration as well.

AIDS

Acquired immune deficiency syndrome (AIDS) results from infection from the human immunodeficiency virus. Although there is no vaccine or cure, experimental treatments continue to evolve. Exercise training is an important adjunct in the management of infection (Spence et al. 1990), but few protocols exist for resistance training programs. Spence and colleagues (1990) reported that during the nonacute stages of AIDS, physiologic adaptation occurred that improved muscle function and improved anthropometric measures. Grinspoon et al. (2000) also showed that resistance training improved muscle mass in men with AIDS wasting. Resistance training guidelines established for healthy adults may be used (table 25.01) with individual modifications as necessary.

Orthopedic Diseases

Normal bone and joint health depends on regular physical activity and load-bearing exercise. Resistance training not only provides normal joint motion but also stimulates collagen and bone growth (Layne and Nelson 1999). Although traditionally used to treat orthopedic diseases, resistance training also may prevent these diseases.

Osteoarthritis

Osteoarthritis is a degenerative disease of joint cartilage, most commonly found in the hand, wrist, hip, and knee. In a systematic review of randomized controlled trials, van Baar et al. (1999) noted that exercise therapy is beneficial in patients with osteoarthritis of the hip or knee. Several studies show that persons with knee osteoarthritis improve in function and report less pain with resistance exercise (Deyle et al. 2000; Ettinger and Afable 1994; Ettinger et al. 1997; Topp et al. 2001). In addition, Sevick et al. (2000) found that resistance training for seniors with knee osteoarthritis was slightly more cost-efficient than aerobic exercise. Low-impact resistance exercise should be prescribed for patients with osteoarthritis. Consequently, elastic resistance exercise is an ideal treatment option for this group of individuals. Elastic resistance exercise has been shown to decrease pain and improve function in individuals with knee osteoarthritis (Deyle et al. 2000; Topp et al. 2001).

Rheumatoid Arthritis

Rheumatoid arthritis is an inflammatory systemic disease affecting multiple joints. Traditionally, rest was prescribed in rheumatoid arthritis to protect the inflamed joints; however, exercise recently has been advocated as a favorable mode of treatment for rheumatoid arthritis. Both low-intensity (40-60% 1 RM; Komatireddy et al. 1997) and high-intensity (80% 1 RM) resistance exercise (Rall et al. 1996; Van den Ende et al. 2000) of major muscle groups have been shown to be safe and effective in increasing strength and reducing pain and fatigue in some rheumatoid arthritis patients.

Osteoporosis

Osteoporosis is characterized by a decrease in bone mineral density. It is particularly common in postmenopausal women and increases the risk of fracture with falls. Recently, resistance training has been recognized as an important preventive and restorative treatment in osteoporosis (ACSM 1995; Layne and Nelson 1999; Nelson et al. 1994).

In a review of the literature, Layne and Nelson (1999) noted that nearly two dozen studies have shown direct and positive relationship between the effects of resistance training and bone density. Appropriate intensity dosing is particularly important in resistance exercise prescription for people with osteoporosis; low-intensity resistance exercise may not be adequate to stimulate bone growth. Nelson et al. (1994) reported that high-intensity (80% 1 RM) strengthening in postmenopausal women prevented the loss of bone density while improving muscle mass, strength, and balance.

Several other researchers have shown significant improvements in strength, balance, and bone density with resistance exercise in subjects with low bone mineral density (Rhodes et al. 2000; Vanderhoek, Coupland, and Parkhouse 2000) in contrast to traditional pharmacological and nutritional approaches (Layne and Nelson 1999). Home programs can be as effective as a supervised program for preventing bone loss and reducing fractures in osteoporosis (Walker et al. 2000). Elastic resistance training is particularly useful for upper extremity strengthening (Bonner 1999) and for improving posture in individuals with osteoporosis.

Neuromuscular Disorders

In addition to cardiovascular exercise, resistance exercise in neuromuscular disorders is essential for maintaining function. Simple tasks such as walking or transfers become difficult as strength declines. Resistance training may help maintain strength to assist in activities of daily living.

Parkinson's Disease

Parkinson's disease is a chronic neuromuscular disease associated with a decrease in the neurotransmitter dopamine. As with other neuromuscular diseases, exercise is important in maintaining function for individuals with Parkinson's disease. People with Parkinson's disease experience symptoms such as rigidity, tremor, and slow movement. Although exercise may not directly affect these primary symptoms, it may improve the associated affects of the disease such as gait, balance, and postural impairments. Recent research has demonstrated exercise to be beneficial to patients in the early stages of Parkinson's disease with mild or moderate symptoms (Formisano et al. 1992; Levine, Brandenberg, and Pagels 2000; Palmer et al. 1986; Schenkman et al. 1998). Resistance exercise, as part of a well-rounded exercise program including cardiovascular and balance training, has been shown to improve cardiovascular fitness, strength, function, and quality of life in people with Parkinson's disease (Levine, Brandenberg, and Pagels 2000).

Multiple Sclerosis

Multiple sclerosis is a progressive neuromuscular disease characterized by destruction of the myelin sheaths surrounding nerves. People with multiple sclerosis are particularly susceptible to fatigue and hyperthermia. Exercise has not been advocated for these patients until recently; therefore, there is little literature on exercise training for individuals with multiple sclerosis. Resistance exercise should complement cardiovascular exercise and balance training as part of a well-rounded program. A moderate resistance training program following the general guidelines in table 25.01 should use the Borg PRE scale (page 331) to avoid excessive fatigue.

Conclusion

Resistance exercise training is an important adjunct in the management and prevention of many chronic diseases. It is important for the health-care professional to have medical clearance from a physician before implementing any exercise program and to maintain communication with all those involved in the patient's health care. There is also a need for more randomized controlled clinical trials to establish the optimal dose-responses of resistance exercise in these special populations. Elastic resistance offers the versatility to perform any number of resistance exercises, it is cost-effective, and it can be an integral part of a home program.

References

"ACSM Position Stand: Exercise and Type 2 Diabetes." 2000. *Medicine and Science in Sports and Exercise* 32: 1345-60.

"ACSM Position Stand: Osteoporosis and Exercise." 1995. *Medicine and Science in Sports and Exercise* 27(4): i-vii.

Adams, K.J., K.L. Barnard, A.M. Swank, E. Mann, M.R. Kushnick, and D.M. Denny. 1999. "Combined High-Intensity Strength and Aerobic Training in Diverse Phase II Cardiac Rehabilitation Patients." *Journal of Cardiopulmonary Rehabilitation* 19(4): 201-15.

American Association of Cardiovascular and Pulmonary Rehabilitation. 1995. *Guidelines for Cardiac Rehabilitation Programs.* 2nd ed. Champaign IL: Human Kinetics.

Aniansson, A., P. Ljungberg, A. Rundgren, and H. Wetterqvist. 1984. "Effect of a Training Programme for Pensioners on Condition and Muscular Strength." *Archives of Gerontology and Geriatrics* 3: 229-41.

Barnard, K.L., K.J. Adams, A.M. Swank, M. Kaelin, M.R. Kushnik, and D.M. Denny. 2000. "Combined High-Intensity Strength and Aerobic Training in Patients With Congestive Heart Failure." *Journal of Strength and Conditioning Research* 14(4): 383-8.

Blair, S.N. 1993. "Physical Activity, Physical Fitness, and Health." *Research Quarterly for Exercise and Sport* 64: 365-76.

Bonner, F. 1999. "Physical Therapy and Rehabilitation of the Osteoporotic Patient." Presented at the American

Academy of Orthopaedic Surgeons, February 6, 1999, Anaheim, CA.

Borg G. 1998. *Borg's Perceived Exertion and Pain Scales.* Champaign, IL: Human Kinetics.

Brilla, L.R., A.B. Stephens, K.M. Knutzen, and D. Caine. 1998. "Effect of Strength Training on Orthostatic Hypotension in Older Adults." *Journal of Cardiopulmonary Rehabilitation* 18(4): 295-300.

Brubaker, P.H., W.J. Rejeski, M.J. Smith, K.H. Sevensky, L.A. Lamb, W.M. Sotile, and H.S. Miller. 2000. "A Home-Based Maintenance Program After Center-Based Cardiac Rehabilitation: Effects on Blood Lipids, Body Composition and Functional Capacity." *Journal of Cardiopulmonary Rehabilitation* 20(1): 50-6.

Centers for Disease Control and Prevention. 2001. "About Chronic Disease." Available: www.cdc.gov/nccdphp/about.htm. [February 7, 2001.]

Christopherson, D.J., W.T. Phillips, D. Louie, R. Wedell, K. Berra, and S. Whaley. 1998. "Effect of Resistance Training With Thera-Band" on Functional Ability and Strength in Cardiac Rehabilitation Participants." Presented at the American Association of Cardiovascular and Pulmonary Rehabilitation, October 1998, Denver, CO.

Damush, T.M., and J.G. Damush. 1999. "The Effects of Strength Training on Strength and Health-Related Quality of Life in Older Adult Women." *Gerontologist* 39(6): 705-10.

Deyle, G.D., N.E. Henderson, R.L. Matekel, M.G. Ryder, M.B. Garber, and S.C. Allison. 2000. "Effectiveness of Manual Physical Therapy and Exercise in Osteoarthritis of the Knee." *Annals of Internal Medicine* 132(3): 173-81.

Dimeo, F.C., M.H.M. Tilmann, H. Bertz, L. Kanz, R. Mertelsmann, and J. Deul. 1997. "Aerobic Exercise in the Rehabilitation of Cancer Patients After High Dose Chemotherapy and Autologous Peripheral Stem Cell Transplantation." *Cancer* 79(9): 1717-22.

Durak, E.P., L. Jovanovic-Peterson, and C.M Peterson. 1990. "Randomized Crossover Study of Effect of Resistance Training on Glycemic Control, Muscular Strength, and Cholesterol in Type I Diabetic Men." *Diabetes Care* 13(10): 1039-43.

Durak, E.P., and P.C. Lilly. 1998. "The Application of an Exercise and Wellness Program for Cancer Patients: A Preliminary Outcomes Report." *Journal of Strength and Conditioning Research* 12(1): 3-6.

Durstine, J.L., ed. 1997. *ACSM's Exercise Management for Persons with Chronic Diseases and Disabilities.* Champaign, IL: Human Kinetics.

Eriksson, J., S. Taimela, K. Eriksson, S. Parviainen, J. Peltonen, and U. Kujala. 1997. "Resistance Training in the Treatment of Non-Insulin-Dependent-Diabetes Mellitus." *International Journal of Sports Medicine* 18(4): 242-6.

Ettinger, W.H., and R.F. Afable. 1994. "Physical Disability From Knee Osteoarthritis: The Role of Exercise As an Intervention." *Medicine and Science in Sports and Exercise* 26(12): 1435-40.

Ettinger, W.H., R. Burns, S. Messier, W. Applegate, W.J. Rejeski, T. Morgan, S. Shumaker, M.J. Berry, M. O'Toole, J. Monu, and T. Craven. 1997. "A Randomized Trial Comparing Aerobic Exercise and Resistance Exercise With a Health Education Program in Older Adults With Knee Osteoarthritis." *Journal of the American Medical Association* 277(1): 25-31.

Faigenbaum, A.D., G.S. Skrinar, W.F. Cesare, W.J. Kraemer, and W.E. Thomas. 1990. "Physiologic and Symptomatic Responses of Cardiac Patients to Resistance Exercise." *Archives of Physical Medicine and Rehabilitation* 71(6): 395-8.

Featherstone, J.F., R.G. Holly, and E.A. Amsterdam. 1993. "Physiologic Responses to Weight Lifting in Coronary Artery Disease." *American Journal of Cardiology* 71: 287-92.

Feigenbaum, M.S., and M.L. Pollock. 1999. "Prescription of Resistance Training for Health and Disease." *Medicine and Science in Sports and Exercise* 31(1): 38-45.

Fleck, S.J., and W.J. Kraemer. 1997. *Designing Resistance Training Programs.* 2nd ed. Champaign, IL: Human Kinetics.

Fletcher, G.F., G. Balady, V.F. Froelicher, L.H. Hartley, W.L. Haskell, and M.L. Pollock. 1995. "Exercise Standards: A Statement for Healthcare Professionals From the American Heart Association." *Circulation* 91: 580-615.

Formisano, R., L. Pratesi, F.T. Modarelli, V. Bonifati, and G. Meco. 1992. "Rehabilitation and Parkinson's Disease. *Scandinavian Journal of Rehabilitation Medicine* 24: 157-60.

Franklin, B.A. 1997. "Myocardial Infarction." Pp. 19-25 in *Exercise Management for Persons With Chronic Diseases and Disabilities,* ed. J.L. Durstine. Human Kinetics: Champaign, IL.

Franklin, B.A., ed. 2000. *ACSM's Guidelines for Exercise Testing and Prescription.* 6th ed. Philadelphia: Lippincott, Williams and Wilkins.

Ghilarducci, L.E., R.G. Holly, and E.A. Amsterdam. 1989. "Effects of High Intensity Training in Coronary Artery Disease." *American Journal of Cardiology* 64: 866-70.

Goldberg, A.P. 1989. "Aerobic and Resistive Exercise Modify Risk Factors for Coronary Heart Disease." *Medicine and Science in Sports and Exercise* 21(6): 669-74.

Grinspoon, S., C. Corcoran, K. Parlman, M. Costello, D. Rosenthal, E. Anderson, T. Stanley, D. Schoenfeld, B. Burrows, D. Hayden, N. Basgoz, and A. Klibanski. 2000. "Effects of Testosterone and Progressive Resistance Training in Eugonadal Men With AIDS Wasting." *Annals of Internal Medicine* 133: 348-55.

Grundy, S.M., G. Blackburn, M. Higgins, R. Lauer, M.G. Perri, and D. Ryan. 1999. "Roundtable Consensus Statement: Physical Activity in the Prevention and Treatment of Obesity and Its Comorbidities." *Medicine and Science in Sports and Exercise* 31 (Suppl): S502-8.

Hambrecht, R., A. Wolf, S. Gielen, A. Linke, J. Hofer, S. Erbs, N. Schonene, and G. Schuler. 2000. "Effect of Exercise on Coronary Endothelial Function in Patients With Coronary Artery Disease." *New England Journal of Medicine* 342(7): 454-60.

Heislein, D.M., B.A. Harris, and A.M. Jette. 1994. "A Strength Training Program for Postmenopausal Women: A Pilot Study." *Archives of Physical Medicine and Rehabilitation* 75(2): 198-204.

Hurley, B.F., J.M. Hagberg, A.P. Goldberg, D.R. Seals, A.A. Ehsani, R.E. Brennan, and J.O. Holloszy. 1988. "Resistive Training Can Reduce Coronary Risk Factors Without Altering VO_2max or Percent Body Fat." *Medicine and Science in Sports and Exercise* 20(2): 150-4.

Ishii, T., T. Ymakita, T. Sato, S. Tanaka, and S. Fuji. 1998. "Resistance Training Improves Insulin Sensitivity in NIDDM Subjects Without Altering Maximal Oxygen Uptake." *Diabetes Care* 21(8): 1353-5.

Kelley, G.A., and K.S. Kelley. 2000. "Progressive Resistance Exercise and Resting Blood Pressure: A Meta-Analysis of Randomized Controlled Trials." *Hypertension* 35(3): 838-43.

Komatireddy, G.R., R.W. Leitch, K. Cella, G. Browning, and M. Minor. 1997. "Efficacy of Low Load Resistive Muscle Training in Patients With Rheumatoid Arthritis Functional Class II and III." *Journal of Rheumatology* 24: 1531-9.

Layne, J.E., and M.E. Nelson. 1999. "The Effects of Progressive Resistance Training on Bone Density: A Review." *Medicine and Science in Sports and Exercise* 31(1): 25-30.

Levine, S., P. Brandenberg, and M. Pagels. 2000. "A Strenuous Exercise Program Benefits Patients With Mild to Moderate Parkinson's Disease." *Clinical Exercise Physiology* 2(1): 43-8.

Maiorana, A., G. O'Driscoll, C. Cheetham, J. Collis, C. Goodman, S. Rankin, R. Taylor, and D. Green. 2000. "Combined Aerobic and Resistance Exercise Training Improves Functional Capacity and Strength in CHF." *Journal of Applied Physiology* 88:1565-70.

McCartney, N. 1998. "Role of Resistance Training in Heart Disease." *Medicine and Science in Sports and Exercise* 30(10) (Suppl.): S396-402.

McCartney, N. 1999. "Acute Responses to Resistance Training and Safety." *Medicine and Science in Sports and Exercise* 31(1): 31-7.

McDonagh, M.J.N., and C.T.M. Davies. 1994. "Adaptive Responses of Mammalian Skeletal Muscle to Exercise With High Loads." *European Journal of Applied Physiology* 52: 139-55.

Miller, W.J., W.M. Sherman, and J.L. Ivy. 1994. "Effect of Strength Training on Glucose Tolerance and Post-Glucose Insulin Response." *Medicine and Science in Sports and Exercise* 16(6): 539-43.

Nelson, M.E., M.A. Fiatarone, C.M. Morganti, I. Trice, R.A. Greenberg, and W.J. Evans. 1994. "Effects of High-Intensity Strength Training on Multiple Risk Factors for Osteoporotic Fractures." *Journal of the American Medical Association* 272(24): 1909-14.

Palmer, S.S., J.A. Mortimer, D.D. Webster, R. Bistevins, and G.L. Dickinson. 1986. "Exercise Therapy for Parkinson's Disease." *Archives of Physical Medicine and Rehabilitation* 67(10): 741-5.

Pollock, M.L., B.A. Franklin, G.J. Balady, B.L. Chaitman, J.L. Fleg, B. Fletcher, M. Limacher, I.L. Pina, R.A. Stein, M. Williams, and T. Bazzarre. 2000. "Resistance Exercise in Individuals With and Without Cardiovascular Disease." *Circulation* 101: 828-33.

Rall, L.C., S.N. Meydani, J.J. Kehayias, B. Dawson-Hughes, and R. Roubenoff. 1996. "The Effect of Progressive Resistance Training in Rheumatoid Arthritis." *Arthritis and Rheumatism* 39(3): 415-26.

Rhodes, E.C., A.D. Martin, J.E. Taunton, M. Donnelly, J. Warren, and J. Elliot. 2000. "Effects of One Year of Resistance Training on the Relation Between Muscular Strength and Bone Density in Elderly Women." *British Journal of Sports Medicine* 34(1): 18-22.

Ross, R., J.A. Freeman, and I. Janssen. 2000. "Exercise Alone Is an Effective Strategy for Reducing Obesity and Related Comorbidities." *Exercise and Sport Sciences Review* 28(4): 165-70.

Schenkman, M., T.M. Cutson, M. Kuchibhatl, J. Chandler, C.F. Pieper, L. Ray, and K.C. Laub. 1998. "Exercises to Improve Spinal Flexibility and Function for People With Parkinson's Disease: A Randomized Controlled Trial." *Journal of the American Geriatrics Society* 46: 1207-16.

Sevick, M.A., D.D. Bradham, M. Muender, G.J. Chen, C. Enarson, M. Dailey, and W.H. Ettinger. 2000. "Cost-Effectiveness of Aerobic and Resistance Exercise in Seniors With Knee Osteoarthritis." *Medicine and Science in Sports and Exercise* 32(9): 1534-40.

Spence, D.W., M.L.A. Galantino, K.A. Mossberg, and S.O. Zimmerman. 1990. "Progressive Resistance Exercise: Effect on Muscle Function and Anthropometry of a Select AIDS Population." *Archives of Physical Medicine and Rehabilitation* 71: 644-8.

Thune, I., T. Brenn, E. Lung, and M. Gaard. 1997. "Physical Activity and the Risk of Breast Cancer." *New England Journal of Medicine* 336(18): 1269-75.

Thune, I., and E. Lund. 1996. "Physical Activity and Risk of Colorectal Cancer in Men and Women." *British Journal of Cancer* 73(9): 1134-40.

Tinetti, M.E., D.I. Baker, G. McAvay, E.B. Claus, P. Garrett, M. Gottschalk, M.L. Koch, K. Trainor, and R.I. Horwitz. 1994. "A Multifactorial Intervention to Reduce the Risk of Falling Among Elderly People Living in the Community." *New England Journal of Medicine* 331(13): 821-7.

Topp, R., S. Woolley, J. Hornyak, S. Khuder, and B. Kahaleh. 2001. In press. "The Effect of Dynamic Versus Isometric Strength Training on Pain and Functioning Among Adults With Osteoarthritis of the Knee." *Archives of Physical Medicine and Rehabilitation*.

United States Department of Health and Human Services. 2001. "Healthy People 2010. Understanding and Improving Health." Available: www.health.gov/healthypeople/default.htm. [February 7, 2001.]

Van Baar, M.E., W.J. Assendelft, J. Dekker, R.A. Oostendorp, and J.W. Bijlsma. 1999. "Effectiveness of Exercise Therapy in Patients With Osteoarthritis of the Hip or Knee." *Arthritis and Rheumatism* 42(7): 1361-9.

Van den Ende, C.H., F.C. Breedveld, S. le Cessie, B.A. Dijkmans, A.W. de Mug, and J.M. Hazes. 2000. "Effect of Intensive Exercise on Patients With Active Rheumatoid Arthritis: A Randomized Clinical Trial." *Annals of Rheumatic Disease* 59(8): 615-21.

Vanderhoek, K.J., D.C. Coupland, and W.S. Parkhouse. 2000. "Effects of 32 Weeks of Resistance Training on Strength and Balance in Older Osteopenic/Osteoporotic Women." *Clinical Exercise Physiology* 2(2): 77-83.

Verrill, D., E. Shoup, G. McElveen, K. Witt, and D. Bergey. 1992. "Resistive Exercise Training in Cardiac Patients." *Sports Medicine* 13(3): 171-93.

Walker, M., P. Klentrou, R. Chow, and M. Plyley. 2000. "Supervised Versus Unsupervised Exercise Program in the Treatment of Osteoporosis" (Abstract). *Clinical Journal of Sports Medicine* 10(3): 227.

Wenger, N.K., E. Froelicher, L.K. Smith, P.A. Ades, K. Berra, J.A. Blumenthal, C.M.E. Certo, A.M. Dattilo, D. Davis, R.F. DeBusk, J.P. Drozda, B.J. Fletcher, B.A. Franklin, H. Gaston, P. Greenland, P.E. McBride, C.G.A. McGregor, N.B. Oldridge, J.C. Piscatella, and F.J. Rogers. 1995. *Cardiac Rehabilitation*. Clinical Practice Guideline No. 17 (AHCPR Publication No. 96-0672). Rockville, MD: Agency for Health Care Policy and Research.

Zion, A.S., R.E. DeMeersman, and D.M. Bloomfield. 2001. "Safely Training Senior Citizens With Orthostatic Hypotension" (Abstract). *Clinical Autonomic Research* 11(3): 179.

Appendix

Table A.01   Thera-Band® Strength Index for Yellow Resistive Bands

Reps	25%	50%	75%	100%	125%	150%	175%	200%	225%	250%
1	1.1	1.8	2.4	2.9	3.4	3.9	4.3	4.8	5.3	5.8
2	2.2	3.6	4.8	5.8	6.8	7.8	8.6	9.6	10.6	11.6
3	3.3	5.4	7.2	8.7	10.2	11.7	12.9	14.4	15.9	17.4
4	4.4	7.2	9.6	11.6	13.6	15.6	17.2	19.2	21.2	23.2
5	5.5	9.0	12.0	14.5	17.0	19.5	21.5	24.0	26.5	29.0
6	6.6	10.8	14.4	17.4	20.4	23.4	25.8	28.8	31.8	34.8
7	7.7	12.6	16.8	20.3	23.8	27.3	30.1	33.6	37.1	40.6
8	8.8	14.4	19.2	23.2	27.2	31.2	34.4	38.4	42.4	46.4
9	9.9	16.2	21.6	26.1	30.6	35.1	38.7	43.2	47.7	52.2
10	11.0	18.0	24.0	29.0	34.0	39.0	43.0	48.0	53.0	58.0
11	12.1	19.8	26.4	31.9	37.4	42.9	47.3	52.8	58.3	63.8
12	13.2	21.6	28.8	34.8	40.8	46.8	51.6	57.6	63.6	69.6
13	14.3	23.4	31.2	37.7	44.2	50.7	55.9	62.4	68.9	75.4
14	15.4	25.2	33.6	40.6	47.6	54.6	60.2	67.2	74.2	81.2
15	16.5	27.0	36.0	43.5	51.0	58.5	64.5	72.0	79.5	87.0
16	17.6	28.8	38.4	46.4	54.4	62.4	68.8	76.8	84.8	92.8
17	18.7	30.6	40.8	49.3	57.8	66.3	73.1	81.6	90.1	98.6
18	19.8	32.4	43.2	52.2	61.2	70.2	77.4	86.4	95.4	104.4
19	20.9	34.2	45.6	55.1	64.6	74.1	81.7	91.2	100.7	110.2
20	22.0	36.0	48.0	58.0	68.0	78.0	86.0	96.0	106.0	116.0
21	23.1	37.8	50.4	60.9	71.4	81.9	90.3	100.8	111.3	121.8
22	24.2	39.6	52.8	63.8	74.8	85.8	94.6	105.6	116.6	127.6
23	25.3	41.4	55.2	66.7	78.2	89.7	98.9	110.4	121.9	133.4
24	26.4	43.2	57.6	69.6	81.6	93.6	103.2	115.2	127.2	139.2
25	27.5	45.0	60.0	72.5	85.0	97.5	107.5	120.0	132.5	145.0

Reprinted by permission from The Hygenic Corporation.

Table A.02   Thera-Band® Strength Index for Red Resistive Bands

Reps	25%	50%	75%	100%	125%	150%	175%	200%	225%	250%
1	1.5	2.6	3.3	3.9	4.4	4.9	5.4	5.9	6.4	7.0
2	3.0	5.2	6.6	7.8	8.8	9.8	10.8	11.8	12.8	14.0
3	4.5	7.8	9.9	11.7	13.2	14.7	16.2	17.7	19.2	21.0
4	6.0	10.4	13.2	15.6	17.6	19.6	21.6	23.6	25.6	28.0
5	7.5	13.0	16.5	19.5	22.0	24.5	27.0	29.5	32.0	35.0
6	9.0	15.6	19.8	23.4	26.4	29.4	32.4	35.4	38.4	42.0
7	10.5	18.2	23.1	27.3	30.8	34.3	37.8	41.3	44.8	49.0
8	12.0	20.8	26.4	31.2	35.2	39.2	43.2	47.2	51.2	56.0
9	13.5	23.4	29.7	35.1	39.6	44.1	48.6	53.1	57.6	63.0
10	15.0	26.0	33.0	39.0	44.0	49.0	54.0	59.0	64.0	70.0
11	16.5	28.6	36.3	42.9	48.4	53.9	59.4	64.9	70.4	77.0
12	18.0	31.2	39.6	46.8	52.8	58.8	64.8	70.8	76.8	84.0
13	19.5	33.8	42.9	50.7	57.2	63.7	70.2	76.7	83.2	91.0
14	21.0	36.4	46.2	54.6	61.6	68.6	75.6	82.6	89.6	98.0
15	22.5	39.0	49.5	58.5	66.0	73.5	81.0	88.5	96.0	105.0
16	24.0	41.6	52.8	62.4	70.4	78.4	86.4	94.4	102.4	112.0
17	25.5	44.2	56.1	66.3	74.8	83.3	91.8	100.3	108.8	119.0
18	27.0	46.8	59.4	70.2	79.2	88.2	97.2	106.2	115.2	126.0
19	28.5	49.4	62.7	74.1	83.6	93.1	102.6	112.1	121.6	133.0
20	30.0	52.0	66.0	78.0	88.0	98.0	108.0	118.0	128.0	140.0
21	31.5	54.6	69.3	81.9	92.4	102.9	113.4	123.9	134.4	147.0
22	33.0	57.2	72.6	85.8	96.8	107.8	118.8	129.8	140.8	154.0
23	34.5	59.8	75.9	89.7	101.2	112.7	124.2	135.7	147.2	161.0
24	36.0	62.4	79.2	93.6	105.6	117.6	129.6	141.6	153.6	168.0
25	37.5	65.0	82.5	97.5	110.0	122.5	135.0	147.5	160.0	175.0

Table A.03   Thera-Band® Strength Index for Green Resistive Bands

Reps	25%	50%	75%	100%	125%	150%	175%	200%	225%	250%
1	2	3.2	4.2	5	5.7	6.5	7.2	7.9	8.8	9.6
2	4.0	6.4	8.4	10.0	11.4	13.0	14.4	15.8	17.6	19.2
3	6.0	9.6	12.6	15.0	17.1	19.5	21.6	23.7	26.4	28.8
4	8.0	12.8	16.8	20.0	22.8	26.0	28.8	31.6	35.2	38.4
5	10.0	16.0	21.0	25.0	28.5	32.5	36.0	39.5	44.0	48.0
6	12.0	19.2	25.2	30.0	34.2	39.0	43.2	47.4	52.8	57.6
7	14.0	22.4	29.4	35.0	39.9	45.5	50.4	55.3	61.6	67.2
8	16.0	25.6	33.6	40.0	45.6	52.0	57.6	63.2	70.4	76.8
9	18.0	28.8	37.8	45.0	51.3	58.5	64.8	71.1	79.2	86.4
10	20.0	32.0	42.0	50.0	57.0	65.0	72.0	79.0	88.0	96.0
11	22.0	35.2	46.2	55.0	62.7	71.5	79.2	86.9	96.8	105.6
12	24.0	38.4	50.4	60.0	68.4	78.0	86.4	94.8	105.6	115.2
13	26.0	41.6	54.6	65.0	74.1	84.5	93.6	102.7	114.4	124.8
14	28.0	44.8	58.8	70.0	79.8	91.0	100.8	110.6	123.2	134.4
15	30.0	48.0	63.0	75.0	85.5	97.5	108.0	118.5	132.0	144.0
16	32.0	51.2	67.2	80.0	91.2	104.0	115.2	126.4	140.8	153.6
17	34.0	54.4	71.4	85.0	96.9	110.5	122.4	134.3	149.6	163.2
18	36.0	57.6	75.6	90.0	102.6	117.0	129.6	142.2	158.4	172.8
19	38.0	60.8	79.8	95.0	108.3	123.5	136.8	150.1	167.2	182.4
20	40.0	64.0	84.0	100.0	114.0	130.0	144.0	158.0	176.0	192.0
21	42.0	67.2	88.2	105.0	119.7	136.5	151.2	165.9	184.8	201.6
22	44.0	70.4	92.4	110.0	125.4	143.0	158.4	173.8	193.6	211.1
23	46.0	73.6	96.6	115.0	131.1	149.5	165.6	181.7	202.4	220.8
24	48.0	76.8	100.8	120.0	136.8	156.0	172.8	189.6	211.2	230.4
25	50.0	80.0	105.5	125.0	142.5	162.5	180.0	197.5	220.0	240.0

Table A.04   Thera-Band® Strength Index for Blue Resistive Bands

Reps	25%	50%	75%	100%	125%	150%	175%	200%	225%	250%
1	2.8	4.6	5.9	7.1	8.1	9.1	10.1	11.1	12.1	13.3
2	5.6	9.2	11.8	14.2	16.2	18.2	20.2	22.2	24.2	26.6
3	8.4	13.8	17.7	21.3	24.3	27.3	30.3	33.3	36.3	39.9
4	11.2	18.4	23.6	28.4	32.4	36.4	40.4	44.4	48.4	53.2
5	14.0	23.0	29.5	35.5	40.5	45.5	50.5	55.5	60.5	66.5
6	16.8	27.6	35.4	42.6	48.6	54.6	60.6	66.6	72.6	79.8
7	19.6	32.2	41.3	49.7	56.7	63.7	70.7	77.7	84.7	93.1
8	22.4	36.8	47.2	56.8	64.8	72.8	80.8	88.8	96.8	106.4
9	25.2	41.4	53.1	36.9	72.9	81.9	90.9	99.9	108.9	119.7
10	28.0	46.0	59.0	71.0	81.0	91.0	101.0	111.0	121.0	133.0
11	30.8	50.6	64.9	78.1	89.1	100.1	111.1	121.1	133.1	146.3
12	33.6	55.2	70.8	85.2	97.2	109.2	121.2	133.2	145.2	159.6
13	36.4	59.8	76.7	92.3	105.3	118.3	131.3	144.3	157.3	172.9
14	39.2	64.4	82.6	99.4	113.4	127.4	141.4	155.4	169.4	186.2
15	42.0	69.0	88.5	106.5	121.5	136.5	151.5	166.5	181.5	199.5
16	44.8	73.6	94.4	113.6	129.6	145.6	161.6	177.6	193.6	212.8
17	47.6	78.2	100.3	120.7	137.7	154.7	171.7	188.7	205.7	226.1
18	50.4	82.8	106.2	127.8	145.8	163.8	181.8	199.8	217.8	239.4
19	53.2	87.4	112.1	134.9	153.9	172.9	191.9	210.9	229.9	252.7
20	56.0	92.0	118.0	142.0	162.0	182.0	202.0	222.0	242.0	266.0
21	58.8	96.6	123.9	149.1	170.1	191.1	212.1	233.1	254.1	279.3
22	61.6	101.2	129.8	156.2	178.2	200.2	222.2	244.2	266.2	292.6
23	64.4	105.8	135.7	163.3	186.3	209.3	232.3	255.3	278.3	305.9
24	67.2	110.4	141.6	170.4	194.4	218.4	242.4	266.4	290.4	319.2
25	70.0	115.0	147.5	177.5	202.5	227.5	252.5	277.5	302.5	332.5

Reprinted by permission from The Hygenic Corporation.

Table A.05   Thera-Band® Strength Index for Black Resistive Bands

Reps	25%	50%	75%	100%	125%	150%	175%	200%	225%	250%
1	3.6	6.3	8.1	9.7	11	12.3	13.5	14.8	16.2	17.6
2	7.2	12.6	16.2	19.4	22.0	24.6	27.0	29.6	32.4	35.2
3	10.8	18.9	24.3	29.1	33.0	36.9	40.5	44.4	48.6	52.8
4	14.4	25.2	32.4	38.8	44.0	49.2	54.0	59.2	64.8	70.4
5	18.0	31.5	40.5	48.5	55.0	61.5	67.5	74.0	81.0	88.0
6	21.6	37.8	48.6	58.2	66.0	73.8	81.0	88.8	97.2	105.6
7	25.2	44.1	56.7	67.9	77.0	86.1	94.5	103.6	113.4	123.2
8	28.8	50.4	64.8	77.6	88.0	98.4	108.0	118.4	129.6	140.8
9	32.4	56.7	72.9	87.3	99.0	110.7	121.5	133.2	145.8	158.4
10	36.0	63.0	81.0	97.0	110.0	123.0	135.0	148.0	162.0	176.0
11	39.6	69.3	89.1	106.7	121.0	135.3	148.5	162.8	178.2	193.6
12	43.2	75.6	97.2	116.4	132.0	147.6	162.0	177.6	194.4	211.2
13	46.8	81.9	105.3	126.1	143.0	159.9	175.5	192.4	210.6	228.8
14	50.4	88.2	113.4	135.8	154.0	172.2	189.0	207.2	226.8	246.4
15	54.0	94.5	121.5	145.5	165.0	184.5	202.5	222.0	243.0	264.0
16	57.6	100.8	129.6	155.2	176.0	196.8	216.0	236.8	252.9	281.6
17	61.2	107.1	137.7	164.9	187.0	209.1	229.5	251.6	275.4	299.2
18	64.8	113.4	145.8	174.6	198.0	221.4	243.0	266.4	291.6	316.8
19	68.4	119.7	153.9	184.3	209.0	233.7	256.5	281.2	307.8	334.4
20	72.0	126.0	162.0	194.0	220.0	246.0	270.0	296.0	324.0	352.0
21	75.6	132.3	170.1	203.7	231.0	258.3	283.5	310.8	340.2	369.6
22	79.2	138.6	178.2	213.4	242.0	270.6	297.0	325.6	356.4	387.2
23	82.8	144.9	186.3	223.1	253.0	282.9	310.5	340.4	372.6	404.8
24	86.4	151.2	194.4	232.8	264.0	295.2	324.0	355.2	388.8	422.4
25	90.0	157.5	202.5	242.5	275.5	307.5	337.5	370.0	405.0	440.0

Table A.06   Thera-Band® Strength Index for Silver Resistive Bands

Reps	25%	50%	75%	100%	125%	150%	175%	200%	225%	250%
1	5	8.5	11.1	13.2	15.2	17.1	18.9	21	23	25.3
2	10.0	17.0	22.2	26.4	30.4	34.2	37.8	42.0	46.0	50.6
3	15.0	25.5	33.3	39.6	45.6	51.3	56.7	63.0	69.0	75.9
4	20.0	34.0	44.4	52.8	60.8	68.4	75.6	84.0	92.0	101.2
5	25.0	42.5	55.5	66.0	76.0	85.5	94.5	105.0	115.0	126.5
6	30.0	51.0	66.6	79.2	91.2	102.6	113.4	126.0	138.0	151.8
7	35.0	59.5	77.7	92.4	106.4	119.7	132.3	147.0	161.0	177.1
8	40.0	68.0	88.8	105.6	121.6	136.8	151.2	168.0	184.0	202.4
9	45.0	76.5	99.9	118.8	136.8	153.9	170.1	189.0	207.0	227.7
10	50.0	85.0	111.0	132.0	152.0	171.0	189.0	210.0	230.0	253.0
11	55.0	93.5	122.1	145.2	167.2	188.1	207.9	231.0	253.0	278.3
12	60.0	102.0	133.2	158.4	182.4	205.2	226.8	252.0	276.0	303.6
13	65.0	110.5	144.3	171.6	197.6	222.3	245.7	273.0	299.0	328.9
14	70.0	119.0	155.4	184.8	212.8	239.4	264.6	294.0	322.0	354.2
15	75.0	127.5	166.5	198.0	228.0	256.5	283.5	315.0	345.0	379.5
16	80.0	136.0	177.6	211.2	243.2	273.6	302.4	336.0	368.0	404.8
17	85.0	144.5	188.7	224.4	258.4	290.7	321.3	357.0	391.0	430.1
18	90.0	153.0	199.8	237.6	273.6	307.8	340.2	378.0	414.0	455.4
19	95.0	161.5	210.9	250.8	288.8	324.9	359.1	399.0	437.0	480.7
20	100.0	170.0	222.0	264.0	304.0	342.0	378.0	420.0	460.0	506.0
21	105.0	178.5	233.1	277.2	319.2	359.1	396.9	441.0	483.0	531.3
22	110.0	187.0	244.2	290.4	334.4	376.2	415.8	462.0	506.0	556.6
23	115.0	195.5	255.3	303.6	349.6	393.3	434.7	483.0	529.0	581.9
24	120.0	204.0	266.4	316.8	364.8	410.4	453.6	504.0	552.0	607.2
25	125.0	212.5	277.5	330.0	380.0	427.5	472.5	525.0	575.0	632.5

Table A.07 Thera-Band® Strength Index for Gold Resistive Bands

Reps	25%	50%	75%	100%	125%	150%	175%	200%	225%	250%
1	7.9	13.9	18.1	21.6	24.6	27.5	30.3	33.4	36.6	40.1
2	15.8	27.8	36.2	43.2	49.2	55.0	60.6	66.8	73.2	80.2
3	23.7	41.7	54.3	64.8	73.8	82.5	90.9	100.2	109.8	120.3
4	31.6	55.6	72.4	86.4	98.4	110.0	121.2	133.6	146.4	160.4
5	39.5	69.5	90.5	108.0	123.0	137.5	151.5	167.0	183.0	200.5
6	47.4	83.4	108.6	129.6	147.6	165.0	181.8	200.4	219.6	240.6
7	55.3	97.3	126.7	151.2	172.2	192.5	212.1	233.8	256.2	280.7
8	63.2	111.2	144.8	172.8	196.8	220.0	242.4	267.2	292.8	320.8
9	71.1	125.1	162.9	194.4	221.4	247.5	272.7	300.6	329.4	360.9
10	79.0	139.0	181.0	216.0	246.0	275.0	303.0	334.0	366.0	401.0
11	86.9	152.9	199.1	237.6	270.6	302.5	333.3	367.4	402.6	441.1
12	94.8	166.8	217.2	259.2	295.2	330.0	363.6	400.8	439.2	481.2
13	102.7	180.7	235.3	280.8	319.8	357.5	393.9	434.2	475.8	521.3
14	110.6	194.6	253.4	302.4	344.4	385.0	424.2	467.6	512.4	561.4
15	118.5	208.5	271.5	324.0	369.0	412.5	454.5	501.0	549.0	601.5
16	126.4	222.4	289.6	345.6	393.6	440.0	484.8	534.4	585.6	641.6
17	134.3	236.3	307.7	367.2	418.2	467.5	515.1	567.8	622.2	681.7
18	142.2	250.2	325.8	388.8	442.8	495.0	545.4	601.2	658.8	721.8
19	150.1	264.1	343.9	410.4	467.4	522.5	575.7	634.6	695.4	761.9
20	158.0	278.0	362.0	432.0	492.0	550.0	606.0	668.0	732.0	802.0
21	165.9	291.9	380.1	453.6	516.6	577.5	636.3	701.4	768.6	842.1
22	173.8	305.8	398.2	475.2	541.2	605.0	666.6	734.8	805.2	882.2
23	181.7	319.7	416.3	496.8	565.8	632.5	696.9	768.2	841.8	922.3
24	189.6	333.6	434.4	518.4	590.4	660.0	727.2	801.6	878.4	962.4
25	197.5	347.5	452.5	540.0	615.0	687.5	757.5	835.0	915.0	1002.5

Reprinted by permission from The Hygenic Corporation.

Index

Page numbers ending in *f* or *t* indicate figures and tables, respectively.

About the Editors

Phillip Page, MS, PT, ATC, CSCS, is a physical therapist, athletic trainer, and certified strength and conditioning specialist. As manager of clinical education and research for Thera-Band Products, he has performed research on elastic resistance exercises. He has lectured internationally on the scientific and clinical use of elastic resistance and developed an educational course on elastic resistance that is being taught in six countries.

Previously, he was team physical therapist for the New Orleans Saints professional football club and Tulane University.

He is certified by the National Athletic Trainers' Association (NATA) and was awarded the NATA's Otto Davis Post Graduate Scholarship in 1991.

He earned a bachelor's degree in physical therapy from Louisiana State University Medical Center in New Orleans and a master's degree in exercise physiology from Mississippi State University. Page is in private practice in Baton Rouge, Louisiana, specializing in sports and orthopedic physical therapy.

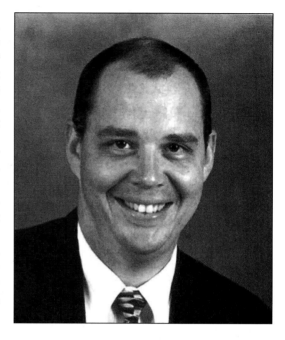

Todd S. Ellenbecker, MS, PT, SCS, OCS CSCS, is the clinic director at the Physiotherapy Associates Sports Clinic, in Scottsdale, Arizona. A licensed physical therapist, he has researched and taught in the field for 16 years.

He co-wrote *The Elbow in Sport, Complete Conditioning for Tennis,* and *Closed Kinetic Chain Exercise.* He also co-edited *Knee Ligament Rehabilitation.*

Ellenbecker has conducted extensive research on exercise and testing in musculoskeletal rehabilitation.

He is certified by the American Physical Therapy Association (APTA) as both a sports clinical specialist and orthopedic clinical specialist. The APTA also awarded him its Sports Physical Therapy Clinical Teaching Award in 1999. He is chairman of the APTA's Shoulder Special Interest Group and a manuscript reviewer for the *Journal of Orthopaedic and Sports Physical Therapy.*

Ellenbecker earned a bachelor's degree in physical therapy from the University of Wisconsin at LaCrosse and a master's degree in exercise physiology from Arizona State University. He also is certified as a strength and conditioning specialist.

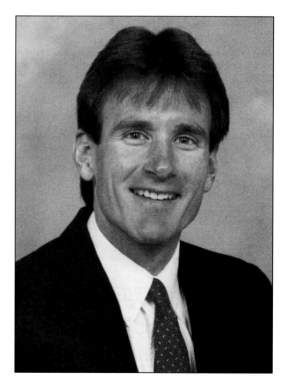